DATE DUE

DE 17 '01			
APR 00 2003			
AG 2 '04			
NO 1 '08			
FE 20 '14			

DEMCO 38-296

THE COLLECTED WORKS OF
L. S. VYGOTSKY

Volume 5
Child Psychology

COGNITION AND LANGUAGE
A Series in Psycholinguistics • Series Editor: R. W. RIEBER

A Continuation Order Plan is available for this series. A continuation order will bring delivery of each new volume immediately upon publication. Volumes are billed only upon actual shipment. For further information please contact the publisher.

THE COLLECTED WORKS OF
L. S. VYGOTSKY

Volume 5
Child Psychology

Translated by
MARIE J. HALL

Prologue by
CARL RATNER
Humboldt State University
Arcata, California

Editor of the English Translation
ROBERT W. RIEBER
John Jay College of Criminal Justice
and the Graduate Center
City University of New York
New York, New York

PLENUM PRESS • NEW YORK AND LONDON

ıloged earlier volumes of this title as follows:

896–1934.
The collected works of L. S. Vygotsky.

(Cognition and language)
Translation of: Sobranie Sochinenii.
Vol. 1– includes bibliographies and indexes.
Contents: v. 1. Problems of general psychology.
1. Psychology I. Rieber, R. W. (Robert W.) II. Carton, Aaron S.

BF121.V9413   1987   150   87-7219

This volume is published under an agreement with the
Russian Authors' Society (RAO)

ISBN 0-306-45707-5

© 1998 Plenum Press, New York
A Division of Plenum Publishing Corporation
233 Spring Street, New York, N. Y. 10013

http://www.plenum.com

10 9 8 7 6 5 4 3 2 1

Printed in the United States of America

Prologue

Carl Ratner
Humboldt State University
Arcata, CA 95521

This volume of Vygotsky's Collected Works contains important writings on the development of human psychology from early childhood to adolescence. The volume is divided into two sections. The first contains about one-half of the chapters of Vygotsky's book, *Pedology of the Adolescent*. This book was published during Vygotsky's lifetime in a limited number of copies. The second section consists of separate articles which were published after Vygotsky died.

The works in this volume reveal some important extensions of Vygotsky's fundamental concepts. In particular, one finds extensive discussions about the transition from elementary psychobiological processes to conscious psychological phenomena. Vygotsky delineates the social and cognitive determinants of this qualitative change. Other concepts which are developed in this volume include the integration of psychological phenomena in consciousness, the relation between structure (or form) and content of psychological phenomena, and the relation between biological processes and psychological functions. Finally, Vygotsky makes a number of methodological points concerning the nature of psychological inquiry. The following prologue will introduce the reader to these concepts.

Higher and Lower Processes

The fundamental principle which drives Vygotsky's developmental psychology is the transition from "lower" psychobiological processes to "higher" conscious psychological functions. The former include reflexes, temperamental traits, and spontaneous, rudimentary conscious processes. The latter include developed, voluntary, mental functions and associated personality characteristics. In Vygotsky's words, psychological development consists in "the transition from direct, innate, natural forms and methods of behavior to mediated, artificial mental functions that develop in the process of cultural development" (p. 168, this volume).

Vygotsky argued that higher and lower functions are fundamentally different from each other in terms of origins, biological mechanisms, and mental features (cf. Ratner, 1991, Chap. 4; Ratner, forthcoming for a discussion of these differences). Consequently, mature psychological functions comprise a novel system which is not derived from lower processes. Elementary psychobiological functions are not the basis of mature, complex, mental psychological phenomena. Nor do the lower processes remain intact and interact with higher processes. Instead, Vygotsky proposed a radical dichotomy between the two which grants real autonomy to higher psychological functions. They develop according to different pathways from lower functions and have their own characteristics. Rather than lower and higher processes forming a continuous gradation in which early processes engender later ones, comprise their components, and affect their character, psychological development requires the introduction of new mechanisms which generate novel, autonomous higher functions.

Vygotsky states this position quite clearly in the present volume. He says, "The circumstance that higher mental functions are not simply a continuation of elementary functions and are not their mechanical combination, but a qualitatively new mental formation that develops according to completely special laws and is subject to completely different patterns, has still not been assimilated by child psychology" (p. 34).

Lower and higher functions rest upon different biological, cognitive, and social foundations. Lower functions are determined by biological mechanisms and they are minimally cognitive. For instance, infantile attention is a simple, involuntary "orientation reflex" that is biologically programmed. Temperamental traits of infants are similarly biologically programmed, involuntary, spontaneous, simple reactions to events. Vygotsky maintains that early, or natural, memory is likewise a spontaneous recollection that is prompted by a direct similarity between a current and prior sensation (p. 98, this volume).

In contrast, higher, mature, complex psychological phenomena are stimulated and organized by social experience and they are mediated by, or depend upon, conceptual thinking. Vygotsky explains this difference in a succinct statement about lower and higher forms of attention:

> the importance of the organic process, which lies at the foundation of the development of attention, decreases as new, qualitatively distinct processes of attentional development emerge. Specifically, we have in mind the processes of *the cultural development of attention*. When we speak of the cultural development of attention, we mean *evolution and change in the means for directing and carrying out attentional processes the mastery of these processes, and their subordination to human control* . . . Voluntary attention emerges owing to the fact that the people who surround the child begin to use various stimuli and means to direct the child's attention and subordinate it to their control . . . and and of itself, the organic, or natural, development of attention never could, and never will, lead to the emergence of voluntary attention (Vygotsky, 1981, pp. 193–194).

Qualitative Change

Vygotsky reiterates the notion of qualitative change throughout this volume. He says that mature psychological functions which are culturally stimulated and organized, and rest upon conceptual thinking, are qualitatively different from biologically based, non-cognitive elementary functions. Another use of the notion of qualitative change is his discussion of the unique character of cognitive concepts. He said that "A concept is not just an enriched and internally interconnected associative group. It is a qualitatively new formation that cannot be reduced to more elementary processes that characterize the development of the intellect at earlier stages (p. 40).

Vygotsky frequently criticized psychologists who recognize only quantitative changes in psychological functioning. One statement expresses this clearly: "if one holds the point of view [that] the process of intellectual changes that occur at adolescence can be reduced to a simple quantitative accumulation of characteristics already laid down in the thinking of a three-year old . . . the word *development* does not apply" (p. 29). Vygotsky was especially critical of Thorndike for whom "higher forms of thinking differ from elementary functions only quantitatively according to the number of associative connections that enter into their composition" (p. 40).

Conceptual Underpinnings of Psychological Phenomena

Mature, complex psychological functions rest upon conceptual thinking. They are "historically based forms of intellectual activity" (this volume, p. 35). Vygotsky expresses this rationalist philosophy forcefully and unmistakably on page 81:

> Development of thinking has a central, key, decisive significance for all the other functions and processes. We cannot express more clearly or tersely the leading role of intellectual development in relation to the whole personality of the adolescent and to all of his mental functions other than to say that acquiring the function of forming concepts is the principal and central link in all the changes that occur in the psychology of the adolescent.

Vygotsky describes how memory changes from a lower to a higher function through the intercession of cognition: "in the child, intellect is a function of memory; in the adolescent, memory is a function of intellect" (p. 96). "We have seen that the child's thinking depends specifically on concrete images, on visual representations. When the adolescent makes the transition to thinking in concepts, his remembering what he perceived and logically comprehended must disclose completely different laws than those that characterized remembering during primary school age" (p. 97).[1]

Perception is another function which is transformed by conceptual thinking:

> Isolated objects of perception become connected because of thinking; they become ordered and acquired sense—a past and a future. Thus, speech leads to thinking about perception, to analysis of reality, to the formation of a higher function in place of an elementary function.
> If we turn to the perception of an adult, we will see that it represents not only a complex synthesis of present impressions and images in memory, but its basis is a complex synthesis of processes of thinking and processes of perception. That which we perceive and that which we know, that which we perceive and that which we think merges into one . . .
> Ordered and comprehended perception, connected with thinking in words, is the complex product of a new synthesis in which visual impressions and processes of thinking are merged in a single alloy that can justifiably be called visual thinking. In contrast to the developed thinking of an adult, a child's thinking unites, orders, and comprehends what is perceived entirely differently. For this reason, the hypothesis of E. Claparède, who says that the child sees differently than the adult, and the statement of K. Koffka that the child lives in another world than we adults do are true in a certain respect. The developed perception of an adult places a net of ordering, logical categories over reality. His is always a comprehended perception (p. 88, this volume; cf. Ratner, 1991, pp. 38–41, 70–76).

Vygotsky says that imagination and fantasy are also intellectualized during adolescence and consequently fulfill a completely new function in the new structure of the adolescent's personality:

> If we correctly defined the higher development of the thinking of the adolescent as a transition from rational to judicious thinking and if we determined correctly the

---

[1]Vygotsky's emphasis on conceptual thinking led him to minimize the importance of non-cognitive factors in determining psychological development. Thus, he criticized psychologists who regard development as due to emotional or sexual changes in adolescence (pp. 30–31, 38, 153–154, this volume).

intellectualization of such functions as memory, attention, visual perception, and willful action, then in the same logical sequence we must reach the same conclusion with respect to fantasy. Thus, fantasy is not a primary, independent and leading function in the mental development of the adolescent; its development is the result of the function of forming concepts, the result which completes and crowns all the complex processes of changes that all of the intellectual life of the adolescent undergoes (p. 154).[2]

Contrary to popular opinion, the intellectualizing of fantasy and imagination enrich them in comparison with their impoverished existence in early childhood. Fantasy and imagination in childhood are bound to real objects and therefore have limited freedom. "The imagination of the adolescent is different from the play of the child in that it breaks the connection with real objects" (p. 161). Utilizing abstract concepts, the adolescent's imagination is more varied than the child's (p. 161; cf. Ratner, 1991, pp. 180–182).

The Integration of Psychological Phenomena

We have just seen how each psychological phenomenon is integrated with conceptual thinking. Their common integration into conceptual thinking also unifies the various phenomena together. Vygotsky expressed this as follows:

> Various functions (attention, memory, perception, will, thinking) do not develop side by side like a bundle of branches placed into a single vessel; they even do not develop like various branches of a single tree that are connected by a main trunk. In the process of development, all of these functions form a complex hierarchic system where the central or leading function is the development of thinking, the function of forming concepts. All the other functions enter into a complex synthesis with this new formation; they are intellectualized and restructured on the basis of thinking in concepts (pp. 84–85).

The fact that psychological phenomena are internally related to each other enables them to modulate and modify one another. Vygotsky emphasized how phenomena change as they become interrelated with new factors. For example, the playing with dolls or tools by a two year old and a four year old seem externally to be very similar; however, they may have completely different foundations and meanings due to the different configuration of factors which permeate them (p. 8).

> The same habits, the same psychophysiological mechanisms of behavior that, from the formal aspect, frequently show no substantial difference at different age levels or at different stages of childhood are included in a completely different *system of tendencies and inclinations* in a completely different force field of direction, and from this arises the deep *uniqueness of their structure, their activity*, and their changes at a *given* definite phase of childhood (p. 4, this volume).

Vygotsky pointed out that qualitative change in psychological characteristics is only recognizable if they are acknowledged to be imbued with new qualities from their internal relationships with other phenomena. Regarding phenomena as discrete atoms (rather than dialectically interrelated) promotes the view that they are autonomous and therefore immune to qualitative change from related phenomena (cf. Ratner, 1997, pp. 15–26 for discussion of this point). Vygotsky repudiated static, atomistic thinking which only notices superficial, overt appearance. He endorsed dialectical thinking which discerns the modulations and transformations of phenom-

---

[2]Donald (1991, p. 212) argues that speech produced distinctive psychological phenomena over the course of human phylogenetic development: "Simultaneously with the appearance of speech there appeared a whole constellation of thought skills that are associated with language . . . Semiotic cultures triggered completely new forms of information processing and storage: semantic memory, propositional memory, discourse comprehension, analytic thought, induction, and verification, among others."

ena that result from their interdependence and interpenetration (p. 196): "the transition from research based on external manifestations, on phenotypic similarity, to a deeper study of the genetic [i.e., changing], functional, and structural nature of thinking at different ages leads us inevitably to rejecting the established traditional view that is inclined to identify the thinking of the adolescent with the thinking of the three year old" (p. 36; cf. Ratner, 1997, Chaps. 2, 4, 5 for application of this concept to psychological research).

The method which

> describes characteristics of behavior according to age was usually reduced to a static characterization, to enumerating a number of features, traits, different characteristics of thinking for a given stage of development. In this case, a static characterization usually substituted for a dynamic consideration of age. Development was lost from sight and the form, characteristic only for a given age, was assumed to be stable, immovable, always equal in itself. Thinking and behavior at each state was considered a thing and not as a process, something at rest and not moving (p. 40).

A given psychological phenomenon changes its nature as it is related to different phenomena across the life span. It does not retain a constant quality, significance, or function. Therefore no single trait, like sexuality, emotionality, aggressiveness, or security can be used to assess (compare) the psychological development of an individual at all ages. The reason is that the trait which is the standardized measure changes. As Vygotsky said, "The importance and significance of any trait change continuously with the transition from age level to age level. This excludes the possibility of dividing childhood into separate periods according to a single criterion for all ages" (p. 188).

Vygotsky believed that all aspects of psychological functioning change through new interrelationships over the life span. Not only do particular phenomena such as thinking, feeling, attention, memory, personality, etc. acquire new characteristics, but even "the driving forces of our behavior change at each age level" (p. 3). Therefore, no one mechanism consistently explains psychological functioning at all age levels. We have seen that intellectual/cognitive processes organize the psychological processes of adolescents and adults, but not infantile or childhood processes. Which mechanisms are central depends upon biological, mental, and social factors. Different constellations (Gestalts) of these factors alter the driving forces of behavior (cf. Asch, 1946, 1952 for brilliant demonstrations of this dialectical standpoint). In Vygotsky's words, "The age levels represent the integral, dynamic formation, the structure, which determines the role and relative significance of each partial line of development" (p. 196). "Processes that are central lines of development at one age become peripheral lines of development at the following age and conversely, peripheral lines of development of one age are brought to the forefront and become central lines since their meaning and relative significance in the total structure of development changes . . ." (p. 197).

Form and Content

According to Vygotsky, it is not only the content of psychological processes which changes over the course of ontogenetic development. The form of psychological operations—or the manner in which information is processed—also changes. This is a break with traditional psychological thinking which postulates certain fixed ways in which thinking, feeling, perceiving, and remembering process information while allowing for new contents to be poured into these unchanging operations. Vygotsky maintained that the very ways of thinking, feeling, perceiving, and remembering change as they confront new contents. The content of thinking is not simply the external data that comprise the subject of thinking; the content that one confronts "moves inward" and becomes an organic component part of psychological operations. The task of mastering new content nudges the youngster along the path of developing psychological operations as well (pp. 32–35, 42 this volume; Ratner, 1991, Chap. 3, especially pp. 131–138 for extended discussion of this point).

Traditional psychology assumes that content is socially organized and variable while operations are biologically determined fixed structures.

> We might say that the fateful break between form and content flows inevitably from the fact that the evolution of content of thinking is always considered as a process of cultural development, primarily facilitated historically socially, and development of the form of thinking is usually considered as a biological process due to organic maturation of the child and the parallel increase in brain weight (p. 37, this volume).

However, the truth of the matter is that operations, structures, and processes are sociocultural phenomena just as much as content is. This is why they change as much as content does. In a powerful statement, Vygotsky explains that only a sociocultural view of human psychology can appreciate the integration of form and content. He says,

> Only with the introduction of the teaching on the higher forms of behavior that are the product of historical evolution, only with the introduction of the special line of historical development or the development of higher mental functions in the ontogenesis of behavior does it become possible to . . . approach the study of the dynamics of form and content of thinking in their dialectical unity (p. 37).

Higher Processes Control Lower Processes

After establishing that higher psychological functions are fundamentally different from lower ones, and that qualitative change is a fundamental law of human psychological development, Vygotsky explains what happens to the lower processes which have been superceded. They do not continue to function in the original state while being supplemented by higher processes. Thus, they do not interact with higher processes. Instead, the lower processes are restructured on a new base: "lower or elementary functions, being processes that are more primitive, earlier, simpler, and independent of concepts in genetic, functional, and structural relations, are reconstructed on a new basis when influenced by thinking in concepts . . ." (p. 81).

This dialectical sublating, surpassing, or *aufhebung* of one level into another requires some explanation. Vygotsky explains how it occurs in psychological and biological phenomena:

> One of the basic laws of development of the nervous system and behavior is that as higher centers or higher formations develop, lower centers or lower formations yield a substantial part of their former functions to the new formations, transferring these functions upward so that the tasks of adaptation that are done by lower centers or lower formations at lower stages of development begin to be done by higher functions at higher stages (p. 83).

In other words, lower centers and formations are controlled by the higher centers and formations and work as subordinate units. They do not maintain an independent existence and original powers. However, if the higher centers and formations should be struck by some disorder, the subordinate unit may resume elements of its old type of functioning and act as a safety valve to provide rudimentary survival activities (pp. 83, 218–220).

The Relative Autonomy of Psychology from Biology

If higher psychological functions are not derived from or continuous with lower psychobiological processes, and if biologically determined lower processes are sublated into, reorganized, and subordinated by socially organized higher processes, then the latter cannot be biologically determined. Of course, higher processes require a biological substratum; however, this substratum is non-determining, in contrast to the biological determination of lower processes. The biological substratum of higher psychological functions—which is primarily the neocortex of the brain—is extremely pliable in response to experience. Thus, the human brain enables, rather than directs or controls, socially organized psychological phenomena (cf. Ratner, 1991, Chaps. 4, 5; Ratner 1989a, b for documentation of these points).

Higher psychological functions actually stimulate neuronal growth in particular directions. They create their own biological mediations. They do not depend upon specialized biological mechanisms which pre-determine them. If they did so, they would not be socially organized and they would not be higher functions. Vygotsky expressed this point as follows: "There is every reason to assume that the historical development of behavior from primitive forms to the most complex and highest did not occur as a result of the appearance of new parts of the brain or the growth of parts already existing" (pp. 35–36, this volume; Donald, 1991, pp. 1–19).

Vygotsky's social explanation of psychological development led him to repudiate biological explanations. He rejected, for example, the notion that psychological development parallels biological maturation. "In comparing the data of onto- and phylogenesis, we did not for a moment take the point of view of biogenetic parallelism, intending to find in the history of the development of the child a repetition and recapitulation of those forms of thinking that prevailed at previous states of human history . . . We did not for a moment identify the process of concrete thinking of the child with the process of concrete thinking in the history of human development" (p. 41). The theory of recapitulation made no sense to Vygotsky because it confused mature, higher psychological processes of primitive adults with lower, elementary childish processes. Concrete thinking of primitive adults and modern children cannot be equivalent because the former is a higher process while the latter is a lower one. Vygotsky repudiated the temptation to compare psychological processes on the basis of superficial, external characteristics. Concrete thinking may appear to be superficially equivalent in primitives and children but a deeper understanding of their characteristics in terms of related biological, social, and cognitive factors reveals that they are really quite different. The sequence of certain kinds of thinking may be similar in ontogenetic and phylogenetic development—in both arenas external signs develop before internal mnemonic devices do (p. 168), and pre-linguistic functions are restructured by language—but the specific characteristics and functions of psychological phenomena are quite different in primitive adults and contemporary children.

Comprehending the Nature of Psychological Phenomena

Vygotsky believed that the way to understand the real (developing) character of psychological phenomena was to look beneath the surface of psychological characteristics: "Changes that occur in the thinking of the adolescent who has mastered concepts are to the utmost degree changes of an internal, intimate, structural nature often not apparent externally, not hitting the eye of the observer" (p. 38). Qualitative features are only recognizable to a dialectical standpoint which seeks out the features and sections of a given stage as varied, or modulated, by each other (pp. 40–41). "The nature of things is disclosed not in direct contemplation of one single object or another, but in connections and relations that are manifested in movement and in development of the object, and these connect it to all the rest of reality" (p. 54).

Vygotsky expressed optimism that

> psychology is moving from a purely descriptive, empirical, and phenomenological study of phenomena to disclosing their internal essence. Until recently, the main problem was the study of symptom complexes, that is, the aggregate of external traits that differentiate the various periods, stages, and phases of child development . . . But the real problem consists of studying what lies behind these traits and determines them . . . (p. 189).

Vygotsky says that the purely descriptive study of external features is fruitless with respect to explanation, prognosis, and practical applications. It can be compared to those medical diagnoses that doctors made at the time when symptomatic medicine prevailed. According to that approach,

> The patient complains of a cough, the doctor makes a diagnosis: the illness is a cough. The patient complains of a headache, the doctor makes a diagnosis: the illness is a headache . . . The matter is precisely the same with respect to symptomatic diagnoses in psychology. If a child is brought in for consultation with complaints that he is developing poorly mentally, has a poor imagination and is forgetful, if after investigation, the psychologist makes the diagnosis: the child has low intelligence quotient and mental retardation, the psychologist explains nothing, predicts nothing, and cannot help in any practical way . . . (p. 205).

Vygotsky would obviously be appalled by the fact that precisely this kind of symptomatic, external assessment is the rule in contemporary psychological science, especially as exemplified by the *Diagnostic and Statistical Manual* for diagnosing psychological disorders (cf. Ratner, 1987; Ratner, 1997, Chap. 1 for additional examples).

Vygotsky argued that psychological phenomena are only truly understood if their internal relations and essential, underlying features are discerned. This, in turn, requires that phenomena be conceptualized in abstract concepts. Consistent with his rationalist philosophy, Vygotsky believed that conceptual thinking is an essential means for comprehending reality. He said, "those who consider abstract thinking as a removal from reality are wrong. On the contrary, abstract thinking primarily reflects the deepest and truest, the most complete and thorough disclosure of reality" (p. 47, this volume). "Recognizing concrete reality with the help of words, which are signs for concepts, man uncovers in the world he sees connections and patterns that are confined in it" (p. 48). "Without thinking in concepts there is no understanding of relations that underlie the phenomena. The whole world of deep connections that underlie external, outward appearances, the world of complex interdependencies and relations within every sphere of activity and among its separate spheres, can be disclosed only to one who approaches it with the key of the concept" (p. 42).

The Socialization of Psychological Phenomena

Vygotsky believed that higher psychological phenomena are stimulated and constituted by social relations. The infant is born into an existing social world and only through participating in this world develops higher mental functions. We have seen that social interactions do not simply elicit pre-formed functions, they literally form the infant's psychology. Vygotsky provides three examples of this process (cf. Ratner, 1991, pp. 28–38 for additional examples).

One example is the manner in which logical thinking develops. Vygotsky, citing the research of James Baldwin, Pierre Janet, and Jean Piaget, states that logical thinking in the child recapitulates the form of social discussion and argumentation between people.

> In the process of developing cooperation and particularly in connection with the appearance of a real argument, a real discussion, the child is first confronted by the need to form a basis, to prove, confirm, and verify his own idea and the idea of his partner in the discussion. Further, Piaget traced that the argument, the confrontation that arises in a children's group is not only a stimulus for logical thought, but is also the initial form in which thought appears . . . P. Janet showed that all deliberation is the result of an internal argument because it is as if a person were repeating to himself the forms and methods of behavior that he applied earlier to others.
>
> Thus, we see that the child's logical deliberation is as if an argument transferred to within the personality and, in the process of the child's cultural development, *the group form of behavior becomes an internal form of behavior of the personality. the basic method of this thinking* (pp. 168–169, emphasis added).

A second example of the sociogenesis of higher psychological phenomena is the development of self-control and voluntary direction of one's own actions:

> The child who learns to modify direct impulse and to subordinate his activity to one rule or another. . . does this initially as a member of a small group . . . Subordination to the rule, modification of direct impulses, coordination of personal and group actions initially, just like the argument, is a form of behavior that appears among children and only later becomes an individual form of behavior of the child himself (p. 169).

A third example of the sociogenesis of individual psychological phenomena is symbolic, or conceptual thinking:

> speech, being initially the means of communication, the means of association, the means of organization of group behavior, later becomes the basic means of thinking and of all higher mental functions, the basic means of personality formation . . . Behind the psychological power of the word over other mental functions stands the former power of the commander and the subordinate (p. 169).

These examples all demonstrate that psychological functions are derived from social relations which exist externally to the individual. Vygotsky summaries his position by saying that "the structures of higher mental functions represent a cast of collective social relations between people. These [mental] structures are nothing other than a transfer into the personality of an inward relation of a social order that constitutes the basis of the social structure of the human personality (pp. 169–170). Vygotsky goes so far as to call this "a law of the development and structure of higher mental functions." This "law of transition of a function from outside inward" means that "all internal higher functions were of necessity external. However, in the process of development, every external function is internalized and becomes internal" (p. 170).[3]

---

[3]Psychological phenomena not only originate in social relations, they are best expressed and understood in social situations: "the social environment is the source for the appearance of all specific human properties of the personality" (p. 203, this volume). Vygotsky recommended that psychological assessment of higher functions be conducted in a social interaction between the subject and tester. In such an occasion, the tester can prompt the subject, demonstrate examples of what he is to do, and ask questions about the reasons for his action. Such social interaction may enable a child to meet higher performance standards than is possible through independent, individual test-taking. And the resulting improvement indicates that this child's psychological competence is different from a child's whose performance is not socially enhanced (pp. 202–203).

Of course, internalized, internal processes then mediate future encounters with the social environment. Encounters do not impinge upon a blank slate, but are refracted by accumulated experiences. As Vygotsky says, "My experience is affected by the extent to which all my properties and how they came about in the course of development participate here at a given moment" (p. 294). However, because psychological properties come about through socialization, as discussed above, we must say that the social environment shapes the experience which an individual has by shaping the psychological properties which comprise experience. In other words, the experience one has depends upon perceptions, emotions, ideals, and imagination which mediate an encounter with the physical or social world. Yet these mediations are all internalized from social relations. Social life is not experienced immediately—anew at each moment—but rather is mediated by psychological functions which have been socialized through previous social encounters. Social life works on us from the outside but also from the inside in the form of higher psychological phenomena. This is why Vygotsky concludes that the researcher must make "a penetrating internal analysis of the experiences of the child, that is, a study of the environment which is transferred to a significant degree to within the child himself and is not reduced to a study of the external circumstances of his life" (pp. 294–295; cf. Ratner, 1997, Introduction and Chap. 4).

The Logical Consistency of Vygotsky's Concepts

A great strength of Vygotsky's psychological system is its logical consistency. The distinction between higher and lower psychological functions, the relative autonomy of psychological functions from biological determinants, the subordination of lower processes to higher ones, the socialization of higher functions, their dependence on conceptual and semiotic symbols, the integration of psychological phenomena—including the unification of form and content, the qualitative changeability of psychological phenomena, and the requirement that they be studied by conceptualizations which penetrate beneath superficial external appearances and disclose essential internal relationships, all support one another. Logical consistency is a hallmark of all great scientific systems (cf. Ratner, 1997, Chap. 5). On this ground, along with the empirical validity of its concepts, Vygotsky's system qualifies as great science.

Sept. 1997, Perm, Russia

REFERENCES

Asch, S. (1946). Forming impressions of personality. *Journal of Abnormal & Social Psychology,* **41**, 258–290.

Asch, S. (1952). *Social psychology.* New York: Prentice-Hall, 1952.

Donald, M. (1991). *Origins of the modern mind: Three stages in the evolution of culture and cognition.* Cambridge: Harvard University Press.

Ratner, C. (1987). Subjective errors in objective methodology. *Contemporary Social Psychology,* **12**, 2, 127–129.

Ratner, C. (1989a). A sociohistorical critique of naturalistic theories of color perception. *Journal of Mind and Behavior,* **10**, 361–372.

Ratner, C. (1989b). A social constructionist critique of the naturalistic theory of emotion. *Journal of Mind and Behavior,* **10**, 211–230.

Ratner, C. (1991). *Vygotsky's sociohistorical psychology and its contemporary applications.* New York: Plenum.

Ratner, C. (1997). *Cultural psychology and qualitative methodology: Theoretical and empirical considerations*. New York: Plenum.

Ratner, C. (forthcoming). The historical and contemporary significance of Vygotsky's sociohistorical psychology. In R. Rieber and K. Salzinger (eds.), *Psychology: Theoretical-historical perspectives*. Washington, D.C.: American Psychological Association.

Vygotsky, L. (1981). The development of higher forms of attention. In J. Wertsch (ed.), *The concept of activity in Soviet psychology* (pp. 189-240). New York: Sharpe.

CONTENTS

Part 1: Pedology of the Adolescent

Part 2: Problems of Child (Developmental) Psychology

PART 1

PEDOLOGY OF THE ADOLESCENT

Selected Chapters[1]

Chapter 1
DEVELOPMENT OF INTERESTS AT THE
TRANSITIONAL AGE

1

The key to the whole problem of the psychological development of the adolescent is the *problem of interests* during the transitional age. All human psychological functions at each stage of development function not without a system, not automatically and not accidentally but within a certain system, directed by certain tendencies, trends, and interests established in the personality.

These driving forces of our behavior change at each age level, and their evolution is the base for change in behavior itself. It would, therefore, be incorrect, as has frequently been done, to consider the development of separate psychological functions and processes only from the formal aspect, in an isolated form, without regard for their direction and independently of the driving forces that these psychophysiological mechanisms bring into play. A purely formal consideration of psychological development is essentially antigenetic[2] since it ignores the fact that with a move to a new age level, not only the mechanisms of behavior themselves change and develop, but also its driving forces. Lack of attention to this circumstance can also explain the lack of results of many psychological studies, especially those pertaining to the transitional age.[3] These studies frequently vainly tried to establish some kind of substantial qualitative differences in the activity of separate behavioral mechanisms, for example, of attention or memory of the adolescent in comparison with the younger, school-age child[4] and the very young child. If such features were established, they usually were limited to purely quantitative description that demonstrated the growth of a function and an increase in its numerical index, but not a change in its internal structure.

Moreover, as we shall see below, of logical necessity, some investigators, depending on a formal consideration of mental development, reached the conclusion that in the adolescent all the basic elements of thinking already are in a set form in the three-year-old child and that intellectual processes at the transitional age level undergo only further development and further growth in the same direction without presenting anything new in comparison with what was observed in early childhood. Charlotte Bühler,[5] who came to this conclusion, cites a much broader parallel between the adolescent during sexual maturation and the three-year-old child, finding, from the formal aspect, a number of similar traits in the psychology of the one and the other. We are inclined to see here a manifestation of an internal insupportability of the purely formal method in pedology and its inability to grasp the developmental process in all its real complexity and to take into account all of

3

those real new formations that arise during the transition of the child from one age level to another.

The key to the understanding of the psychology of age, as has been said, is based in the problem of direction, in the problem of driving forces, in the structure of *tendencies and aspirations of the child*. The same habits, the same psychophysiological mechanisms of behavior that, from the formal aspect, frequently show no substantial difference at different age levels or at different stages of childhood are included in a completely different *system of tendencies and inclinations* in a completely different force field of direction, and from this arises the deep *uniqueness of their structure, their activity*, and their changes at a *given* definite phase of childhood.

Specifically because of this failure to take into account the indicated circumstances, for many decades child psychology was not able to find even one essential trait that would distinguish the child's perception from the adult's perception and would indicate the content of processes of development in this area. For this reason, a serious turning point in the history of the study of child behavior was the realization that formal consideration alone was inadequate and there was a need to study those basic points of *direction, points with a unique configuration whose structure we find at each given stage, within which all mechanisms of behavior find their place and their significance.*

A point of departure for scientific study in this area is admitting that not just the child's habits and psychological functions (attention, memory, thinking, etc.) are developing—at the base of mental development lies, first of all, an evolution of the child's behavior and interests, a change in the structure of the direction of his behavior.

2

Psychology came to realize this idea only recently. We are no longer speaking of the old subjective psychology in which interests were either identified with mental activity and considered as a purely intellectual phenomenon (J. Herbart),[6] or ascribed to the sphere of emotional experiences and defined as joy from an effortless functioning of our powers (W. Jerusalem and T. Lipps),[7] or derived from the nature of human will, converging with action and constructed on the basis of wishes; but even in objective psychology, which strived to construct studies about interest on a biological base, the problem of interest was greatly clouded for a long time by multiple and, for the most part, completely erroneous attempts to present relations existing between interest and mechanisms of our behavior in a proper light.

Edward Thorndike[8] defines interest as a *striving*, calling attention to its driving, impelling force, to its dynamic nature, to the decisive factor of direction that it contains. The striving to devote one's thoughts and actions to some kind of phenomenon the author terms an interest in this phenomenon. Thorndike states that the feeling of enthusiasm, mental excitation, and attraction to a subject is termed an interest.

Even in this formula, together with a more or less clearly expressed new view of interest, we find a number of undefined points (a feeling of enthusiasm, mental excitation, attraction to a subject) from the aggregate of which the author tries by means of summation to reach a definition of interest.

Developing these thoughts further, Thorndike wrote that interests may be either innate or acquired. In this respect, interests are no exception to the general rule that our behavior is comprised of both innate reactions and acquired reactions built up on their base. In an attempt to divide interests into innate and acquired, objective psychology again confronts all the differences between interest and mechanisms of behavior or mental functions and, not without reason, at this point many divergences arise among opinions and views of interest.

The central question for all of these teachings is this: are new interests acquired in the process of human development or can they be reduced to innate interests promoted by biological factors? This problem can be expressed differently: should psychology differentiate between interest and tendency, and what relation do they have to each other? As we have seen, Thorndike gives a positive answer to this question, distinguishing between innate and acquired interests. But he is inclined to identify the relation between tendency and interest with the relation between innate and acquired reactions.

That this point of view in its logical development compels identifying interests with reactions is easy to see from the conclusions drawn from this position by representatives of the new dynamic psychology in America. R. Woodworth, for example, believes that the ability of the human mind to acquire new mechanisms is at the same time an ability to acquire new tendencies, since each mechanism that is at the stage of development at which it has reached a certain effectiveness, but is not yet automatic, is in itself a striving and can be a motive for action that lies outside its direct functioning.

For partisans of dynamic psychology, the tendencies themselves represent only a mechanism in action in dynamic connection with other mechanisms, and for this reason, as the same author says, the process of developing secondary or acquired motives will be a part of the general process of developing habits. In other words, on the basis of their studies, the authors are inclined toward the conclusion that together with the formation of habits, new conditioned reflexes and new mechanisms of behavior, new interests and new driving motives are created that are subject mainly to the same laws that govern the development of conditioned reflexes. From this point of view, every activity creates a new interest. On this basis, striving arises toward certain objects that are also essentially interests.

The world would be boring, these authors maintain, if objects in themselves did not attract us and only hunger, fright, and other innate instinctive reactions would always wholly determine our relation to one object or another.

A mechanical conception of the development of interests as if they accompany, like a shadow, the development of habits that arise as simple practices and are essentially nothing more than a tendency to repeat actions done over and over again, being simple inertia of behavior, casts a negative aura over what is at the base of this teaching about interest, the inertia and inertness of the driving forces of our behavior, including both the innate and the acquired directions of our reactions.

The whole trouble with this teaching lies in its reducing the mechanism of acquiring interests to a simple mechanism of dressage and training, the basis of which is a simple force of inertia, a mechanical action of habitual repetition. Thus, the theory blunders in a series of internal contradictions attempting, on the one hand, to understand the rise of new tendencies in the process of development and, on the other hand, to dissolve new inclinations in a general tendency toward repetition and to reduce them to a single common denominator with the formation of new habits. This is the source also of the mechanical conception that newly acquired interests do not differ at all from innate or instinctive tendencies. H. English, for example, believes that dispositions developed through habit provide for us the same kind of authentic force of striving as the instinctive. In this claim the theory under consideration essentially confronts rejection of its own basic position, declining to establish a difference between instinctive striving and developed disposition.

Psychologists who do not believe it possible to identify interest or striving with a mechanism in action defend the opposite point of view. Thus, on the basis of his research, W. MacDougall concludes that at the base of all striving, of every interest there is essentially an innate, instinctive inclination that is manifested only in habit and is promoted by one set of mechanisms or another. He says that habits do not contain in themselves any inherent striving; they determine how we must carry out our tasks but are not the driving forces of the process and do not sustain it. As MacDougal demonstrates with a simple experimental example, in itself habit does not contain interest, but is always an inherent factor in the unfolding of a psychological process, a factor that must be strictly distinguished from the driving force, from the prompting motive that sets in motion and sustains the whole process of a given operation.

Let us imagine that we are saying the alphabet beginning with the first letter and continuing to the last and suddenly break this task in the middle. Naturally an urge arises to continue this unfinished or interrupted action. One may easily have the impression that habit itself evokes this urge, that in it is based, so to speak, the interest in saying the whole series of letters to the end. Actually, we can easily be convinced that this is not so. The interest that we perceive as striving when our task is interrupted, is actually based in the original purpose for which we undertook the task in the first place. Let us imagine that we again say the whole alphabet to the same letter at which our first recitation was interrupted, but this time with a different intention—not to say the whole alphabet to the end, but to determine where a given letter is in the order. Here the intention is different, the different purpose leads to completely different results: coming again to the same letter and, consequently, interrupting the habit at the same place, we, however, cannot find even the least tendency to continue this same habit since the motivating striving itself was exhausted at a given point.

Analysis of similar cases, says the author, leads us to the unavoidable conclusion that habit does not include in itself any kind of striving.

MacDougall, observing two boys whom he enticed with competition and an appeal to their pride to undertake the uninteresting and heavy work of uprooting a stump, showed that this complete absorption in an object, this deep interest in activity that at first glance might have been taken for an independently and newly acquired interest in that work actually displays a closer dependence on basic instinctive interests (pride, competition, etc.) and disappears as soon as the latter are satiated and satisfied. In this way, the author comes to a decisive rejection of the position that interests are acquired and arise the same way habits do.

If the second theory of interests occupies an advantageous position in comparison with the first in one respect (it can penetrate more deeply into the structure of behavior and understand complex and multistage relations that exist between interest and habit), then in another respect, this theory takes a great step backward in comparison with the teaching of Thorndike and Woodworth, admitting that all interests, all impelling forces of our activity are innate and in the last analysis are dependent on the biological nature of instincts.

The argument about whether new tendencies are acquired or not acquired led, as frequently happens in scientific arguments, to a new precision and a new formulation of the problem itself and consequently to elucidation of the relative truth contained in both the one theory and the other and toward overcoming the serious errors that dilute the portion of truth that is in each of them. Both theories are supportable in a critical part where they attempt to disclose the error of the opposite teaching, and both are equally insupportable in the positive part, equally impotent in overcoming the mechanistic view of behavior and the development of interest.

Partisans of the first theory, MacDougall's, say that the world would be boring if all our behavior were directly determined by the instincts of hunger, fright, etc. Here they are absolutely right: the actual picture of an interested relation to the world does not at all coincide with that which would be drawn on the basis of MacDougall's theory, but the latter might justifiably respond to critics in their own words; he could say: the world would be just as boring if our relations to one object or another were determined exclusively by the force of habit or the tendency toward inertia.

A new formulation of the problem demonstrated that, on the one hand, the authors who consider acquisition or development of new tendencies and interests possible are right, and on the other, that there is some element of truth favoring partisans of the point of view that not every habit in itself is really a striving or really an interest, that there are broader spheres of personality, deeper and more stable tendencies; there are permanent tendencies, there are as if basic lines of our behavior that can be essentially and completely justifiably termed interests which in their turn determine the functioning of one set of habits or another.

Actually, if we take the point of view of those who believe that every habit because of its origins is provided with its own driving force, we inevitably come to a behavioral picture that is monstrous in its mechanistic and atomistic qualities, in its explosiveness and chaotic nature, which in this case would resemble not an organic whole formation, but an "insane machine" in which every screw would move according to its own laws and the forces contained within it. With this understanding it becomes absolutely impossible to explain scientifically the basic problem: what is the origin of the connectedness, orderliness, fusion, and mutual compatibility of separate processes of behavior, the development of whole systems of behavior, and what is the explanation of the difference between the process of psychological development and the simple process of dressage that facilitates the development of ever newer habits.

But if we take the opposite point of view and identify interests with instinctive tendencies, we are confronted by a no less monstrous and hopeless picture of each new generation endlessly trampling along the circle of innate, instinctive tendencies; and how man goes beyond the limits of his animal nature, how in the process of societal life he develops as a cultural and working being, again becomes inexplicable and beyond understanding.

But from both points of view equally hopeless is the solution of the problem of how behavior develops and its central question—how do new formations arise in the process of psychological development: the problem of the origin of the new in the process of development remains equally inaccessible to both theories. Overcoming the basic errors of both theories, we come to the possibility of a new, synthetic approach to the problem of interests which gives us a structural theory of interests forming before our eyes.

3

The structural theory of interests, as has already been said, attempts to rise above the extremes of both one-sided points of view. Complex and penetrating experimental studies done to solve the problem of the relation between interest and habit compel the new psychology to reach a conclusion that the old point of view, which saw a driving force in the associative connection between two elements, a driving force that activated psychological processes, cannot be supported in the face of new facts. K. Lewin[9] says that an experimental study of habit showed that connections created by habit as such never are the driving force for a psychological process.

A single formation of association, it seems, is still inadequate for setting into motion any kind of nerve mechanism. The habits, customs, associative connections and combinations that are formed can exist as a series of potentially ready mechanisms, but in themselves, owing only to the fact of their existence, they do not have any primordial inducing force and thus do not contain any special, inherent tendency.

Lewin's studies showed that facts fully correspond to MacDougall's conclusions, which we mentioned above. Habit in itself does not elicit any tendency to continue activity, on the contrary—a tendency to continue activity is relatively independent of a number of habits in which it finds its realization. Thus, when we experimentally interrupt the flow of some activity, the urge to complete it finds its resolution, its discharge, in some other replacing, surrogate activity that has nothing in common with the former activity according to associative mechanisms. But when any activity exhausts the interest it evoked and results in satiety and the test subject's refusal to continue the work, it is very easy to induce continuation of the same activity without a break if a new tendency, a new interest, is created for the subject that involves a given habit in a different structure, gives him another direction.

We may consider it to be an experimentally established fact that habits and associative mechanisms do not act without system, automatically, chaotically, each with the force of a special, inherent striving toward action, but that they all really are induced to activity only as subordinate points in some general structure, a common whole, some common dynamic tendency only within which they acquire their functional significance and their sense. The combination itself of habits, the order of their coming into action, their structure and methods of activity—all of this is determined primarily by that orderliness, those complex relations that exist within a given dynamic tendency. Such *integral dynamic tendencies that determine the structure of the direction of our reactions can justifiably be termed interests.*

The relation of separate kinds of activities to the whole dynamic tendency that encompasses them may be explained with examples cited by Lewin. He says that a small child experiences joy in throwing various objects; later he begins to tuck objects behind a cabinet or under the rug; when he gets older, he gladly begins to hide and to play hide and seek, frequently even when he tells a lie, hiding plays a significant role in his lie. Another example: at first a small child has a great urge to open and close any box; then while still in his mother's arms, he begins delightedly to open and shut a door; later when he learns to walk, he tirelessly continues the same game with door and subsequently opens and shuts all doors. Under similar circumstances, not only capabilities with respect to certain actions develop, but it is easy to detect the development of tendencies, needs, and interests.

In this way, we see that *needs, tendencies, and interests* are more broadly encompassing, integral processes than any separate reaction. Reactions different in themselves may evoke one and the same tendency and, conversely, completely different interests frequently find expression and satisfaction in reactions that are externally identical. Lewin believes that actions of a two- or four-year-old that seem externally to be very close to each other, like playing with dolls or playing with a tool box, or playing streetcar may have completely different foundations.

Human activity is not simply the sum of unregulated working habits; it is structurally encompassed and regulated by integral dynamic tendencies—strivings and interests. Together with establishing the structural relation between interest and habit, the new theory comes with a logical sequence to a completely new formulation of the old problem of innate and acquired interests; it poses the question not as it was posed formerly: are interests exclusively innate and given together with basic instinctive tendencies of man or are they acquired in parallel to the formation of new habits in the process of simple training.

Interests are not acquired, but *develop*—this introduction of the concept of *development* into the teaching on interests includes the most important word enunciated by the new theory pertinent to the whole problem of interests. For the first time, a real possibility was opened for overcoming the mechanistic point of view of interest, inherent in the same way in both opposed directions that earlier psychology took with respect to this problem.

Interests understood as integral, structural, dynamic tendencies are considered by the new psychology in the light of this understanding as vital organic processes, deeply rooted in the organic, biological base of personality, but developing as the whole personality develops. These processes, like all vital processes, manifest a completely overt development, growth, and maturation. This clearly expressed ontogenesis of needs, tendencies, and interests discloses, in the words of Lewin, the same kind of rhythm as, for example, the biological development of the egg. Lewin believes it is made up of a series of dynamic phases of which each is relatively autonomous. The concepts of maturation and crisis are most essential here.

In light of the new theory, which includes the fate of interests in the general context of ontogenesis, the problem of the relation of the biological and the social in the development of interests is presented to us in a new form. The impelling force of human activity or striving is also a simple mechanical sum of separate arousal or of instinctive impulses. These inclinations are rooted as if in special clusters that might be termed needs since we ascribe to them, on the one hand, a stimulating force for action, we consider them a source from which tendencies and interests take their beginning, and, on the other hand, we emphasize the fact that needs have a recognized objective meaning in relation to the organism as a whole.

In this way, we come to a general conclusion that human behavior is moved by needs, but the structural theory,[10] in contrast to the theory of MacDougall, far from reduces all needs only to innate or instinctive. Needs disclose completely clearly expressed ontogenesis. Together with needs rooted in innate tendencies, the structural theory distinguishes needs that arise in the process of the child's personal development that are required in his adaptation to the environment, primarily the social environment. By the same token, the circle of basic needs is immensely extended, but the matter is not limited to this: together with real needs that arise in the process of long-term development, this theory also distinguishes so-called artificial needs, quasi-needs, that comprise the true sphere of interests of the person. In the first place, these quasi-needs display a very important analogy to real needs and dependency on them.

The basis for this rapprochement is not only the analogy purely external to real needs, but also the genetic connection consisting of the fact that the new needs arise on the basis of real needs and use innate mechanisms that set our reactions in motion. In other words, a temporary need or interest acts within certain limits exactly as do real needs. Quasi-needs do not simply imitate basic real needs in a new form, but are newly formed in the true sense of the word. These new formations exhibit real interactions with real needs and are closely or distantly related to them; sometimes they contradict them and sometimes they facilitate them. When a temporary need arises, the system of habits or thinking operations that must lead to a satisfaction of this need has not yet been created and formed. Only a general attitude develops, a tendency, a direction of behavior toward solving the problem and, as Lewin says, only a combination or coincidence of the temporary need and a concrete situation determines what concrete actions will be produced.

We come to establishing the last point that marks the new theory of interests, specifically, to establishing their two-sided, objective–subjective nature. Let us recall that the argument regarding whether interests are created or not created was, to a significant degree, an argument about what is the driving force of our behavior—is it subjective satisfaction connected with instincts, an internal tendency, or objective attractiveness of objects and activities themselves.

Thus, a serious problem arose that was actually not eliminated over the whole course of the development of teaching on interests: does interest have an objective or subjective character?

An indication of the dialectic resolution of the question is already contained in Hegel.[11] He believed that the true path toward a solution lies not in confirming some single side of interest, subjective or objective, but in admitting the complex and indivisible union of both sides. The structural theory proceeds along the path marked out by Hegel. Hegel says that whoever manifests activity with respect to anything is not only interested in the thing, but is also stimulated by it. Together with inclinations and needs, interest is a tendency that stimulates activity.

In other words, an exceptionally unique relation between man and the objective activity arises. Lewin finds this unique relation in the fact that on the basis of such temporary need or interest, the structure of man's environment, or, as the investigator puts it, the structure of the field,[12] changes radically. Even with real needs, we note that they do not directly lead us to certain actions; most often their direct influence is that they change for us the character of the things around us.

In the presence of need, certain things or processes of a stimulating character are external to us. All things related to food have this character for the hungry animal. Objects in the environment are not neutral for us. As Lewin says, they not only create difficulties for us in our actions to a greater or lesser degree or, conversely, facilitate actions, but many things and events that we meet manifest for us a more or less determined will, they stimulate us to certain actions: beautiful weather or a lovely landscape move us to take a walk, the steps of a staircase stimulate a two-year-old to climb and slide, doors stimulate him to open and close them, a dog—to tease it, a tool box, to play, a chocolate or piece of pancake arouses a desire to eat it, etc.

The stimulating character of things may be positive or negative, stimulating us directly or indirectly, strong or weak, etc., but the sense of the basic laws remains always one and the same: specifically, on the basis of arising needs, objects can be divided into neutral or stimulating, and the latter actively affect our behavior by their presence. The same is true with respect to temporary needs. They also bring about a change in the structure of the environment. A temporary need also leads to objects in the environment beginning to have a stimulating effect on us, they seem to require certain actions from us, elicit, provoke, draw or repel us, demand, attract or alienate, they play an active, not a passive role with respect to the need itself. Just as gunpowder explodes only when a spark falls into it, need acts when it meets external things that excite it and have the power to satisfy it.

The circle of things that have a stimulating character is determined more or less closely biologically with respect to actual needs; but it is more flexible, indeterminate, and pliant with respect to temporary needs. For this reason, Lewin formulates a general position in this form: to a certain degree, he says, the expressions "one need or another arose," and "one sphere of things or another stimulates certain actions" are equivalent. Thus, in structural theory, the stimulating effect things have on us is ascribed its proper place. What kind of stimulating forces influence each need as it arises is far from indifferent for the development and fate of that need. The barrenness of the old formulation of the problem of interest lay in the fact that the objective and subjective aspects of the process were separated, whereas the real basis of the process is specifically its two-sided nature in which subjective and objective factors are complexly synthesized.

4

The most important and substantial inadequacy of the structural theory of interests is that it does not detect the most serious difference that distinguishes interests from instinctive needs: it establishes a series of functional and structural differences between temporary needs and real needs, but does not take into account the principal difference in the essence itself, in the very nature of both phenomena; more simply speaking, it does not consider the social, historical nature of human interests. In essence, only man in the process of historical development has risen to creating new driving forces of behavior, only in the process of historical, social life of man did his new needs arise, form and develop; the most natural needs underwent a deep change in the process of man's historical development.

Structural psychology does not take into account this kind of change in human nature in the process of historical development nor does it consider the historical character of new formations that might be termed interests. It approaches interests as a natural and not a historical category; it considers the process of development of interests as analogous to biological, organic processes of maturation and growth; for it, the development of interest is similar to the development of an egg and for this reason, it looks to the physics of a living organism for analogy and considers needs and temporary needs primarily as the sources of organic energy, forgetting that human needs are often refracted through the prism of complex social relations. It is inclined to consider the ontogenesis of needs and interests mainly as an organic, vital process, forgetting that development of interest in the true sense of the word is the content of the social-cultural development of the child to a much greater degree than of his biological formation. For this reason, it simplifies the complex relations between the biological, organic basis of interests and the complex process of the development of their higher formation, a process that is a part of the general growth of the child into the life of the social whole to which he belongs.

It forgets the words of Karl Marx that the need of a man becomes a human need, and for this reason structural theory is most well grounded where development of interests is accomplished at the least distance from the development of their biological base; but this complex merging of two lines of development, the biological and the social-cultural, which actually lies at the base of ontogenesis, from the point of view of this theory, seems to be without a solution, and the lines that form the theory are not distinguished with adequate clarity. Specifically, as we have already indicated in a preceding chapter,[13] for a proper understanding of the basic cluster of biological needs from which the development of interests begins at the transitional age, it is necessary to take into account the historical nature of human attraction, the historical form of human sexual love. F. Engels, it seems, was the first to call attention to it in the phylogenetic plan of development.

"Modern sexual love differs substantially from simple sexual attraction, from the Eros of the ancients. First, it presupposes a mutual love on the part of the loved being; in this respect, a woman is on even footing with a man, while for ancient Eros, far from always was her consent required. Second, the force and du-

ration of sexual love are such that impossibility of possession or possibility of separation present themselves to both sides as great if not the greatest misfortune; they
take great risk, even put their lives on the line, in order only to belong to each
other, something which happened in ancient times perhaps only in cases of violation
of conjugal fidelity. And finally, a new moral criterion appears for judging and jus-
tifying sexual union; people ask not only whether it was marital or extramarital,
but also whether it arose as mutual love or not?" (K. Marx and F. Engels, *Works*,
Vol. 21, pp. 79-80).

Engels speaks of a newer, individual love between two persons of different
sex, of this high, moral process: initially a historical form of this individual sexual
love arose only in the middle ages, that is, the higher form of human need is a
historical form.

In the ontogenetic plan that is of interest to us now, we must also make a
distinction between the social-cultural line in the development and formation of
needs of the child and the adolescent and the biological line of development of
his organic tendencies. This is especially important with respect to the transitional
age. Here, during a time of extremely sharp acceleration of both the biological and
the cultural wave of development, here, during a time of maturation of both biological and cultural needs, we cannot find the key to a true understanding of the
changes taking place if we do not take into account that not only the content of
human thought, not only the higher forms and mechanisms of human behavior, but
the driving forces of behavior themselves, the very motors that set these mechanisms
into action, and the direction of human behavior undergo complex social-cultural
development.

In this sense, interests represent a specifically human state that distinguishes
man from animals: the development of interests lies at the base of all cultural and
mental development of the adolescent; in a higher form, becoming conscious and
free, interest stands before us as a realized striving, as an attraction for itself, in
contrast to instinctive impulse, which is an attraction to itself.

A better real indicator of everything that has been said about the nature of
our interests and their development, a better confirmation of all the powerful aspects of the structural theory and the most convincing refutation of its errors, the
best visual and real illustration of the truly scientific teaching on interest is the
history of the development of interests during the transitional age.[14]

5

The teaching on interests during the transitional age may serve as the best
illustration of Lewin's position cited above on the fact that interests cannot be understood outside the process of development, that concepts of growth, crisis, and
maturation are the basic concepts in the approach to this problem. It is enough to
consider the history of the development of interests at this age to be definitively
convinced of how erroneous it is to identify interests with habits and driving forces
with mechanisms of behavior.

Here, in the course of a comparatively small period of time, in the course of
five years, such intensive and deep changes in the driving forces of behavior take
place that they absolutely clearly form a special line of development that does not
coincide with the line of development of the mechanisms of behavior themselves.
If in the mental development of the adolescent we do not distinguish the process
of habit formation from the process of unfolding of interests, we will not at all be

able to explain the fact, central to all of this age, that habits change in a very substantial way in the course of one or two years.

Mechanisms of behavior formed earlier continue to exist, new mechanisms arise on their base, and interests, that is, needs that set these mechanisms in motion, change in a most radical way. We shall understand nothing in the mental development of the adolescent if we do not take into account this basic fact. And, as we have indicated above, many difficulties evident in the fact that psychologists did not know how to find substantial changes in the thought processes of adolescents but limited themselves to verifying further development of the same mechanisms that even a three-year-old child has can be explained first of all by the following: psychology failed to distinguish with adequate clarity the difference between the development of the line of direction and the stimulating motives of thinking and the mechanisms themselves of intellectual processes.

Without considering this fact, we will not later understand that in the process of the adolescent's development, at its most critical stage, there is usually a decline in school progress, a weakening of formerly established habits, particularly when productive work of a creative nature unfolds before the child.

But the transition of behavioral mechanisms to a lower level, a drop in the curve of development of intellectual processes, is not observed if the adolescent is confronted with a task that requires using habits that are more or less mechanical. It is difficult to find more clear evidence for the fact that habit itself may undergo comparatively little change, as is apparent in the mechanical work of the adolescent; nevertheless the method of his activity in the new structure of interests may undergo substantial changes.

We can say without exaggeration that at this age, the line of development of interests and the line of development of behavioral mechanisms are so clearly separated, each of them individually moving so complexly, that we can only manage to understand the main features of development correctly specifically from the relationship of the two lines.

Moreover, at exactly this age, the relations of the real biological needs of the organism and the higher cultural needs, which we term interests, appear in all their distinctness. Nowhere in the development of the child can we see with such clarity the fact that maturation and formation of recognized vital tendencies are an indispensable prerequisite for a change in the interests of the adolescent.

We shall subsequently see how both mutually connected processes—maturation of new tendencies and reconstruction on this basis of the whole system of interests—are clearly disconnected in time and form the initial and indispensable point of an essentially single developmental process.

Finally, the relation of subjective and objective factors within the structure itself of tendencies and interests, a change in the internal system of needs, and the stimulating force of the things in the environment find distinct expression in the history of interests of the transitional age. Here we can again trace with experimental clarity how maturation and the appearance of new internal tendencies and needs immeasurably broadens the circle of things that have stimulating power for adolescents, how whole spheres of activity that were formerly neutral in the relations of the child now become basic points that determine his behavior, how together with a new internal world, an essentially and completely new external world arises for the adolescent.

Without understanding that all behavioral mechanisms of the adolescent begin to operate in a completely different internal and external world, that is, with a radically changed system of internal interests and a system of stimulating actions originating externally, we will not be able to understand those really deep changes that are taking place in the adolescent during this period. But nowhere does the difference between interests and habits appear as clearly as in the fact that reconstruction of systems of interests at the transitional age allows us to distinguish more internally the intimate structure of every complex developmental process about which we spoke in one of the first chapters[15] of our course. Using a graphic comparison, we said there that the developmental processes in childhood and in the transitional age frequently resemble the conversion of a caterpillar to a pupa to a butterfly. Here, with a qualitative change in forms, with the appearance of a new formation in the developmental process, the very process discloses its complex structure. It is made up of processes of dying off, reverse development or a curtailment of the old form, and construction and maturing of a new form through processes of birth. Conversion of the pupa to butterfly similarly assumes both the demise of the pupa and the birth of the butterfly; all evolution is at the same time involution. This is how James Baldwin[16] formulates this basic law of development. The complex merging of processes of dying and being born interwoven one with the other can be traced with particular clarity in the development of interests.

Even at the first superficial glance it is easy to note that not only new interests develop in the adolescent, but the old die off; he not only begins to be interested in a number of things completely new to him, but also loses interest in things that occupied him previously. With the rise to a new level, the old dies off, and this especially distinct, long-term, and frequently excruciating process of dying off of childhood interests at the transitional age, as we shall see later, fills a whole chapter in the history of the development of interests of the adolescent. Moreover, curtailment of the old interests that prevailed in the preceding period is not accompanied to any degree by the dying off of the old habits acquired during early school years or earlier or by the dying off of old behavioral mechanisms that took shape and were formed in childhood.

Of course, these mechanisms also undergo substantial changes, but the fate of the changes, the line of their unfolding and refolding, hardly coincides with the line of unfolding and refolding of childhood interests, with their fate. Specifically for this reason the problem of interests at the transitional age was usually posed as a purely empirical problem with no theoretical basis; specifically for this reason, it is the key problem for all of the psychology of the adolescent; finally, specifically for this reason it contains a clear expression of the whole basis of the law of development of interests in general; without knowledge of these, the fate of interests at the transitional age remains completely obscure and incomprehensible. We considered it indispensable to precede the analysis of interests of the adolescent with a general analysis of the problem of interests.

Explaining the general bases of the teaching on interest is half the job of analyzing interests of the transitional age. We have already said that psychologists who do not consider the changes and shifts in the area of interests subject themselves willy-nilly to the illusion that in the mental development of the adolescent there is absolutely nothing substantially new in comparison with what is present in a three-year-old. In their opinion, there is simply a further improvement of the same apparatus, a further movement along one and the same line.

In the following chapter on the problem of thinking during the transitional age, we will consider this view in detail. Now, in connection with the problem of interest, of central significance for us is the analogous prejudice according to which in the area of interests, the transitional age represents a single whole that is not divided into separate phases and stages, that is, as if with respect to interests, that age is characterized as a single static whole.

The idea of denying more serious shifts in the area of interests of the adolescent is waiting for a classical study of the transitional age. Such authors, for example, as T. Ziehen (1924) are inclined in general to speak against establishing separate phases in the transitional years and trust that development during this period continues evenly. Actually such a point of view means nothing other than rejection of understanding the development that the interests of the adolescent undergo. All successes of modern psychology are connected with overcoming specifically this prejudice; they are all directed toward isolating, analyzing, and describing as precisely as possible the separate phases and stages that comprise the process of sexual maturation as a whole. Using the recognized analogy, we might say that the most characteristic feature of modern psychology of the adolescent is its attempt to understand the personality of the adolescent not as a thing, but as a process, that is, to approach it dynamically and not statically, and this is inevitably connected with distinguishing separate phases and periods in the development of the interests of the adolescent.

6

The principal position of the new psychology of the adolescent in this area is that the basic phases in the development of interests coincide with the basic phases of biological maturation of the adolescent. This alone tells us that development of interests is closely and directly dependent on the processes of biological maturation and that the rhythm of organic maturation determines the rhythm in the development of interests.

With respect to this, Oswald Kroh[17] justifiably expressed a new point of view on the phases in the development of the adolescent radically different from the views of Ziehen. The basic idea in his work is the following: development does not occur evenly and regularly; the development of the adolescent, including development of his interests, occurs as an arithmetical progression in which separate phases are clearly evident. These are determined bilaterally—both by the rhythm of internal maturation and changes in the glandular system of internal secretions and by the fact that the adolescent, maturing biologically, loses connections with his environment.

After the explanation that interests develop on the basis of development of tendencies and together with the development of interest, the whole character of relations to the environment changes, we do not find it at all surprising that the phases comprising the arithmetical progression during the period of sexual maturation are marked not only by a series of internal organic changes, but also by a reconstruction of the whole system of relations to the environment. After the explanation that development of interests includes an involution of former interests, we are not at all surprised that the transition of development from one phase to another is directly manifested mainly in the demise of old connections to the environment and that there are whole periods in the development of the child in which he rejects his environment.

Kroh distinguishes two periods of rejection[18] particularly clearly: (1) at the age of three approximately, and (2) at approximately 13, at the beginning of sexual maturation. From this, many authors, including Charlotte Bühler, have made a far reaching analogy between the process of development of the adolescent and processes of development of the three-year-old. We will put this idea aside to be considered later.

Now we are interested only in the fact that in summarizing the data of modern teaching on phases of sexual maturation, we see that all authors establish a complex arithmetical progression and the presence of phases at that age. Thus, discredited are both the idea of Ziehen of even and regular development during this period and another traditional view that assumed the critical processes of involution of the psychology of the adolescent to be the absolute content of the period of development as a whole and lost from sight the phenomena of growth and maturation behind the phenomena of crisis. Moreover, growth, crisis, and maturation—these three points basically determine the three stages of sexual maturation and only in their aggregate give a true representation of the process of development as a whole. For this reason, P. L. Zagorovskii,[19] summing up contemporary teaching on the breaking up of the period of sexual maturation into separate phases, completely correctly states that a number of studies of adolescence done recently significantly limit the view of the period of sexual maturation to an age of fluctuation of moods, a period of contrasts in development (S. Hall),[20] etc. The negative phase takes a certain limited time, and after it ends, the adolescent enters the next phase of development.

We note that quite often the argument in contemporary literature on the essence of the transitional age—is it a tragic unfolding crisis or a positive and multifaceted synthesis that forms the base of maturation—is due partly to an incorrect static posing of the problem that attempts to encompass within a single formula the transitional period as a ready-made and concluded thing with firm, established, and determined properties. In movement, in dynamics, and in development of the transitional age, both polar points find a real, vital coincidence.

The process of maturation is composed of crisis and of synthesis that represent various points in one and the same wave of development. If we move to the content of the basic phases that comprise the development of interests during the transitional age, we will have to indicate that the basis for this whole development is the organic changes connected with the processes of sexual maturation. Sexual maturation means the appearance in the system of organic tendencies, of new needs and stimulations—this is what lies at the base of the whole change in the system of interests in the adolescent. A better indication of this is the fact that processes of change in interests usually coincide exactly in time with the time of onset of organic changes. When sexual maturation is delayed, the crisis of interests is postponed; when sexual maturation occurs early, the crisis of interests occurs near the initial stage of this period.

This is why we can precisely track what seem like two basic waves in the development of interests during the transitional age: the wave of new tendencies that form an organic base for a new system of interests and then a wave of maturation of this new system built onto the new tendencies. In this respect, W. Peters (1927) completely justifiably proposed to distinguish two basic phases during the transitional period, the first of which he termed the phase of tendencies, and the second, the phase of interests.[21] It is understood that the distinguishing and designation are very conditional, but basically they completely accurately convey one of the main results to which a series of studies on the transitional age lead us. The first phase, the phase of tendencies, usually lasts about two years. It is characterized by Peters as a phase of negative display of interests, a phase of rebellion against authority, rapid and sharp change in moods, and sharp fluctuations in direction.

For us, this phase is characterized mainly by the fact that it contains two basic points: first, the unfolding and dying off of formerly established systems of interests (the basis for the negative, protesting, rejecting character), and, second, the processes of maturation and appearance of the first organic tendencies that signify the onset of sexual maturation. Specifically, the combination of both points taken together characterizes what at first glance is a strange fact, that in the adolescent we can see as if a common general decrease, and sometimes even a complete absence of interests. The disruptive, devastating phase during which the adolescent finally concludes his childhood caused L. N. Tolstoy[22] to term this period the "desert of adolescence."

Thus, the period as a whole is characterized by two basic traits: first, this is a period of a breaking away from and demise of old interests and, second, a period of maturing of a new biological base on which new interests develop later.

7

The demise of the old interests and maturing of tendencies leaves the impression of a desert. This circumstance provided a reason for Peters to call this a stage in the whole phase of tendencies and contrast it with the following phase of maturation, the phase of interests. We know that all interests are built on a certain instinctive base on which alone their further development is possible, but an essential trait of development is exactly the fact that the biological base, or subsoil of interests, which over the course of other growth periods remains more or less constant, itself shifts and undergoes substantial changes in the transitional age, disrupting the formerly established harmony of tendencies and disclosing new, first-to-mature instinctive impulses.

It is not surprising that the whole superstructure, like present buildings during an earthquake, is shaken to its roots. The period of disruption of the superstructure and disclosure of new layers of tendencies is the phase that Peters terms the phase of tendencies. For him this phase is characterized mainly by a general indeterminate and diffuse irritability, increased excitability, rapid onset of fatigue and exhaustion, abrupt and sharp fluctuations in mood, protest and rebellion against authority.

Thus, for him also, another process goes hand in hand with the disclosure of new tendencies: the process of devastation or destruction of old interests. The new replacement phase is characterized according to Peters mainly by the presence of contradictory traits, specifically, by the maturing and establishing of new interests that unfold on a completely new basis.

Typical for the beginning of the process is a multiplicity of interests that the adolescent manifests as he enters the second phase. From this multiplicity of interests, a certain basic nucleus of interests is gradually developed through differentiation and continues to develop during the second phase, characterized by a polar relation of the initial and the final points. If initially, the phase of development of interests is marked by romantic aspirations, then the final phase is marked by a realistic and practical selection of one most stable interest, usually directly linked to the basic vital line selected by the adolescent. It must be noted that Peters' observations relate to the course of these two phases of interests in a working-class adolescent. Peters, like many other authors, establishes that for the proletarian adolescent, youth begins later and ends earlier and that the passage of this whole period of development is either compressed or extended depending on unfavorable or favorable economic and social-cultural conditions. Peters' observations, like those of other authors in other countries, pertain to the working-class adolescent in capitalist countries. Peters says that a 14-year-old is still a child and an 18-year-old, already an adult.

According to Peters' observations, in the working-class adolescent, the first phase is usually as long as in the bourgeois adolescent, differing sometimes, depending on conditions of life, by being more stormy. The second phase of interests is, on the other hand, greatly abbreviated and compressed in time, limited in natural development, impeded by early vocational work and difficult conditions of life.

Another trait of the phase—specifically, the involution of former interests—was the reason for describing this phase in the development of the adolescent as negative or the phase of rejection. Using this phrase, Charlotte Bühler notes that the phase is characterized primarily by negative tendencies and a drop in school interests together with other purely negative symptoms typical of the onset of this phase; absence of any definite and stable interests is the main trait of the whole phase. Essentially, in describing the negative phase, Bühler is describing the same stage in the development of the adolescent as is Peters, but placing more emphasis on a different trait.

If for Peters, the stimulation of new tendencies against a background of demise of childhood interests is most important in the symptomatic complex of the period under consideration, for Bühler, the rejection of former interests against a background of springing up of new tendencies is most important. Actually, among the symptoms that characterize onset of the negative phase, Bühler includes a keen sexual curiosity that appears most frequently in the adolescent during this period. She considers it not accidental that, according to data of Berlin statistics, sexual transgressions of girls occur most frequently during just this phase.

It is extremely interesting to note that specifically at the beginning of sexual maturation, during the negative phase, sexual tendencies appear least disguised, in an open form, and as sexual maturation proceeds, we can observe not an increase, but a decrease of these symptoms in this form. Specifically for the negative phase, their lack of disguise and an unprocessed, bare manifestation is characteristic. Together with the negative symptoms, Bühler notes not only the appearance of tendencies as basic traits from which the entire picture of the phase as a whole is made up, but she goes even further, trying to place all the points of rejection of this phase, everything that makes it negative, in direct biological relation to sexual maturation, to the formation of sexual attraction.

Here Charlotte Bühler bases her thinking on the biological analogy of F. Doflein, and certain other investigators indicate that animals before the onset of sexual maturity display agitation, increased excitability, and urges toward isolation. Noting further that the period of negativism in girls usually occurs before the first menstruation and ends with its onset, Bühler is inclined to consider the whole complex of negative symptoms as the real onset of sexual maturation.

Bühler marks the beginning of the phase with a completely distinct drop in productivity and capacity for activity even in the area of special giftedness and interests. (We note that in this case we have a beautiful illustration of the extent to which development of mechanisms of behavior, habits, and abilities does not parallel the development of interests, and we observe in the negative phase how deep the divergence is between the one process and the other.) Further, together with this decrease, we see inner discontent, anxiety, striving for isolation, self-isolation, sometimes accompanied by a hostile attitude toward those around. The decrease in productive activity, demise of interests, and a general anxiety constitute the main distinct traits of the phase as a whole. The adolescent as if repels his environment, that which recently was the subject of his interest; sometimes negativism passes more smoothly and sometimes it manifests itself in the form of disruptive activity. Together with subjective experiences (depressed state, repression, and melancholy revealed in entries in diaries and other documents that disclose the internal, intimate life of the adolescent), this phase is characterized by hostility and a tendency toward arguments and infractions of discipline.

The whole phase might be called the phase of a second negativism, since such a negative attitude usually is manifested in early childhood at the age of approximately three years. As we have noted, Bühler uses this as a basis for making a far-reaching analogy between the first and the second phase of negativism. But it is to be understood that this similarity is limited to a purely formal likeness of the one period to the other; evidently, the negative attitude characterizes every alteration, every break, every transition of the child from one stage to another, being a requisite bridge over which the child rises to a new level of development. According to Bühler's data, in girls this phase begins on average at 13 years 2 months and lasts several months.

8

Similar observations were made by other investigators. For example, O. Sterzinger turned his attention to the fact that teachers had for a long time complained of the decrease in degree of school success and productivity of the students, of the difficulty they meet in their school work usually in the fifth class in 14- and 15-year-old adolescents. This same circumstance was also noted by Kroh: in the first phase of sexual maturation, there is a seeming decrease in ability and productivity in mental work of the students. Kroh indicates that the disturbingly poor school success that is usually observed in the middle school in the fifth class even in adolescents who were until then good students can be explained by the fact that at this point a change occurs in purpose from visualization and learning to understanding and deduction. The transition to a new and higher form of intellectual activity is accompanied by a temporary decrease in capacity to work.

On a firm basis, Kroh characterizes the whole stage as a stage of disorientation in internal and external relations. At the point of transition, when the traits of the past which is dying off are mixed in the personality of the adolescent with traits of the imminent future, there is a certain change in the basic lines and direction and a certain temporary state of disorientation. Specifically at this time there is a certain divergence between the child and his environment. Kroh believes that in the course of the whole process of development there is never a greater separation between the human "I" and the world than during this period.

Otto Tumlirz (1931)[23] characterizes this phase in the development of interests similarly. For him, the period of sexual maturation also begins with the phase whose central point is a breaking of formerly established habits. This is a period of collision of various psychological directions, a period of uneasiness, of internal and external rejection and protest. This period in which there are no positive and stable interests is marked by opposition and a negative attitude. The first phase of rejection is replaced by another, positive phase, which Tumlirz terms a time of cultural interests.

We see that the most diverse investigators, regardless of their divergence in individual determinations, concur in admitting that there is a negative phase at the beginning of the transitional age. In the work of various authors, we find valuable additions to this position from the factual aspect. Thus, A. Busemann, who studied the problem of the reflection of basic traits of youth in the opinions of young people themselves, notes that particularly in girls, the onset of symptoms of discontent occurs at approximately 13 years of age, and in boys, at approximately 16 years of age.

E. Lau, whose research draws our attention mainly because it is concerned with working-class adolescents, notes that at the age of about 15 or 16, there is a decrease in the adolescent's interest in his work, and a negative attitude toward his vocation frequently appears suddenly. This attitude usually passes quickly and yields to a positive attitude.

Studies of other authors[24] helped to make more precise the differences in the course of the phase in boys and in girls and to explain individual symptoms of this phase. The research of K. Reininger showed that the negative phase was observed in girls usually between the ages of 11 years 8 months and 13 years. The phase continues for eight to nine months. Reininger concludes that the negative phase is a normal and necessary period through which the adolescent must pass. In Reininger's opinion, absence of this phase is observed only when development of the adolescent departs from the normal in one respect or another or with premature onset of maturity.

The end of the phase is marked by the following basic symptom: increase in success and productivity of intellectual activity. Among the symptoms that characterize this stage, the investigator notes instability, anxiety and depressed mood with negative coloring, passivity, and decrease in interests. Among girls in social classes without means, the same phase can be observed; it takes the same course basically, but occurs somewhat later, at approximately 13-14 years of age.

L. Vecerka did a similar study of this phase in girls in which she studied the development of social relations among adolescents, their relations with adults and different forms of family life in childhood. According to her data, the evolution of social relations and interests connected with them clearly discloses two polar phases of which the first phase is characterized by a disintegration of group bonds, a disruption of formerly established relations among children, a sharp change in relations with other people, and the second phase, which Vecerka termed the phase of unions, is characterized by the opposite traits, most of all an extension and strengthening of social bonds.

H. Hetzer observed the passage of the same phase in boys. The phase usually occurred somewhat later than in girls, between ages 14 to 16. The symptoms were the same as those in girls: a drop in productivity and pessimistic moods. A substantially different trait is a more stormy and longer negative phase and a more active nature of the negativism, a certain decrease in apathy and passivity in comparison with girls in the same phase, and somewhat greater manifestation of disruptive activity in the most various forms.

9

We can find exceptionally interesting data on the genesis of this phase and its characteristics as applied to the Soviet adolescent in two remarkable studies of P. L. Zagorovskii (1929). The first was a systematic study of seven school groups in classes IV, V, VI, and VII. The observations continued for a whole school year. From 274 students 11.5 to 16 years of age, 52 were selected who exhibited negativism in an especially clear and distinct form. Of the total number of adolescents in the study, 19% were in the negative phase of development. While among the group being observed, there was an approximately equal number of each sex, the group of 52 adolescents in the negative phase of development was made up of 34 girls and 18 boys. Of the group, 82% of the children (43 individuals) belonged to families of white-collar or intellectual employees and only 18% (9 individuals) were children of workers. The average age of the girls going through the negative phase was 14 years, 2 months (ranging from 13 years 2 months to 14 years 9 months); the average age of the boys was 14 years 6 months.

With respect to symptoms that characterize the passage of the negative phase, this study generally confirmed what was noted earlier.

Zagorovskii considers the first feature observed in adolescents in the negative phase to be a decreased success rate and work capacity. Following a period of normal rate of success and work capacity, there are lapses in work and a sudden failure to do assignments; students who had done certain work with enthusiasm suddenly lose interest in it; to the teacher's questions as to why one assignment or another had not been done, frequently the answer is: I didn't want to do it. Rate of success decreases especially markedly in some cases. Infractions of discipline among the adolescents are noted (mainly among boys); opposition to the group of friends, "verbal negativism" and negativism in acts, breaks in friendships, contempt for rules established by the group, a tendency toward solitude—these are the adolescent's behavioral features most frequently accompanying this phase. A passive, apathetic, dreamy state is observed more often in girls.

In some cases (in eight adolescents) a keen interest in reading was noted in which the adolescents made a transition to books with a different content, specifically to stories that contain an erotic factor. In a number of cases, we may assume the presence of keen sexual interest, but Zagorovskii's observations could not clearly illuminate this side of the adolescent's life.

The decrease in capacity to work and in rate of success can be described identically for boys and for girls in the negative phase. Zagorovskii states that work capacity decreases especially in creative assignments (composition, problem solving). Moreover, sometimes no deterioration is noted in mechanical tasks.

What is essentially new in Zagorovskii's studies is the description of adolescent behavior in the family during the negative period. The general conclusion that can be reached on the basis of these data is that the negativism of the adolescent is not as marked within the family as it is in school; conversely, in some adolescents, negative manifestations that are sharply obvious in the family are almost indiscernible in the school situation.

Thus, two points catch our attention in this study: first, the decrease in work capacity predominantly in creative tasks, which is understandable in connection with the transition of the adolescent to new still not firmly established forms of intellectual activity, and which is linked to the fact that these kinds of work, more than work of a mechanical nature, must be based on creative interests of the adolescent which are at a low ebb during this period of changing interests; second, the closer dependence of negative attitudes on environmental conditions (not all children displayed negative attitudes to the same degree, and they manifested different forms of these attitudes in the family and in school).

A second study with 104 adolescents entering the period of sexual maturation led the author to greater precision with respect to a number of questions connected with this problem and made possible a more valuable and serious qualitative analysis of the phenomena observed. The average age of the girls in the study was 13 years 3 months (from 12 years to 13 years 9 months), average age of boys, 14 years 4 months (from 13 years 6 months to 15 years 8 months).

The data obtained was subject to qualitative analysis which identified the type of pupils with respect to their passage through the negative phase of development. The author proposes that instead of "types," the designation "forms of behavior of the Soviet pupil" be used since the concept "type" presumes something stable, unchangeable, which cannot be said about children according to the data Zagorovskii obtained. The forms that the negative phase took in the adolescents can be reduced to three basic variants: in the first, sharply expressed negativism was manifested in all areas of the child's life, old interests dropped off sharply and took new directions, for example, in questions of sex life; the behavior of the adolescent in some cases changed to some extent within several weeks.

In some cases, the negativism was startlingly stable. The pupil drops out of the family completely; he is not receptive to the persuasions of elders; in school he is increasingly excitable or, conversely, dull, that is, it is easy to see schizoid traits in him. There were 16 such children (nine boys and seven girls), and among these, four were from working-class families. Among the girls, melioration of negative traits occurred significantly sooner than in boys. In describing these children the author says that the initial period of sexual maturation is difficult and severe.

The second variant of the passage of the negative phase is remarkable for its milder traits of rejection. The adolescent, the potential negativist, to use Zagorovskii's expression, could be said to display a negative attitude only under certain life situations, under certain conditions of the environment; his negativism arises mainly as a reaction to a rejecting effect of the environment (oppressive effects of the school situation, family conflicts), but these reactions are unstable and short-lived. It is characteristic specifically for these children that they behave differently in different social situations, for example, in school and in the family. This type includes a significant majority of the pupils studied (68 of 104).

Finally, the third variant of passage through the first phase of sexual maturation, negative manifestations, cannot be fixed at all. Here no decrease at all is noted in rate of success; there is no disruption of friendships, dropping out of the group, or change in relations with the teacher or the family. Also, Zagorovskii notes that a change in interests is apparent: an interest in the other sex is exhibited, interest in different books is evident, but there is a decrease in interest in school social life. This group includes approximately 20% of the children observed. A certain positive attitude to life situations was noted in the whole group and these children pass through the same biological phases of development as do the children who are open negativists. As the author expresses it, the third group of children exhibit no negative phase at all, and their positive emotional state does not decline over the course of the long period. Most of the children without the negative phase come from working-class families (11 of 20).

On the basis of his studies, Zagorovskii concludes that a substantial correction must be made in the positions of the authors who describe the negative phase. In his opinion, there is no doubt that negativism as a recognized phase in the development of the adolescent's interests, characterized by a detachment of the adolescent from his environment, does occur in human development. But Zagorovskii believes that the purely biological formula derived by Charlotte Bühler must be rejected. He thinks that the insupportability of this formula lies in the fact that negative reflexes with respect to the environment observed in higher mammals may in the human social sphere be inhibited or modified and may assume unique forms of expression. Further, negativism may not appear in every life situation. To a significant degree, a sharp exhibition of these symptoms may be due to inadequacies of the pedagogical approach.

Zagorovskii believes that we know little about the pedagogy of adolescents, that we have not yet developed definite methods with adolescents-negativists, but the fact noted by all investigators that the negative phase in the normal adolescent is not long, that it can be manifested in various forms of behavior, that is, be subject to influences, speaks for a conclusion favoring pedagogical optimism.

It seems to us that in describing the negative phase together with properly noted symptoms that characterize the early onset of sexual maturation, most authors simplify the problem exceedingly, and because of this, a contradictory picture develops of the various forms of manifestation of the negative stage under various conditions of the social environment and education.

10

It is impossible to limit the analysis of this phase to biological forms alone, as Zagorovskii correctly indicates. However, it seems to us that even his objection does not cover the whole problem: in the development of the adolescent's interests, even he is inclined to ascribe to the environment only the role of a factor that may inhibit, moderate, or provide various external expression, but not newly create and form the interests of the adolescent. Also, the most essential trait of this period is that the period of sexual maturation is a period of social maturation of the personality as well. Together with the awakening of new tendencies that provide the biological soil for reconstruction of the whole system of interests, there is a reconstruction and formation of interests from the top, from the aspect of the maturing personality and the world view of the adolescent.

Authors-biologizers lose sight of the fact that the human adolescent is not only a biological and natural, but also a historical and social being and of the fact that together with social maturation and a growing of the adolescent into the life of the community that surrounds him, his interests are not poured into him mechanically like a liquid into an empty vessel, into the biological forms of his tendencies, but, in the process of internal development and reconstruction of the personality, themselves reconstruct the very forms of the tendencies, carrying them to a higher level and converting them into human interests, and themselves become internal component factors in the personality.

Ideas surrounding the adolescent and present at the beginning of his maturation outside him become his internal property, an inalienable part of his personality.

A second correction that must be introduced into the teaching on the negative phase is that from biological and sociopsychological aspects, it is just as wrong to describe this period as a homogeneous stage and to imagine the whole melody of this critical stage to be made up of a single note. Actually, the processes of development in general and this process in particular are distinguished by an immeasurably more complex construction and immeasurably finer structure.

A. B. Zalkind[25] speaks of the serious pedagogical error that is the source of a number of absurdities in applications of the educational approach to this critical period. The error is due mainly to the fact that the critical stage is assumed to be a homogeneous stage in which there are ostensibly only processes of stimulation, ferment, and outbursts—in a word, phenomena that can be dealt with only with incredible difficulty. Actually, the critical period, regardless of all its complexity and difficulty, is not at all distinguished by the tragic element that was ascribed to it in the old pedology; it is completely heterogeneous: three types of processes occur simultaneously in it, and each of these types requires its own timely and integral consideration in conjunction with all the others in developing methods of education.

These three types of processes that comprise the critical period in the development of the adolescent are the following according to Zalkind: (1) increasing stabilizing processes that fix former acquisitions of the organism, making them ever more fundamental and ever more stable; (2) processes that are actually critical and completely new and changes that develop very rapidly and energetically, and (3) processes that result in the setting up of emerging elements of the adult person that are the basis for further creative activity of the developing person. The internal heterogeneity and the unity of the critical stage, in the thinking of Zalkind, are encompassed in the following claim: this stage concludes and arrests childhood, it creates something completely new, and it bears in itself elements of ripening in the full sense of the word.

It seems to us that specifically the consideration of the heterogeneity of the critical phase together with consideration of the transformation of tendencies into interests, that is, the cultural setting up and formulation of tendencies, presents in a really true light the problem of the negative phase.

The interests of the adolescent are the central point that determines the structure and dynamics of each phase.

Zalkind states that at the transitional age, the problem of interests becomes exceptionally complicated. It is quite clear that if we do not create in adolescents positive attitudes toward certain impressions that interest them, we will not be able to master by pedagogical action the main part of those biological things of value that are involved at the transitional age. We can quite confidently point out that the problem of education and training at the transitional age is a problem of proper building of interests of the age, dominants of the age in the opinion of the author.

11

In this respect, the teaching of Thorndike on the pedagogical significance of interests is of exceptional theoretical and practical interest. His teaching consists basically of three ideas, each of which separately and all taken together assume major significance for the problem of interests at the transitional age.

The first idea is that education is linked to interests in two respects. The purpose of education is to create certain positive interests and to eliminate undesirable interests since essentially education can never form in advance *all* future features of behavior of a person; it forms and creates only the basic interests that move and direct a person in later life. Thus we see how erroneously from the psychological aspect the process of education is formed when attempts are made to reduce it to simple development of new conditioned reflexes without regard for the development and education of the driving forces of behavior. Creation of habits alone or mechanisms of behavior alone without cultivating interests will always remain a purely formal education that will never solve the problem of the required direction of behavior.

The formation of interests acquires primary significance in comparison with the formation of habits especially at the transitional age, during the period of maturation when the basic attitudes of future life are determined to a greater degree by the formation of interests than by conclusive development of habits. Moreover, in education interests play the role of means since all motivation for activity and for acquiring habits and knowledge is based on interest. Thorndike ascribes great significance to this distinction since in teaching, the main errors with respect to interests are due to confusing means with goals.

Thorndike's second idea is that interest as a driving force that puts in motion the mechanism of behavior unavoidably—whether we want it or not—accompanies and determines the unfolding of every psychological process.

Thorndike maintains that all work presupposes interest. No physical or mental work is possible without interest, the least interesting work is still done because of interest, interest in avoiding punishment, in maintaining position in class, or in preserving self-respect; there must be some interest here. The problem of interest in teaching is whether or not children learn with interest; they never learn without interest: the question is what kind of interest will it be, what will its source be.

Finally, Thorndike's third idea, without which a correct understanding of interests in the transitional age is impossible, is that with respect to all instincts and habits just as with respect to interests, we must not consider nature as a reliable guide to ideals of education. For this reason, we can and must change interests, change their direction, switching the interests from one area to another, and we must cultivate and create new interests.

12

From these positions it becomes clear from historical and practical aspects that the second phase in the development of interests in the transitional age is a phase of affirmation, a positive phase, a phase of interests, as Peters terms it, or a phase of cultural interests according to Tumlirz.

Before we consider this phase in detail, we must very briefly and schematically consider the process of development of interests during the transitional age as a whole and for this, we must remember that, essentially speaking, in addition to the two phases noted by almost all the authors—the phases of negation and affirmation—a third phase must be identified, in essence even more correctly identified as the first, the preparatory phase. Previously we presented the opinion of A. E. Biedl[26] on the biological three-part division of the period of sexual maturation. With respect to psychology, there is no reason to reject this division, all the more so because in the development of interests we clearly distinguish still another, a preparatory phase. From the biological aspect it is characterized by an intensified activity of the hypophysis and the thyroid gland, which influence the growth of the sex glands and in this way prepare for sexual maturation. Thus we have a kind of latent period of sexual maturation during which the internal, deepest system of the organism is being prepared for sexual maturation that has not yet involved the other systems of the organism. A. B. Zalkind terms the latent period of sexual maturation the consolidation-preparation period since in it, on the one hand, elements of the future crisis are being prepared and, on the other hand, processes of childhood development are fixed and concluded.

This relatively calm, latent period of sexual maturation occurring in the very depths is, from the aspect of interests, characterized by absence of any particularly clear dominant attitudes or especially keen interests. How can the seeming paleness of the preparatory stage be explained? Mainly by a certain lack of general stimulation. During the latent period, we have a prologue of further development, a prologue which contains in an embryonal, undeveloped, and unseparated form all three basic periods which make up that age—demise of childhood, crisis, and maturation. The most unique forms and the richest development are characteristic for interests in the second stage of the transitional age. Here the law of switching of interests assumes special significance; we must use the effect of this switching to explain why the stormy and negative phenomena of the negative phase in adolescents are replaced by a positive direction and a favorably organized social atmosphere.

Zalkind enumerates several basic foci (groups) of dominants, or interests of the age, the aggregate of which comprises the nucleus of interests in the second stage. All the dominants may be a difficult, morbific factor that causes irritability, distractedness, dullness, and certain manifestations of negativism, but in switching the drive to dominant paths, to paths of keen interests, they are an invaluable source that feeds positive direction and transforms the negative phase into a creatively rich and valuable phase of development.

The first group of interests or dominants may be termed the egodominant or egocentric attitude of the adolescent. This dominant consists of the fact that the adolescent's developing personality is one of the central foci of interests, the point of departure for the approach to the second stage as a whole. Zalkind says that we should also be interested in the unique attitude of the adolescent toward the future, toward the broad, large dimensions that for him are much more subjectively acceptable than the more imminent, current, everyday matters. The *dominant of the distant future*, as the author terms it, is a specifically age-related trait of the second stage of the transitional age. Hence the author does not deny that the adolescent during this period is in conflicting relations with his environment, dissatisfied with it, seemingly leaping out of it, looking for something outside it, seeking the distant, greater dimensions, rejecting the mundane, the current.

However, it would be incorrect to understand both these foci of interests as made up and formed definitively at the very beginning of the stage. Proceeding from the personal, touching on and saturating the personal, it is necessary to switch it to social tracks; proceeding from the distant, from great dimensions of the adolescent, it is necessary, rousing him in this respect, to gradually reconstruct his work processes, his interests, involving them more and more in the routine, in the current, in everyday work. Zalkind believes that if we do not take these two basic dominants into account, then neither our routine nor our everyday matters will interest the adolescent or be used in his general development.

Among the basic interests, the author includes the thrust toward opposition and mastery, toward strong-willed pressure, which sometimes is resolved in stubbornness, hooliganism, struggle against educational authority, protest and other manifestations of negativism. The effort dominant approaches directly to the other, also basic, purposeful attitude of the adolescent, specifically the romance dominant that is expressed in especially strong thrusts of the child toward the unknown, the risky, toward adventures and toward social heroism.

It is easy to see that these dominants are dual and, in essence, are manifested both in the negative and in the positive phase. It would be more correct to say that according to psychological structure itself, they include both factors of rejection that precede attitudes internally necessary to the process of development and factors of affirmation that replace them. Negation and affirmation understood in this way appear to be two internal requisite factors of a single process of development of interests during the transitional age.

13

In conclusion, it remains for us to speak of an exceptionally widespread theory in modern pedagogical literature on the positive phase in the development of interests of the adolescent. Our exposition would be incomplete without a critical illumination of the theory. We have in mind the theory of serious play developed by William Stern[27] pertaining to the positive phase in the development of the adolescent's interests. Stern believes that we can correctly understand all the more important manifestations of the transitional age if we consider them in the light of the biological theory of play that Karl Groos[28] developed at one time. As we know, Groos considers children's play as it relates to the future. The biological function of play is to serve as a natural school of self-education, self-development, and exercise of natural instincts of the child. Play is the best preparation for future life; in play the child exercises and develops capabilities that will be useful to him in the future; in this way, play is a kind of biological supplement to the pliable instincts and capabilities of the child, a kind of specially organized, prolonged extrauterine process of functional development and perfecting of basic instincts and capabilities, according to Groos.

In preschool years, play encompasses almost all the behavior of the child; during school years, play and work or play and school tasks, becoming separate, form two basic streams along which the activity of the schoolchild flows and finally, in the transitional age, as Kroh and other investigators correctly note, work moves to first place, putting play in a subordinate and secondary position. Stern believes, however, that the matter is not quite like this. Just as the transitional age as a whole is a time of transition from childhood to a mature state, just as a number of features are evidence of such a transitional, mixed, middle state of the personality and its functions, precisely so interests of the adolescent and basic forms of his behavior, in the opinion of Stern, may best be described as serious play. By this combination of words, seemingly paradoxical at first glance, Stern wants to stress that the adolescent's behavior occupies a middle ground between the play of the child and serious activity of adults. The fluctuating, intermediate, mixed state also is that unique age-related form in which the interests of the adolescent are expressed.

Just as a child's play, according to the theory of Groos, anticipates and foreshadows future forms of life activity, precisely so does the adolescent in serious play exercise and develop the functions that are maturing at this time. According to Stern, serious play of the adolescent is manifested in two basic areas—in the erotic and in the area of social relations. Subjectively, the adolescent perceives this play completely seriously; sexual daydreams, erotic fantasy, flirtation, reading erotic literature, playing at love—at all points the difference between the actual and the seeming is erased. Satisfaction consists not in the result of activity, but in the process of its functioning. Stern believes that the eroticism of the adolescent is an unconscious school of love, the concept of "eternal love" disappears after a short time and the adolescent makes a transition to new objects of love; this is only a preliminary feeling, a preparation for the future love of the adult person; however, this is already not the play of a child but serious play in which catastrophic moments can suddenly appear.

Another form of serious play, according to Stern, is serious play in social relations. He believes that the adolescent conducts serious play in life relations; the whole transitional age appears to the author from the point of view of a period of introduction to the problem of relations between people. Friendship and enmity, colored by affectivity characteristic for children's play, the creation of various associations, circles, and societies, frequently with empty rules, purely external forms of personal contact—all of this, from the point of view of the theory of serious play, cannot be understood other than in the light of the middle, transitional form between purely childish imitation in play of the activity of adults and the real, serious relations of mature people.

The theory of serious play elicits very substantial objections. True, its factual basis does not seem to us to be completely false; on the contrary, undoubtedly the recognized intermediate form of activity appearing genetically between the play of the child and the serious activity of the adult can be observed in the adolescent; undoubtedly to a significant degree, it fills the transitional age; further, there is every factual basis for accepting the idea that the initial forms of amorous relations among adolescents actually do resemble playing at love.

Many have objected to Stern's theory. Zagorovskii, taking the theory as a whole, objected to attaching recognized steps in the development of social behavior to a certain age; for example, the phase in social development which, according to

Stern, the adolescent goes through at age 14-14.5 years, children of the city schools in the USSR go through in older school groups in the first level, and collectivistic reactions and collectivistic attitudes can be developed significantly earlier than the adolescent years.

It seems to us that this objection to Stern's theory is far from the only one and not the most substantial, although it is completely justified. The most important objection is roused by the purely mechanistic attempt to consider the transitional age as a certain arithmetical average, as a simple replacement of immature traits by traits of maturity. It is true that in every transitional form there are still traits of the preceding period while traits of the following period are maturing but, in addition, the process of development is far from being reduced to a simple transition from one step to another through a step that connects them and represents their arithmetical average. Also, Stern's theory is essentially a purely biological theory of the transitional age, a purely naturalistic theory of play; the teaching of Groos on play in early childhood suffers from the same defect; it also is a purely naturalistic teaching that cannot establish the principal difference between the play of an animal and the play of a human child.

Inability to differentiate the two lines in the developmental process in the child—the line of natural, biological, organic evolution and the line of social-cultural formation—in the complex synthesis that makes up the real process leads to the problem of tendency–interest, the central problem of the whole period of sexual maturation, being resolved extremely simplistically by deriving an arithmetical average of both components in the form of serious play. Play is self-education; what corresponds to it in the adolescent is a complex and long process of transforming tendencies into human needs and interests. Not the arithmetical average between them, but a complex and real synthesis of the one and the other, a transformation of tendency into interest is the true key to the problem of the transitional age.

Chapter 2
DEVELOPMENT OF THINKING AND FORMATION OF CONCEPTS IN THE ADOLESCENT[29]

1

The history of the development of thinking in the transitional age is itself undergoing a certain transitional stage from the old construction to a new understanding of maturation[30] of the intellect. This understanding arises on the basis of new theoretical views of the psychological nature of speech and thinking, of development, and of the functional and structural interrelation of these processes.

In the area of the study of thinking in the adolescent, pedology is overcoming the basic and radical prejudice and a fateful error that stands in the way of developing a correct conception of the intellectual crisis and maturation that are the content of the development of thinking in the adolescent. This error is usually formulated as a conviction that there is nothing essentially new in the thinking of the adolescent compared with the thinking of the younger child. Some authors, defending thinking, come to the extreme view that the period of sexual maturation does not mark the appearance in the sphere of thinking of any kind of new intellectual operation that a child of three cannot already do.

From this point of view, development of thinking is not at all at the center of the processes of maturation. Substantial, violent shifts taking place during the transitional period in the whole organism and the personality of the adolescent, revelation of new, deep layers of personality, maturation of higher forms of organic and cultural life—all of this, from the point of view of these authors, does not affect the thinking of the adolescent. All changes occur in other areas and spheres of the personality. Thus, the intellectual changes in the whole process of crisis and maturation of the adolescent are diminished and reduced to almost zero.

On the one hand, if one holds this point of view, the process itself of intellectual changes that occur at this age can be reduced to a simple quantitative accumulation of characteristics already laid down in the thinking of a three-year-old ready for further purely quantitative increase to which, strictly speaking, the word *development* does not apply. Charlotte Bühler has expressed this point of view most consistently in the theory of the transitional age where, among other things, further uniform development of the intellect during the period of sexual maturation is set up. In the general system of changes and in the general structure of processes of which maturation is made up, C. Bühler ascribes an extremely insignificant role to intellect, not perceiving the enormous positive significance of intellectual development for the fundamental, most profound reconstruction of the whole system of the adolescent personality.

In general and on the whole, this author believes that during the time of sexual maturation, there is a very strong separation of dialectic and abstract thinking from visual thinking since the opinion that any one of the intellectual operations in general appears anew only at puberty is one of the tales that have long since been exposed by child psychology. Even in a three- or four-year-old child, all potentials for later thinking are present. To support this thinking, the author cites the studies of Karl Bühler,[31] which present the point of view that intellectual development in its most essential traits, in the sense of maturation of basic intellectual processes, is already set up in early childhood. According to Charlotte Bühler, the difference in the thinking of the young child and that of the adolescent is that in the child visual perception and thinking are usually much more closely connected.

She says that the young child seldom thinks purely verbally and purely abstractly. Even the most talkative and verbally gifted children always start from some concrete experience, and when they yield to the tendency to talk, they usually chatter without thinking. The mechanism is trained without pursuing any other function. The fact that children make deductions and judgments only within a circle of their concrete experiences and that the goals of their plans are contained in a tight circle of visual perception is well known and has provided grounds for the false conclusion that children cannot think abstractly at all.

C. Bühler believes that this opinion has long since been refuted since it has been established that a child perceives very early, abstracting and selecting, and fills in such concepts as "good," "evil," etc. with some vague, general content; the child forms other concepts by abstraction and makes judgments. But we must not deny that all of this is very dependent on the child's visual perceptions and representations. In the adolescent, on the contrary, thinking is freer of the sensible base and is less concrete.

Thus, we see that the denial of substantial changes that occur in the adolescent's intellectual development inevitably leads to admitting simple growth of the intellect during the years of maturation and greater independence from perceptible material. We might formulate the idea of C. Bühler thus: the thinking of the adolescent acquires a certain new quality in comparison with the thinking of the young child; it becomes less concrete and, in addition, "it becomes stronger and firmer," "grows and increases" in comparison with the thinking of the three-year-old, but not a single intellectual operation arises anew during the whole transition, and for this reason thinking itself during this period has no substantial or determining significance for the processes of development of the adolescent as a whole and occupies no more than a modest place in the general system of crisis and maturation.

This point of view should be considered as the traditional and, unfortunately, the most widespread and uncritically accepted of the contemporary theories on the transitional age. In light of contemporary scientific data on adolescent psychology, this opinion seems to us to be very wrong: its roots are in the old teaching that of all the mental changes that occur in the child that turn him into an adolescent, it noted the trait that is only the most external, superficial, and obvious, specifically the change in emotional state.

Traditional psychology of the transitional age is inclined to see the central nucleus and main content of the whole crisis in the emotional changes and to compare the development of the emotional life of the adolescent to the intellectual development of the schoolchild.[32] We see this as everything being turned on its head; in light of this theory, everything seems to us to be turned inside out: specifically, the young child seems to be the most emotional being; in his general structure, emotion plays the pre-eminent role and the adolescent appears before us primarily as a thinking being.

The traditional point of view is expressed most fully, yet tersely, by F. Giese. In his words, while the mental development of the child before sexual maturation involves primarily the functions of perception, a store of memory, intellect, and attention, emotional life is representative of the time of sexual maturation.

Subsequent development of this point of view leads to the banal view which is inclined to reduce all mental maturation of the adolescent to an increased emotionality and dreaminess, to outbursts and similar somnolent products of emotional life. The fact that the period of sexual maturation is a period of a powerful rise of intellectual development and that during this period, thinking moves to the forefront for the first time, not only remains unnoticed when the question is posed in this way, but is even completely enigmatic and unexplained from the point of view of this theory.

Other authors also express the same point of view, for example, O. Kroh, who, like C. Bühler, sees all differences between the thinking of the adolescent and the thinking of the young child in the fact that the visual base for thinking, which plays such a significant role in childhood, moves to the background during the period of maturation. Kroh diminishes the significance of this difference when he completely properly indicates that, between concrete and abstract forms of thinking, an intermediate step frequently appears in the process of development that is also characteristic of the transitional age. This author gives the most complete positive formulation to the theory, shared also by C. Bühler, who said that we must not expect the child of school age to make a transition in the area of judgment to completely new forms. Differentiation, appreciating nuances, great confidence and awareness in using forms available now and before must be considered here as the most essential tasks of development.

Generalizing the position that reduces development of thinking to further growth of forms already present, Kroh assumes that in both the area of processes that work on perception (selecting, directing, perception of categories, and reordering classification) and in the sphere of logical connections (understanding, judgment, deduction, criticism), during the on-going school age, no new forms of mental functions and acts arise. They all existed previously, but during school age, they undergo significant development that is apparent in their more differentiated and nuance-sensitive and frequently more conscious application.

If the content of this theory can be expressed in a single sentence, it might be said that the appearance of new shades or nuances, greater specialization, and conscious application is all that distinguishes thinking during the transitional age from the thinking of the young child.

In essence this same point of view is developed in our literature by M. M. Rubinstein,[33] who considers sequentially all the changes that occur during the transitional age in the areas of thinking as further movement along the paths that were already in place in the thinking of the very young child. In this sense, the views of Rubinstein wholly agree with the views of C. Bühler.

Rejecting the position of E. Meumann,[34] who finds that the ability to make deductions is formed entirely at age 14, Rubinstein asserts that not one of the forms of intellectual activity, including making deductions, appears initially during the transitional years. This author points to the extreme error of the idea that childhood differs from youth in the area of mental development only in that the central act of thought—deduction—properly appears only during the transitional age. Actually, this is completely incorrect; there is absolutely no doubt that thought and its central act—deduction—is present in children. For Rubinstein, the whole difference between the thinking of the child and that of the adolescent is only the following: children accept as essential traits what for us adults is objectively nonessential, accidental, and external. Rubinstein believes that, in general, in both determinations and judgments, only during adolescence and youth does the major premise begin to be filled in by essential traits or, in any case, is a tendency to find specifically these and not to be guided by the first external trait clearly delineated.

The whole difference, it seems, can be reduced to the fact that these forms of thinking are themselves filled in with different contents in the child and in the adolescent. Rubinstein says the following about judgments: in the child, these forms are filled in with nonessential traits, but in the adolescent a tendency develops to fill them in with essential traits. Thus, the whole difference is in the material, in the content, in the filler. The forms remain the same and at best undergo a process of further accumulation and strengthening. Among such new shades or nuances, Rubinstein includes the ability to think in essentials and a significantly greater stability in directed thought, a greater flexibility, greater extent, agility in thinking and similar such traits.

The central idea of this theory can be understood easily from the objections that its author addresses to those who are inclined to deny the sharp rise and intensification in mental development of the adolescent and youth. Defending the idea that intellectual development of the adolescent is characterized by a sharp rise and intensification, Rubinstein writes that this is borne out by the observation of facts and theoretical considerations; otherwise we would have to assume that the inflow of new experiences, new content, and new interrelations contributes nothing: the cause remains without effect. Thus, typical traits of increased mental development must be sought not only in new interests and demands, but also in intensification and broadening of the old, in their range, in the whole breadth of vital interestedness.

In this defense, Rubinstein reveals an internal contradiction that is equally present in all theories that are inclined to deny the appearance of anything substantially new in thinking during the period of sexual maturation. All authors who deny the appearance of new forms of thinking during the transitional age agree, however, that filling in this thinking, its content, the material with which it operates, the objects to which it is directed—all of this undergoes a real revolution.

2

The break in the evolution of forms and content of thinking is very characteristic for any dualistic and metaphysical system in psychology that does not know how to present them in dialectical unity. Thus, it is deeply symptomatic that the most consistent, idealistic system of the psychology of the adolescent, presented in Edward Spranger's book (1924),[35] is silent on the development of thinking during the transitional age. In this work, there is no chapter devoted to this problem; moreover, all the chapters of the book, imbued with one common idea, are devoted to disclosing the process which, in Spranger's opinion, is the basis of the whole process of maturation and which is termed the adolescent's growing into the culture of his time. Chapter after chapter considers how the content of adolescents' thinking changes, how the thinking is filled with completely new material, how it grows into completely new spheres of culture. The adolescent's growing into spheres of law and politics, professional life and morality, science and world view—for Spranger, all of this is the central nucleus of processes of maturation, but intellectual functions of the adolescent in themselves, the forms of his thinking, the composition and structure of his intellectual operations, remain unchanged, eternal.

If we think deeply about all these theories, we cannot dismiss the idea that at their base there is a serious, very simple, very elementary psychological conception of the forms and content of thinking. According to this conception, the relations between the form and content of thinking resemble the relation between a vessel and the liquid that fills it. This is the same mechanical filling of the form with sex, the same potential for filling this same unchangeable form with ever newer content, the same internal disconnectedness, mechanical contrasting of the vessel and the liquid, of the form and what fills it.

From the point of view of these theories, the most serious revolution in the completely reformed content of the adolescent's thinking is in no way connected with the development of the intellectual operations themselves, which are solely responsible for the appearance of one content of thinking or another.

This revolution, according to the conceptions of many authors, is derived either from outside in such a way that those same, unchangeable forms of thinking, always equal to each other at each new stage of development, depending on enrichment of experience and broadening of connections with the environment, are filled with ever newer content, or the flowing spring of this revolution is hidden in the wings of thinking in the emotional life of the adolescent. It mechanically turns on the processes of thinking in a completely new system and directs them, like simple acts, to a new content.

In both cases, evolution of the content of thinking seems to be an impassable chasm separated from the evolution of intellectual forms. Through the power of facts, every theory that consistently takes off in this direction comes up against this kind of an internal contradiction. This can be easily demonstrated with a simple example: not one of the theories cited above denies, nor can it deny, the very serious, fundamental revolution in the content of the thinking of the adolescent, the complete reformation of the whole material content that fills the empty forms. Thus C. Bühler, who finds in the three-year-old all the basic intellectual operations proper to the adolescent, limits her claim exclusively to the formal aspect of the problem under consideration. Bühler would, of course, call it a tale if someone should claim that there is essentially nothing new in the thinking of the adolescent in comparison with what is already present in the thinking of the three-year-old.

Bühler cannot deny the fact that only when adolescence is reached is there a transition to formally logical thinking. She cites the studies of H. Ormian (1926), who demonstrated that only at the age of approximately 11 is a turning to purely formal thinking noted. As to the content of thinking, she, like Spranger, devotes a significant part of the work to explaining new layers of the content of ethical, religious conceptions and the rudiments of a world view in the development of adolescents.

Precisely so, together with new nuances to which he reduces the development of thinking during school years, Kroh indicates that only in the adolescent does the possibility of operating logically with concepts arise. Citing the studies of F. Berger, on the problem of perception of categories and its pedagogical significance, Kroh asserts that the perceiving and ordering function of psychological categories initially appears in all distinctness in experiences and memories during the period of sexual maturation.

Thus, all the authors agree that, while denying new formations in the area of intellectual forms, they must inevitably admit a complete reformation of the whole content of thinking during the transitional age.

We are considering the analysis and criticism of this point of view in such detail because without overcoming it decisively, without disclosing its theoretical bases, and without contrasting it with new points of view, we will not see any possibility of finding the methodological and theoretical key to the whole problem of the development of thinking during the transitional age. For this reason, it is very important for us to understand the theoretical bases on which all of these various theories, different in details, but similar in central nucleus, are constructed.

3

We have already said that the main root of all this theoretical blundering is the break between the evolution of form and content of thinking. The break in its turn is due to another basic defect of the old psychology, especially child psychology; specifically, child psychology until recently lacked a proper scientific conception of the nature of higher mental functions. The circumstance that higher mental functions are not simply a continuation of elementary functions and are not their mechanical combination, but a qualitatively new mental formation that develops according to completely special laws and is subject to completely different patterns, had still not been assimilated by child psychology.

Higher mental functions, the product of the historical development of humanity, have a special history in ontogenesis also. The history of the development of higher forms of behavior discloses a direct and close dependence on organic, biological development of the child and on the growth of his elementary psychophysiological functions. But the connection and dependence are not identity. For this reason, in research, we must identify the line of development of higher forms of behavior in ontogenesis also, tracing it in all its unique patterns, not forgetting for a moment its connection with the overall organic development of the child. We said at the beginning of the course that human behavior is not only the product of biological evolution that resulted in the appearance of a human type with all the psychophysiological functions proper to it, but also a product of historical or cultural development. The development of behavior did not stop with the beginning of the historical existence of humanity, but neither did it simply continue along the same paths along which biological evolution of behavior proceeded.

The historical development of behavior was carried out as the organic part of societal development of man, subject basically to all the patterns that determine the course of the historical development of humanity as a whole. Similarly to this, in ontogenesis also, we must distinguish both lines of development of behavior presented in an intertwined form, in a complex dynamic synthesis. But actually, a study that meets the true, real complexity of this synthesis, not intent on simplifying it, must take into account all the uniqueness of the formation of higher types of behavior that are the product of the cultural development of the child.

In contrast to Spranger, deep, scientific studies show that in the process of cultural development of behavior, not only the content of thinking changes, but also its forms; new mechanisms, new functions, new operations, and new methods of activity arise that were not known at earlier stages of historical development. Exactly so, the process of the cultural development of the child includes not only a growing into one area or another of culture, but also, step by step, together with the development of content, there is a development of forms of thinking and those higher, historically developed forms and abilities of activity whose development is the requisite condition for growing into a culture.

Actually, every really serious study teaches us to admit the unity and indivisibility of form and content, structure and function; it shows how every new step in the development of thinking is inseparably connected with the acquisition of new mechanisms of behavior and a rise to a higher step of intellectual operations.

A known content may be adequately represented only with the help of known forms. Thus, the content of our dreams cannot be adequately represented in the forms of logical thinking, in the forms of logical connections and relations; it is inseparably connected with the archaic, ancient, primitive forms or methods of thinking that are proper to it. And conversely: the content of one science or another, assimilation of a complex system, mastery, for example, of modern algebra, presupposes not simply filling with appropriate content the same forms that are already present in a three-year-old—new content cannot develop without new forms. The dialectical unity of form and content in the evolution of thinking is the alpha and omega of the modern scientific theory of speech and thinking. Actually, is it not enigmatic from the point of view of the theories set out above, which deny the development of new qualitative steps in the thinking of the adolescent, that modern studies have developed standards of mental development that require, for example, in the Binet–Simon tests[36] (edited by C. Burt and P. P. Blonsky),[37] a description and explanation of a picture from a 12-year-old, a solution to a life problem from a 13-year-old, defining abstract terms from a 14-year-old, indicating the difference between abstract terms from a 15-year-old, and catching the sense of a philosophical argument from a 16-year-old? Can these empirically established symptoms of intellectual development be understood from the point of view of a theory that admits only new nuances arising in the thinking of the adolescent? From the point of view of nuances, can we explain that the average 16-year-old adolescent attains a degree of mental development of which an indicative trait or symptom is capturing the sense of a philosophical argument?

Only a failure to distinguish between the evolution of elementary and higher functions of thinking, between biologically based and historically based forms of intellectual activity can lead to denying a qualitatively new stage in the development of the adolescent's intellect. Elementary new functions actually do not arise in the transitional age. This circumstance, as K. Bühler correctly indicates, agrees completely with biological data on the weight increase of the brain. L. Edinger, one of the eminent experts on the brain, established the following general position: whoever knows the structure of the brain in a living being will conclude that the appearance of new abilities is always connected with the appearance of new sections of the brain or with the growth of those that existed previously (1911).

This position, developed by Edinger with respect to phylogenesis of the mind, is now very frequently and readily applied to ontogenesis as well in an attempt to establish a parallel between the development of the brain, since this is evidenced by the increase in its weight, and the appearance of new abilities. Forgotten here is the fact that the parallel may be true only with respect to elementary functions and abilities that are, like the brain itself, the product of biological evolution of behavior; but the essence of historical development of behavior also consists specifically in the appearance of new abilities not connected with the appearance of new parts of the brain or with the growth of parts that are present.

There is every reason to assume that the historical development of behavior from primitive forms to the most complex and highest did not occur as a result of the appearance of new parts of the brain or the growth of parts already existing. This is the essence of both the transitional age and the age of cultural development or development of higher mental functions for the most part. P. P. Blonsky is absolutely right in thinking that the childhood of permanent teeth can be considered to be the time when the child becomes civilized, the time when he assimilates modern science, beginning with writing and modern technology. Civilization is a somewhat recent acquisition of humanity in order that it might convey itself by inheritance.

Thus, it is difficult to expect that evolution of higher mental functions would proceed parallel to the development of the brain, being accomplished mainly and specifically under the influence of inheritance. According to the data of O. Pfister, in the first three-quarters of a year, the brain doubles its original weight, by the end of the third year, it triples it; in all, in the process of development, there is a fourfold increase in the weight of the brain.

K. Bühler assumes that one of the phenomena of child psychology agrees completely with this. The child acquires all basic mental functions in the first three or four years of life and during all subsequent life, does not achieve such basic inner successes as he does, for example, at the time when he learns to speak.

This parallel, we repeat, may be valid only for maturation of elementary functions that are the product of biological evolution and develop together with the growth of the brain and its parts. For this reason, we must limit the position of Charlotte Bühler, who expects that sometime it may be possible to find physiological bases in the development of brain structure for each major shift in the inner life of the normal child.

We must limit her position: basically, it is applicable to shifts in mental development due to heredity, but the complex syntheses that arise in the process of the child's and the adolescent's cultural development are based on other factors—mainly on societal life, cultural development, and work activity of the child and adolescent.

True, there is the opinion that during the transitional age, the brain develops more intensively and owing to this development, the more serious intellectual shifts that are observed during the transitional time may occur. Blonsky developed the hypothesis that the phase of milk teeth in childhood, as distinct from the preceding and succeeding phases, is not a phase of intensive development of thinking and speech; more likely it is a phase of development of motor habits, coordinations, and emotions. Blonsky links this circumstance to the fact that during the milk teeth phase there is intensive growth of the spinal cord and the cerebellum in contrast to the toothless and school-age phase of childhood, which are mainly phases of intensive cortical (intellectual) development. Observation of the intensive transformation of the head during the prepuberty age leads the author to think that during the school age, there is mainly a development of the frontal part of the cortex. However, from the point of view of the data on which Blonsky relies and which he himself terms shaky and unreliable, we are justified in reaching conclusions only with respect to the prepuberty age, that is, early school age.

Regarding the transitional age, with respect to the adolescent, these hypotheses have no factual data. True, according to the reports of N. V. Vyazemskii, the whole brain increases quite significantly at age 14-15, then, after a certain pause and slowing down, makes a new slight rise at age 17-19 and 19-20. But according to newer data, during the whole period of development from age 14 to 20, the whole brain increases very insignificantly.

We must seek new ways to explain the intensive intellectual development that occurs during the period of sexual maturation.

Thus, the transition from research based on external manifestations, on phenotypic similarity, to a deeper study of the genetic, functional, and structural nature of thinking at different ages leads us inevitably to rejecting the established traditional view that is inclined to identify the thinking of the adolescent with the thinking of the three-year-old. Moreover, even in the part where these theories are ready to admit a qualitative difference between the thinking of a young child and of an adolescent, they erroneously formulate the positive achievement, the really new that occurs during this time.

As new studies show, the claim that the abstract thinking of the adolescent breaks away from the concrete, and the abstract from the visual, is incorrect: the movement of thinking during this period is characterized not by the intellect's breaking the connections to the concrete base which it is outgrowing, but by the fact that a completely new form of relation between abstract and concrete factors in thinking arises, a new form of their merging and synthesis, that at this time elementary functions long since established, functions such as visual thinking, perception, or the practical intellect of the child appear before us in a completely new form.

Thus, the theory of C. Bühler seems insupportable not only with respect to what it denies, but also with respect to what it claims, not only in its negative, but also in its positive part. And conversely, in the thinking of the adolescent, not only completely new complex synthetic forms that the three-year-old does not know arise, but even those elementary, primitive forms that the child of three has acquired are restructured on new bases during the transitional age. During the period of sexual maturation, not only new forms arise, but specifically due to their arising, the old are restructured on a completely new base.

Summarizing what has been set forth, we may say that the principal methodological obstacle for the traditional theory is the glaring internal contradiction between admitting a very serious revolution in the content of the adolescent's thinking and denying any substantial shift in the evolution of his intellectual operations, in the inability to correlate the changes in the development of the content and the form of thinking. As we tried to show, the break, in its turn, is due to the failure to distinguish the two lines in behavior—the development of elementary mental functions and the development of higher mental functions. On the basis of conclusions reached, we can now formulate the principal idea that always guides our critical research.

We might say that the fateful break between form and content flows inevitably from the fact that the evolution of content of thinking is always considered as a process of cultural development, primarily facilitated historically and socially, and development of the form of thinking is usually considered as a biological process due to organic maturation of the child and the parallel increase in brain weight. When we speak of the content of thinking and its changes, we have in mind a quantity historically changeable, socially facilitated, arising in the process of cultural development; when we speak of forms of thinking and their dynamics, we have in mind either the metaphysically fixed mental functions or biologically determined, organically arising forms.

Between the one and the other, a chasm develops. The historical and the biological in the child's development seem to be severed; no bridge exists between the one and the other that would enable us to unite the facts of the dynamics of form of thinking with the facts of the dynamics of the content that fills these forms. Only with the introduction of the teaching on the higher forms of behavior that are the product of historical evolution, only with the introduction of the special line of historical development or the development of higher mental functions in the ontogenesis of behavior does it become possible to fill this chasm, to throw a bridge across it, to approach the study of the dynamics of form and content of thinking in their dialectical unity. We can correlate the dynamics of content and form through the common factor of historicity that distinguishes equally both the content of our thinking and the higher mental functions.

Based on these views, which in their aggregate make up the teaching on the cultural development of the child, which we presented elsewhere,[38] we find the key to the correct formulation, and consequently to the true solution of the problem of the development of thinking during the transitional age.

4

The key to the whole problem of development of thinking during the transitional age is the fact, established by a series of studies, that the adolescent masters for the first time the process of forming concepts, that he makes the transition to a new and higher form of intellectual activity—to thinking in concepts.

This is the central phenomenon of the whole transitional age, and underestimating the significance of intellectual development of the adolescent and the attempt of most modern theories on the transitional age to place changes of an intellectual nature in the background in comparison with emotional and other aspects of the crisis can be explained for the most part by the fact that the formation of concepts is a highly complex process and is not at all analogous to the simple maturation of elementary intellectual functions and for this reason cannot easily be subjected to external verification, to crude, visual determination. Changes that occur in the thinking of the adolescent who has mastered concepts are to the utmost degree changes of an internal, intimate, structural nature often not apparent externally, not hitting the eye of the observer.

If we limit ourselves to changes of an external nature only, we will have to agree with investigators who assume that nothing new arises in the thinking of the adolescent, that it grows evenly and gradually in a quantitative respect, being filled with always new content and becoming ever more correct, more logical, closer to actuality. But if we only move from purely external observations to deep internal investigation, this whole claim disintegrates to dust. As has already been said, the formation of concepts stands at the center of the development of thinking during the time of sexual maturation. This process signifies truly revolutionary changes both in the area of content and in the area of forms of thinking. We have said that from the methodological point of view, the break between the form and content of thinking, which is the tacit assumption at the base of most theories, is completely insupportable.

Actually, the form and content of thinking are two factors in a single whole process, two factors internally linked to each other by an essential, not accidental bond.

There is a certain content of thoughts that can be understood adequately only in certain forms of intellectual activity. There are other contents that may be adequately communicated in those same forms, but necessarily require qualitatively different forms of thinking that comprise an indissoluble whole with them. Thus, the content of our dreams cannot be adequately communicated within the system of logically structured speech, in forms of verbal, logical intellect; all attempts to communicate the content of graphic dream-thinking in the form of logical speech inevitably distorts the content.

The same is true of scientific knowledge. For example, mathematics and the natural and social sciences cannot be adequately communicated and presented other than in the form of logical verbal thinking. The content is closely connected with the form, and when we say that the adolescent rises to a higher level in thinking and masters concepts, by the same token, we indicate forms of intellectual activity that are actually new and content of thinking that is just as new opening before the adolescent at this time.

Thus, in the very fact of formation of concepts, we find a solution to the contradiction between the abrupt change in content of thinking and the immobility of its forms during the transitional time which flowed inevitably from the theories considered above. Many modern studies compel us to reach the incontrovertible conclusion that specifically the formation of concepts is the basic nucleus which is the center for all changes in the thinking of the adolescent.

N. Ach,[39] the author of one of the most serious studies of the formation of concepts, whose book (1921) constituted an epoch in the study of this problem, in developing the complex picture of the ontogenesis of the formation of concepts, identifies the transitional age as this kind of crucial boundary that signifies a decisive qualitative turning point in the development of thinking.

In the words of Ach, we can establish yet another rapidly passing phase in the process of intellectualization of mental development. As a rule, it comes at the period bordering on sexual maturation. Before the onset of sexual maturity, the child has no potential for forming abstract concepts, as has been explained, for example, in the observations of H. Eng (1914), but due to the effect of training when educational material is assimilated that consists for the most part of general positions that express some law or rule, through the influence of speech, attention is diverted more and more in the direction of abstract relations and thus leads to the formation of abstract concepts. .

N. Ach notes the influence of the content of assimilated knowledge on the one hand and the directing influence of speech on the attention of the adolescent on the other hand as two basic factors that lead to the formation of abstract concepts. He refers to the studies of A. Gregor (1915) that demonstrated the great influence of knowledge on the development of abstract thinking.

We see here an indication of the genetic role of the new content that is opened before the thinking of the adolescent and which of necessity requires his transition to new forms, and places before him problems that can be resolved only through the formation of concepts. At the same time, we can observe functional changes in the direction of attention made with the help of speech. The crisis in the development of thinking and the transition to thinking in concepts is thus prepared from both aspects: from the aspect of change in function and from the aspect of new problems that arise in the thinking of the adolescent relating to the assimilation of new material for thought.

In conjunction with the transition to a higher level, according to Ach, the process of intellectualization, like the transition to thinking in concepts, narrows more and more the circle of visual thinking in concepts and thinking in graphic representations. This leads to a demise of the method of thinking which the child uses, with which the child must part, and to the construction of a completely new kind or type of intellect in its place. To this, Ach links the problem to which we must turn in the following chapter. He asks whether the transition from graphic thinking to thinking in concepts is the basis of the fact that eidetic tendency, studied by E. Jaensch,[40] is found significantly less frequently at this stage than in the child.

25*

Thus, as a result of our studies, we have found that the adolescent makes a most important step along the path of intellectual development during the time of sexual maturation. He makes the transition from complex thinking to thinking in concepts. Forming concepts and operating with concepts—this is the essentially new ability that he acquires at this age. In concepts, the intellect of the adolescent finds

*Sections 5-24 are repeated in full in Chapter 5 of the book, *Thinking and Speech,* published in Volume 2 of the present edition, and are omitted for this reason in the present volume. The numbering of the sections is retained.—Editor's note.

not simply a continuation of preceding lines. A concept is not just an enriched and internally interconnected associative group. It is a qualitatively new formation that cannot be reduced to more elementary processes that characterize the development of the intellect at earlier stages. Thinking in concepts is a new form of intellectual activity, a new method of behavior, a new intellectual mechanism.

In this unique activity, the intellect finds a new, previously nonexistent *modus operandi* (mode of action—Ed.); a new function different in both composition and structure as well as in method of action develops in the system of intellectual functions.

The traditional view that is inclined to reject the appearance of essentially new formations in the intellect of the adolescent and strives to consider his thinking simply as a continuation, extension, and deepening of the thinking of the three-year-old, as is reflected most clearly in the work of C. Bühler, actually does not note the qualitative differences between concepts, complexes, and syncretic formations. This view is based on purely quantitative conceptions of the development of the intellect strangely similar to the theory of E. Thorndike, according to which higher forms of thinking differ from elementary functions only quantitatively according to the number of associative connections that enter into their composition. Specifically because this view prevails in traditional psychology of adolescence, we considered it necessary to trace carefully the whole course of the development of thinking and to show three different qualitative states through which it passes in all their uniqueness. The principal subject of our study was the thinking of the adolescent. However, we always used genetic sections in studying thinking just as an anatomist-investigator makes sections at various stages of development of any organ and compares these sections with each other and establishes the course of development from one stage to another.

In modern pedological studies, as A. Gesell[41] correctly points out, the method of genetic sections is the central method for studying behavior and its development. The former method—describing characteristics of behavior according to age—was usually reduced to a static characterization, to enumerating a number of features, traits, different characteristics of thinking for a given stage of development. In this case, a static characterization usually substituted for a dynamic consideration of age. Development was lost from sight and the form, characteristic only for a given age, was assumed to be stable, immovable, always equal in itself. Thinking and behavior at each age stage was considered as a thing and not as a process, something at rest and not moving. In addition, the essence of each form of thinking can be disclosed only when we begin to understand it as a certain, organically indispensable factor in a complex and merged process of development.

The only adequate method for disclosing this essence is the method of genetic sections for comparative genetic study of behavior at different stages of development.

This is the way we tried to proceed; we tried to disclose the uniqueness of the thinking of the adolescent. We were interested not simply in a cross section of the characteristics of thinking during the transitional age, an inventory of methods of intellectual activity found in the adolescent, and not in listing the forms of thinking in their quantitative relation to each other. We were interested primarily in establishing what is substantially new, in what the transitional age brings with itself to the development of thinking; we were interested in thinking and its coming into being. Our goal was to capture the process of crisis and maturation of thinking that is the basic content of this age.

To do this, we had to present the thinking of the adolescent in comparison with preceding stages, find the transition of one form of thinking to another and by comparison establish the decisive change, the fundamental reconstruction, the radical reorganization that occurs in the thinking of the adolescent. For this, we had to make as if sections of the process of the development of thinking at different stages and always following the comparative-genetic path, try to connect these sections with each other to establish the real process of movement that occurs in the transition of thinking from one stage to another.

In the future, we will proceed in precisely this way because the comparative-genetic method of examination, the method of genetic sections, is the basic and principal method of pedological research.

True, in subjecting the results of our comparative study to functional checking, we always brought in data not only on the ontogenesis of thinking, but also its phylogenetic development, data on the breakdown and involution of thinking in abnormal processes. Proceeding in this way, we were governed by the principle of unity of higher forms of intellectual activity no matter how various the processes in which this unity found its concrete expression. We assumed that the basic laws of structure and activity of thinking remain the same, the basic patterns directing them—the same in the normal and abnormal state, but only that these patterns acquire different concrete expression depending on different conditions.

Just as modern pathology considers illness as life in special, changed conditions, we are justified in considering the activity of thinking affected by one abnormality or another as a manifestation of general patterns of thinking under special conditions created by the abnormality.

In modern psychoneurology, the idea that development is the key to understanding the breakdown and involution of mental functions is firmly rooted, and the study of the breakdown and disintegration of these functions, the key to understanding their structure and development. Thus, general and pathological psychology mutually enlighten each other if they are constructed on a genetic base.

In comparing the data of onto- and phylogenesis, we did not for a moment take the point of view of biogenetic parallelism, intending to find in the history of the development of the child a repetition and recapitulation of those forms of thinking that prevailed at previous stages of human history. We followed the same comparative method by which K. Groos properly identified the task as consisting not only in finding similarity, but also in establishing differences; the word "comparison" here means not isolating only coinciding traits, but even more it means finding the differences in the similarity.

For this reason, we did not for a moment identify the process of concrete thinking of the child with the process of concrete thinking in the history of human development. We were always interested in the most complete elucidation of the nature of the phenomenon that was the object of our research. This nature is disclosed in the diverse connections and forms of manifestation of essentially one and the same type of thinking. Of course to say that logical thinking arises at a certain stage in the development of human history and at a certain stage in the development of the child is to claim an incontrovertible truth and at the same time not in any way to indicate that the one who claims this takes the point of view of biogenetic parallelism. Precisely so, comparative analysis of complex thinking in its phylogenetic and ontogenetic aspects does not in the least presuppose the idea of parallelism between the one process and the other or the idea of identity of the one form and the other.

We tried to emphasize one factor especially in the phenomenon that interests us, because it is preeminent in a comparative study of different manifestations of one and the same form of thinking. That factor is the unity of form and content in the concept. Specifically because of the fact that in the concept, form and content are given as a unity, the transition to thinking in concepts signified a real revolution in the thinking of the child.

26

Now it remains for us to consider what the basic traces are of the fact that the adolescent makes a transition to thinking in concepts. What we would like to bring to the forefront is the deep and fundamental changes in the content of the thinking of the adolescent. Without overstating, we could say that the whole content of thinking is reformed and reconstructed in conjunction with the formation of concepts. The content and form of thinking do not relate to each other as water does to a glass. The content and form are in an indissoluble relationship and mutual dependence.

If we understand content of thinking to be not simply the external data that comprise the subject of thinking at any given moment, but the actual content, we will see how, in the process of the child's development, it constantly moves inward, becomes an organic component part of the personality itself and of separate systems of its behavior. Convictions, interests, world view, ethical norms and rules of behavior, inclinations, ideals, certain patterns of thought—all of this is initially external, and becomes internal specifically because as the adolescent develops, in conjunction with his maturation and the change in his environment, he is confronted by the task of mastering new content, and strong stimuli are created that nudge him along the path of developing the formal mechanisms of his thinking as well.

The new content, which confronts the adolescent with a series of problems, leads to new forms of activity, to new forms of combining elementary functions, and to new methods of thinking. As we shall see, specifically during the transitional age, the new content itself creates new forms of behavior, mechanisms of a special type about which we will speak in a later chapter. Together with the transition to thinking in concepts, the adolescent is confronted by a world of objective, societal consciousness, a world of societal ideology.

Cognition in the true sense of that word, science, art, various spheres of cultural life may be adequately assimilated only in concepts. True, even the child assimilates scientific facts, and the child is imbued with a certain ideology, and the child grows into separate spheres of cultural life. But an inadequate, incomplete mastery of all of this is characteristic for the child, and for this reason, the child, perceiving the established cultural material, does not yet actively participate in its creation.

On the contrary, the adolescent, making the transition to an adequate assimilation of this content which can be presented in all its completeness and depth only in concepts, begins actively and creatively to participate in various spheres of cultural life that open before him. Without thinking in concepts there is no understanding of relations that underlie the phenomena. The whole world of deep connections that underlie external, outward appearances, the world of complex interdependencies and relations within every sphere of activity and among its separate spheres, can be disclosed only to one who approaches it with the key of the concept.

This new content does not enter mechanically into the thinking of the adolescent, but undergoes a long and complex process of development. Owing to this extension and deepening of the content of thinking, a whole world with its past and future, nature, history, and human life opens before the adolescent. Blonsky correctly states that the whole history of the child is a gradual broadening of his environment, beginning with the mother's womb and the crib and continuing with the room and the home with its immediate environment. Thus, by the extension of the environment, we can determine the development of the child in its onward course. The extension of the environment during the transitional age leads to the fact that for the adolescent, the world becomes the environment for thinking. As we know, F. Schiller expressed this idea in a certain couplet where he compared the infant for whom his crib was boundless, with the youth whom the whole world could not contain.

Most of all, as Blonsky correctly notes, the basic change in the environment consists of the fact that it expands to participation in societal production. On this basis, in the content of thinking, societal ideology is represented most of all as connected with one position or another in societal production.

Blonsky says that we must also present class psychology not as suddenly arising, but as gradually developing. It is understood that we have its full development as early as during youth when a man already occupies or is preparing to occupy one position or another in societal production. The history of the school-age child and the youth is the history of very intensive development and formulation of class psychology and ideology.

In conjunction with this, Blonsky correctly indicates the widespread error concerning how class psychology and ideology arise and develop. Usually reference is made to the instinct of imitation as the basic mechanism for the origin and formulation of the content of thinking in the adolescent. Moreover, reference to the instinct of imitation, as the author correctly notes, undoubtedly obscures understanding of the formation of class psychology in the child.

Blonsky indicates that even authors who consider it possible to speak of class psychology of the child frequently present its formation thus: through imitation class psychology is created, class ideals are created, and class ethics are created. If we understand imitation as it is usually understood in psychology, then this claim is completely unwarranted.

Class psychology cannot, of course, be created by external imitation. The process of its formation is undoubtedly deeper. Class psychology in the child is created as a result of his working with those around him, or, stated more simply and directly, as a result of common life with them, common activity, common interests. Let us repeat, class cohesion is formed as a result not of external imitation, but by shared life, activity, and interests.

We agree completely that the process of formation of class psychology is incomparably deeper than authors who refer to instinct of imitation believe it to be. Further, we believe that we cannot argue with Blonsky's position that shared life, activity, and interests are the basic and central factor in this process. We think, however, that in this case an essential link in explaining the process as a whole has been omitted. For this reason, Blonsky's statement does not solve the problem, which remains open even after we reject the reference to the instinct of imitation.

It is understood that sharing of life, work, and interests places before the adolescent a number of problems; in the process of solving them, class psychology develops and takes shape. But we must not lose sight of that mechanism, those methods of intellectual activity that facilitate the completion of this process. In other words, we can never give a genetic explanation of the phenomenon of which Blonsky speaks specifically because the transitional age is a time of intensive development and formulation of class psychology and ideology. If we do not consider the formation of concepts as a basic intellectual function whose development opens a new content for the adolescent's thinking, we will not understand why shared life and interests do not result in such an intensive development in that area during the early or preschool age in which we are interested. Obviously, with genetic analysis of development of the content of thinking, we cannot for a moment lose sight of the connection between the evolution of content and the evolution of form of thinking. In particular, we cannot for a single moment forget the basic and central position of all of adolescent psychology: the function of formation of concepts lies at the base of all intellectual changes at this age.

In this sense, the attempt of some authors to ignore wholly the factor of formation of concepts in the development of forms of thinking and to proceed from direct analysis of content is of exceptional interest. Thus, W. Stern in his work on the development of the formation of ideals in the maturing youth comes to the conclusion that metaphysical world understanding instinctively becomes a part of the adolescent during sexual maturation, that it is as if hereditarily fixed at this age. We find similar attempts in the work of other authors who devote several pages or several lines to the development of thinking, and sometimes simply bypass it in silence, but instead try to reconstruct directly the structure of the content of thinking in various spheres of consciousness. It is natural that in this case the structure of thinking acquires a metaphysical character. In the exposition itself, in the characterization of the consciousness of the adolescent, they rush to idealization as the basic method of representation, and it is not surprising that for such authors as Stern and Spranger the adolescent seems to be a natural-born metaphysicist because where the deep changes and alterations in the content of his thinking originate, what moves the flood of his ideas, remains a mystery.

Moreover, if we do not follow the path of those authors who accept the metaphysics of their own constructs for the metaphysical structure of the thinking of the adolescent, we must consider, as we have already said, the evolution of the content of thinking in conjunction with the evolution of its form, and we must trace in detail the kind of changes in the content of thinking that formation of concepts elicits. We will see that the formation of concepts discloses before the adolescent a world of social consciousness and leads inevitably to intensive development and formulation of class psychology and ideology. For this reason it is not surprising that the adolescent that Stern and Spranger study stands before the investigators as a metaphysicist. The whole crux of the matter is that the metaphysical nature of thinking of the adolescent is not an instinctive peculiarity of the adolescent, but is the inevitable result of the formation of concepts within the sphere of a specific societal ideology.

Specifically the higher forms of thinking, especially logical thinking, open up before the adolescent in their significance. Blonsky says: if the child's intellect at the stage when teeth are replaced is still quite markedly eidetic, then the intellect of the adolescent is marked by a striving to be logical. This striving is manifested primarily in criticism and in greater demands that what is said be proven. The adolescent urgently requires proofs.

The mind of the adolescent is more likely to be burdened by the concrete, and concrete natural history, botany, zoology, and mineralogy (one of the favorite subjects in step I in school) take a secondary place for the adolescent, yielding to philosophical questions of natural history, the origin of the world, man, etc. In the same way, interest in the numerous historical concrete stories is also relegated to a secondary position. Their place is taken more and more by politics, which is of great interest to the adolescent. Finally, all of this is very closely connected to the fact that the average adolescent loses interest in art and drawing, which the child so loves during prepuberty. The most abstract art—music—is the greatest favorite of the adolescent.

The development of social-political world view does not account for all the changes that occur during the time of maturation of thinking in the adolescent. This is only one, perhaps the most clear and significant part of the changes that are occurring.

It is completely right that the decisive event in the life of the average adolescent is entry into societal production and by the same token, into full class self-determination. In Blonsky's opinion, the adolescent is not only the son of his social class, but is already himself an active member of that class. Correspondingly, the years of adolescence are the years of forming the adolescent, primarily his social-political world view. In these years, in their basic outlines, the views on life, people, and society are worked out, and one kind or another of social sympathies and antipathies are formed. The years of adolescence are the years of intensive racking of the brain over problems of life, as Blonsky maintains (1930, pp. 209-210). Problems that life itself poses for the adolescent and his decisive entry as an active participant into this life require for their solution the development of higher forms of thinking.

In describing the adolescent, we have thus far bypassed in silence a most essential trait that has been noted several times by investigators and which it would be strange to find at other stages of the child's development. It is typical and characteristic specifically for the adolescent. We have in view the contradictoriness that is the basic trait of that age, the contradictoriness that is expressed also in the content of the adolescent's thinking, specifically: the content of his thinking includes seemingly contradictory factors.

The intellect of the adolescent, according to Blonsky, is marked by an inclination toward mathematics. Although, according to a widespread point of view, adolescents are not very much in the habit of mastering mathematics, the author refers to school experience in defending his opinion. Blonsky believes that the interval from age 14 to 17 is usually the stage of maximally intensive mathematical formation in school practice and specifically during this time, a person usually acquires the greatest part of his mathematical baggage. In precisely the same way, there is an increased inclination toward physics. Finally, this is the age of philosophical interests and is logically sequential in tendencies toward argument. But how can love of mathematics, physics, and philosophy, love of logic, balance of judgment, and proof be reconciled with what E. Kretschmer terms "romanticism of thought," which also is undoubtedly present in the adolescent? Blonsky answers this contradiction with the words of Kretschmer: both complements of thinking, regardless of the external differences, are closely connected with each other in biological relation.

We think that the fact that Blonsky notes is pointed out quite correctly. The explanation, however, that he tries to give for the contradictoriness of intellectual tendencies and interests of the adolescent is essentially inadequate for solving the problem that confronts us. Blonsky explains the inclination toward mathematics, physics, and philosophy with characteristics of the schizothemic temperament for which a certain splitting between poles is characteristic: inordinate acuteness, increased impressionability, sensitivity, and excitability on the one hand and an affective dullness, coldness, and indifference, on the other.

We think, however, that the deep biological relationship between the two types of thinking to which Kretschmer refers can scarcely serve as a real base for the unique combination of "romanticism of thought" and excessive drive toward logic that is observed during the transitional age. We believe that specifically the genetic explanation[42] will be the most correct in this case. If we take into account the great broadening of activity, the serious deepening in connection and relation between

TABLE 1

| Age, years | Questions | | Ratio, % |
	Regressive	Progressive	
12-13	108	11	9.8
14-15	365	49	7.4
15-16	165	35	4.7
16-17	74	19	3.9
Students	46	36	1.3

things and phenomena that the thinking of the adolescent masters for the first time, we will also understand the basis for the increased logical activity and the basis for the "romanticism of thought" that is present in the adolescent.

The fact of formation of concepts, novelty, and youth and the character of this new form of thinking, which is inadequately fixed, unstable, and underdeveloped, explain the contradiction that observers have noted. This contradiction is a contradiction of development, a contradiction of a transitional form, a contradiction of the transitional age.

We are inclined to use youth and the not yet fully established character of the new form of thinking to explain still another feature noted by Blonsky—the inadequate dialectics of the adolescent, his tendency to hone every question into the form of alternatives: either/or.

We think that here too what is at work primarily are not the characteristics of the temperament of the adolescent, but the simple circumstance that dialectical thinking is a higher level in the development of mature thinking and cannot, it is understood, become the property of the adolescent, who has just arrived at the formation of concepts. Moreover, with the formation of concepts, the adolescent enters the path of development that sooner or later will bring him to mastering dialectical thinking. But it would be improbable to expect that this necessary and higher level of development will already be present at the first steps that the adolescent takes who has just mastered a new method of intellectual activity.

The studies of Groos (1916) can be a good illustration of the radical change and the radical reconstruction in the content of thinking of the adolescent; these studies show in an isolated, pure form the effects of age on directedness of thinking, on the separate content of intellectual activity of the adolescent.[43] Resorting to experiment, Groos attempted to explain what kind of questions arise at different age levels in the developing human being in connection with one process of thinking or another. The subjects were given different themes for consideration. After reading the themes, the subjects were asked each time: what would you want to learn most of all? The responses elicited in this way were recorded, collected, and classified with respect to logical interest that was evident in them. The study established the dominant logical interests in their age dynamics and in their increment.

One of the principal points of the study is an elucidation of whether interest of the thinking person is directed toward causes or effects. While in adult subjects of almost all ages, there is a predominance of movement of thought forward to consequences, in children questions relating to other circumstances predominate. Groos reached the conclusion that interest in consequences increases with growth in intellectual development (see Table 1).

In the data obtained, Groos is completely justified in seeing an important indication of the development of interests in the mind of the child and the youth because the relative growth of progressive and regressive positions at different ages

TABLE 2

Age, years	Ratio, %
11-13	2
14-15	13
15-16	12
16-17	42
Students	55.5

while the themes remain identical undoubtedly indicates the role of age in the change of direction of logical interests in thinking.

Another study pertains to the nature of questions that arise in the thinking of the child and the adolescent. Groos assumes that judgment is always preceded by a state of uncertainty coupled with the need to know that we often express with a question even if we ask it of ourselves (we have in mind not a question asked aloud, but an internal question).

Groos believes that even in the internal, verbal formulation there are two kinds of questions corresponding to our motives of judging, specifically, questions of determination and questions of decision. The question of determination corresponds to simple not knowing with its complete uncertainty. It is similar to an empty vessel that may be filled only with the answer. For example: What is it? Where did it come from? Who was that? When? Why? Why was this done? Such a question cannot be answered with a simple "yes" or "no." On the other hand, questions of decision can be answered "yes" or "no," since the potential for decision is contained in the question itself. For example: Is this a rare plant? Was this rug brought from Persia? Such a question, especially if posed to oneself, is identical to the expression of a state of conscious expectation from which a hypothetical conclusion can be reached in some cases.·

Since it is obvious that more mental activity is expressed in questions of decision than in questions of determination and since this division also masks a deeply rooted difference between the two motives of judgment, studying the results of our experiments directed toward eliciting questions from schoolchildren must be of interest. According to the data of Groos, as children grow, the number of questions of judgment increase more than the empty questions. Their ratio is presented in Table 2.

In the increase of progressive thinking as in the development of inherent assumptions and presuppositions internally related to it, the essential trait of the transitional age undoubtedly is apparent: not only an enormous enrichment of the content of thinking, but also new forms of movement, new forms of operating with this content. In this sense the decisive significance, it seems to us, is that of the unity of form and content as a basic trait in the structure of a concept. There are areas of reality, there are connections and phenomena that can be adequately represented only in concepts.

For this reason, those who consider abstract thinking as a removal from reality are wrong. On the contrary, abstract thinking primarily reflects the deepest and truest, the most complete and thorough disclosure of the reality opening up before the adolescent. Regarding the changes in content of the thinking of the adolescent, we cannot bypass one sphere that appears at this outstanding time of reconstruction of thinking as a whole. We are speaking of the awareness of one's own internal activity.

27

Kroh maintains that the mental world opens before the maturing adolescent, and his attention is initially directed toward other people to an ever increasing degree. The world of internal experiences, closed to the very young child, now opens before the adolescent and presents an extremely important sphere in the content of his thinking.

In the penetration into internal activity, into the world of his own experiences, the function of concept formation, which appears during the transitional age, again plays a decisive role. Just as the word is a means for understanding others, it is the means for understanding oneself. From birth, for the speaker, the word is a means for understanding himself, for the apperception of one's own perceptions. Because of this, only with the formation of concepts does an intensive development of self-perception, self-observation, intensive cognition of internal activity, the world of one's own experiences, occur. According to the correct note of W. Humboldt,[44] thought becomes clear only in concepts, and only together with the formation of concepts does the adolescent begin to truly understand himself and his internal world. Lacking this, thought cannot attain clarity and cannot become concept.

Conception, being an important means of cognition and understanding, results in basic changes in the content of the adolescent's thinking. First, thinking in concepts leads to discovery of the deep connections that lie at the base of reality, to recognizing patterns that control reality, to ordering the perceived world with the help of the network of logical relations cast upon it. Speech is a powerful means of analysis and classification of phenomena, a means of ordering and generalizing reality. The word, becoming the carrier of the concept, is, as one of the authors correctly noted, the real theory of the object to which it refers. The general in this case serves as the law of the particular. Recognizing concrete reality with the help of words, which are signs for concepts, man uncovers in the world he sees connections and patterns that are confined in it.

In our experiments, we repeatedly found an extremely interesting close tie between different concepts. The mutual transition and linking of concepts, reflecting mutual transition and linking of phenomena of reality, means that every concept arises already connected with all others and, having arisen, seemingly determines its place in a system of previously recognized concepts.

In our experiments, the subject was confronted with the task of forming four different concepts. We saw how the formation of one concept was the key to the formation of the other three and how the latter three usually developed in the adolescent not in the same way as the first developed, but through the concept that had already been worked out and with its help. The course of thought in developing the second, third, and fourth concepts always differed profoundly from the course of thought in developing the first, and only in exceptional cases were the four concepts developed with the help of four identical operations. The mutual connection of concepts, their internal relation to one and the same system also make the concept one of the basic means of systematization and recognition of the external world. But the concept not only results in a system and serves as a basic means of recognizing external reality. It is also a basic means for understanding another, for adequate assimilation of the historically constituted social experience of humanity. Only in concepts does the adolescent systematize and comprehend the world of social consciousness for the first time. In this sense, Humboldt's definition is completely correct; he said that to think in words is to join one's own thinking to thought in general. Complete socialization of thought is contained in the function of concept formation.

Finally, the third sphere that arises anew in the adolescent's thinking in connection with the transition to forming concepts is the world of his own experiences, the systematization, cognition, and ordering of which becomes possible only at this point. On a firm basis, one of the authors says that consciousness is a phenomenon that is completely different from self-consciousness, which develops late in man, whereas consciousness is a normal attribute of his mental life.

"Self-consciousness is not given initially. It develops gradually to the extent that man, by using words, learns to understand himself. It is possible to understand oneself in various degrees. The child at an early stage of development understands himself very little."* His self-consciousness develops extremely slowly and in strict dependence on the development of thinking. But a decisive step along the path to understanding oneself, on the path toward the development and shaping of consciousness, is taken only during the transitional age together with the formation of concepts.

In this sense, completely consistent and justified is the analogy, made by thinking in concepts, between understanding and ordering things and the internal reality, an analogy cited by many authors. "Man subjects all his actions to such legislative plans. Strictly speaking, arbitrariness is possible only in deed and not in thought, not in words with which man explains his motives. The need to explain his behavior, to disclose it in words, to present it in concepts inevitably leads to subjecting his own actions to these legislative plans. A willful person summoned unexpectedly to account for the basis of his willfulness will say: 'That's what I want'; rejecting any measure of his actions, he cites his 'I' as law. But he himself is dissatisfied with his answer and only answered so because he had no other answer. It seems difficult to imagine *sic volo* (that's what I want—Ed.) said not as a joke but with no anger. Together with this attribute of self-consciousness, freedom and purpose are also established."

We will treat these complex problems in a subsequent chapter and will not discuss them in detail here. We will only say that, as we shall see later, separating the world of internal experiences from the world of objective reality is something that is constantly developing in the child, and we will not find this separation between self and the world in the child who is beginning to speak as we will in the adult. For the child in the first days of life, everything he senses and the whole content of his consciousness is still an undifferentiated mass. Self-consciousness is acquired only through development and is not given to us together with consciousness.[45]

Thus, understanding reality, understanding others, and understanding oneself—this is what thinking in concepts brings with itself. This is the kind of revolution that occurs in the thinking and consciousness of the adolescent; this is what is new, what distinguishes the thinking of the adolescent from the thinking of the three-year-old.

We think that we shall express completely correctly the problem of studying thinking in concepts for the development of personality and its relation to the surrounding world if we compare it with the problem that confronts the history of language. A. A. Potebnya[46] believed that showing the actual participation of the word in the formation of a sequential series of systems that encompass the relation of the personality to nature is the basic problem of the history of language. In general outline, we will truly understand the significance of this participation if we accept the basic premise that language is not the means to express an already pre-

---

*L. S. Vygotsky does not indicate the source of this and the following citation. We could not establish who the author was.—Editor's note.

pared thought, but to create it, that it is not a reflection of world contemplation that has developed, but an activity that composes it. In order to perceive one's own mental movements, in order to interpret one's own internal perceptions, man must objectivize them in a word and must join this word to other words. For understanding even one's own external nature, it is not at all indifferent how this nature presents itself to us, by means of specifically which comparisons its separate elements are as perceptible to the mind as these same comparisons are real for us, in a word, Potebnya assumes that the primary property and degree of obliviousness of the internal form of the word are not indifferent for thought.

If we are speaking here of the formation of a number of systems that encompass the relation of the personality to nature mediated by speech, then together with this, we must not forget for a moment that both knowing nature and knowing personality is done with the help of understanding other people, understanding those around us, understanding social experience. Speech cannot be separated from understanding. This inseparability of speech and understanding is manifested identically in both social use of language as a means of communication and in its individual use as a means of thinking.

28

We elaborated material that was collected by our colleague, E. I. Pashkovskaya, which involved several hundred adolescents studying in a factory-trade apprenticeship school (FAS) and in the School for Christian Youth (SCY). The purpose of the study was to elucidate what in similar studies in younger children was called a study of the stock of ideas.

Actually in Pashkovskaya's studies more extensive problems were solved: we were interested here not so much in the stock of ideas, not so much in the inventory of the knowledge that an adolescent commands, not so much in a cross section of those points of which his thinking is made up—in general, not in the quantitative aspect of the stock of ideas as primarily in the structure of the content of thinking and the complex connections and relations established in the thinking of the adolescent between different spheres of experience. We were interested in elucidating the qualitative difference between the structure of one thought content or another in the adolescent and the corresponding idea of a child and how various spheres of reality are connected with each other in the thinking of the adolescent. On this basis, the word "idea" seems scarcely appropriate. We were not speaking of ideas at all in this case. If this word expresses more or less precisely the subject of study when it is directed toward the thinking of the young child, in applying it to an adolescent, it loses almost all meaning, all sense.

The unit (or the aggregate of units that comprise the content of the thinking during the transitional age), the simplest action with which the intellect of the adolescent operates, is, of course, not a representation, but a concept. Thus, Pashkovskaya's study encompassed the structure and connection of concepts pertaining to the various aspects of reality, external and internal, and formed as if a natural supplement to preceding research, the results of which we presented above.[47] We were interested in the thinking of the adolescent from the aspect of content; we wanted to take a look at concept from the point of view of the content that it represented and to see whether the theoretical connection that we assumed between the development of a new form of thinking—the function of forming concepts—and a radical reconstruction of the whole content of intellectual activity of the adolescent really exists.

The research encompassed various spheres of experience of the adolescent and included a study of concepts that relate to phenomena of nature, technical processes and tools, phenomena of social life, and concepts related to abstract ideas of a psychological nature. Basically, the research confirmed the presence of connections that we expected and showed that together with functions of concept formation, the adolescent also acquires something completely new in structure and in method of systematization, in scope and depth of the content of the aspects of reality reflected in it. Because of this research, we can disclose how the content of his thinking is enriched and new forms are acquired.

In *this* we see the basic and central results of the whole work and the direct confirmation of the hypothesis which we mentioned above. We believe that one of the basic errors of modern psychology of concepts is not taking this circumstance into account, a failure that leads either to a purely formal consideration of concepts, ignoring the new areas and new system presented in the content of the concepts, or to a purely morphological phenomenological analysis of the content of thinking from the material aspect without taking into account the fact that morphological analysis alone is always insupportable and requires cooperation with functional and genetic analysis because the given content may be adequately presented only in a certain form, and mastery of the given content becomes possible only with the appearance of specific functions of thinking, specific methods of intellectual activity.

We have already indicated that the function of forming concepts during the transitional age is a young and unstable acquisition of the intellect. For this reason, it would be a mistake to imagine that all thinking of the adolescent is imbued with concepts. On the contrary, here we observe concepts only in the process of their being established; they will not be a dominant form of thinking until the very end of the transitional age, and the intellectual activity of the adolescent is still done for the most part in other, genetically earlier forms.

On this basis we tried to explain this inadequacy in the adolescent's thinking and the romanticism of his thinking which many investigators indicate. From the aspect of content, we find a complete parallel to this position. It is curious that a significant number of the adolescents studied, when confronted with the task of defining an abstract concept, respond on the basis of completely concrete determinations. Thus, to the question, what is good, they answer: "To buy the best, that is good" (14-year-old, FAS); "Good is when a man did something good for another man, this is good" (15-year-old, SCY). But even more often they give a worldly, practical definition of this term: "Good is what one acquires, for example, very good earrings, watches, trousers, etc." (13-year-old, SCY); "What you get, that is good" (13-year-old, SCY); or even more concretely: "Finery when a girl is given in marriage, a hope chest" (13-year-old, SCY); "Good is what we have, that is, notebook, pen, ballpoint, etc." (14-year-old, FAS), or finally: "Valuable things" (13-year-old, SCY), etc.

If the subjects give other definitions for this concept based on its meaning as a certain psychological and moral quality, then the character of these definitions very often, especially at the beginning of the transitional age, remains just as concrete. They take the word in its worldly meaning and explain it with the help of the most concrete example. The definition of such concepts as "thought," "love," etc. have a similar character at the beginning of the transitional period. To the question, what is love, they answer: "love is that a person likes another person who touched his heart" (14-year-old, SCY); "Love is a name, a man loves a woman" (13-year-old, SCY); "Love is someone who wants to get married, then he sits with a girl and proposes that she marry him" (13-year-old, SCY); "Love happens between relations and acquaintances" (13-year-old, SCY).

Thus, even from the aspect of content of thinking at the beginning of the transitional age, we find the same predominance of the concrete, the same attempt to approach an abstract concept from the point of view of the concrete situation that manifests it. Essentially, these definitions differ in no way from the definition cited above from the material of A. Messer,[48] which is typical for early school age also. But here we must make an important reservation: what we have noted as a frequently encountered phenomenon in the first half of the transitional age is not an essential, not a specific, not a new, and for this reason from the genetic aspect, not a characteristic trait of the transitional age. It is a remnant of the old. Although this form of thinking now predominates, as the adolescent moves ahead, it will be involuted, curtailed, and will disappear.

There is a transition toward more abstract thinking; although it is not now a quantitatively dominant form, it is specific for the transitional age: as the adolescent moves ahead, it will develop. The past belongs to concrete thinking and most of the present, to the abstract—the smaller part of the present, but to make up for it, all of the future.

We will consider the studies of Pashkovskaya in detail on other pages. We will only say that two points are in the foreground in the analysis of the rich factual material. First, connection and relations that exist between concepts come through. Each of the 60 answers* was internally and organically linked with every other answer. The second point is that we observe how the content enters the internal composition of thinking, how it stops being its external, directing factor, how it begins to be expressed in the speaker's own name.

According to the Latin expression *communia proprio dicere* (literally: to express the general through the particular—Editor), the content of thinking becomes an internal conviction of the speaker, the directedness of his thoughts, his interest, the norm of his behavior, his desire and intention. This occurs especially markedly when we deal with the adolescents' answers to actual questions on contemporary events, politics, social life, plans for their own life, etc. It is characteristic that in the answers, the concept and the content reflected in it are not given as given by a child, as assimilated from outside, something completely objective; it is merged with complex internal factors of the personality, and at this time it is difficult to determine where the objective statement ends and where the manifestation of personal interest, conviction, and direction of behavior begins.

In general, it would be difficult to find more distinct evidence for the position that content does not enter into thinking as a factor external and peripherally related to it, that it does not fill one form or another of intellectual activity the way water fills an empty glass, that it is organically connected with intellectual functions, that every sphere of the content has its specific functions and that content, becoming a property of the personality, begins to participate in the general system of movement of the personality, in the general system of its development as one of its internal factors.

Thought, clearly assimilated, being the personal thought of the adolescent, in addition to its own logic and its own movement, begins to be subject to the general patterns of development of the personal system of thinking in which it is included as a certain part, and the task of the psychologist is to trace this process exactly and know how to find the complex structure of the personality and its thinking, which includes clearly assimilated thought. Like a ball, which when thrown against the deck of a ship moves along the diagonal of a parallelogram of two forces,

*Each subject answered 60 questions, and the answers were analyzed.—Editor's note.

thought assimilated at this time moves along the diagonal of some kind of complex parallelogram reflecting two different forces, two different systems of movement.

29

Here we come close to establishing one of the central points that must be explained if we are to overcome the usual error relative to the break between form and content in the development of thinking. From formal logic, traditional psychology adopted the idea of the concept as an abstract mental construct extremely remote from all the wealth of concrete reality. From the point of view of formal logic, the development of concepts is subject to the basic law of inverse proportionality between the scope and content of a concept. The broader the scope of a concept, the narrower its content. This means that the greater the number of objects that the given concept can be applied to, the greater the circle of concrete things that it encompasses, the poorer its content, the emptier it proves to be. The process of forming concepts according to formal logic is extremely simple. The points of abstracting and generalizing are internally closely connected with each other from the point of view of one and the same process, but taken from different aspects. In the words of K. Bühler, what logic terms an abstraction and generalization is completely simple and understandable. A concept from which one of the traits is taken away becomes poorer in content, more abstract and augmented in scope, and becomes general.

It is completely clear that if the process of generalizing is considered as a direct result of abstraction of traits, then we will inevitably come to the conclusion that thinking in concepts is removed from reality, that the constant represented in concepts becomes poorer and poorer, scant and narrow. Not without reason are such concepts frequently termed empty abstracts. Others have said that concepts arise in the process of castrating reality. Concrete, diverse phenomena must lose their traits one after the other in order that a concept might be formed. Actually what arises is a dry and empty abstraction in which the diverse, full-blooded reality is narrowed and impoverished by logical thought. This is the source of the celebrated words of Goethe: "Gray is every theory and eternally green is the golden tree of life."

This dry, empty, gray abstraction inevitably strives to reduce content to zero because the more general, the more empty a concept becomes. Impoverishing the content is done from fateful necessity, and for this reason psychology, proceeding to develop the teaching on concepts on the grounds of formal logic, presented thinking in concepts as the system of thinking that was the poorest, scantiest, and emptiest.

Moreover, the true nature of a concept was seriously distorted in the formal presentation. A real concept is an image of an objective thing in its complexity. Only when we recognize the thing in all its connections and relations, only when this diversity is synthesized in a word, in an integral image through a multitude of determinations, do we develop a concept. According to the teaching of dialectical logic, a concept includes not only the general, but also the individual and particular.

In contrast to contemplation, to direct knowledge of an object, a concept is filled with definitions of the object; it is the result of rational processing of our experience, and it is a mediated knowledge of the object. To think of some object with the help of a concept means to include the given object in a complex system of mediating connections and relations disclosed in determinations of the concept.

Thus, the concept does not arise from this as a mechanical result of abstraction—it is the result of a long and deep knowledge of the object.

Together with overcoming the formal-logical point of view of the concept, together with exposing the incorrectness of the law of inverse proportionality between scope and content, the new psychology is beginning to grope for a correct position in the study of concepts. Psychological research is disclosing that in a concept, we always have an enrichment and deepening of the content that the concept contains. In this respect, the Marxist equating of the role of abstraction with the power of the microscope is completely correct.[49] In genuine scientific research, with the help of the concept, we are able to penetrate through the external appearance of phenomena, across the external form of their manifestations, and see the hidden connections and relations lying at the base of the phenomena to penetrate into their essence, just as with the aid of a microscope, we disclose in a drop of water a complex and rich life, or the complex internal structure of a cell hidden from our eyes.

According to the well-known definition of Marx, if the form of a manifestation and the essence of things coincided directly, then all science would be superfluous (see K. Marx and F. Engels, *Works*, Vol. 25, Part II, p. 384). For this reason, thinking in concepts is the most adequate method of knowing reality because it penetrates into the internal essence of things, for the nature of things is disclosed not in direct contemplation of one single object or another, but in connections and relations that are manifested in movement and in development of the object, and these connect it to all the rest of reality. The internal connection of things is disclosed with the help of thinking in concepts, for to develop a concept of some object means to disclose a series of connections and relations of that object with all the rest of reality, to include it in the complex system of phenomena.

Also, the traditional representation of the intellectual mechanism itself that is the basis for the formation of the concept changes. Formal logic and traditional psychology reduce the concept to a general representation. The concept differs from the concrete representation according to this teaching in the same way that the group photograph of F. Galton[50] differs from the individual photographic portrait. Or another comparison is frequently made: it is said that instead of general representations, we think by means of their substitutes—words which play the role of credit cards that substitute for gold coins.

In the most developed form, modern psychological research assumes that if both of these points of view are insupportable, then everything must still exist, as K. Bühler maintained, as some equivalent logical operation—abstraction and generalization—if not directly in a separate representation, then in any case in the course of representation in abstract thinking, since the real course of mental phenomena is closely linked to these operations. In what does Bühler see the psychological equivalent of these logical operations? He finds it in orthoscopic thinking and perception, in the development of invariants, that is, in the fact that our perceptions and other processes of reflection and cognition of reality have a certain constancy (a stability of perceived impressions). In Bühler's opinion, anyone who could indicate more precisely how this happens, how, independently of the changing position of the observer and the changing distances relative to the impressions of form and size, a kind of absolute impression develops, would render a decisive service to the teaching on the formation of concepts.

By referring to orthoscopic or absolute perceptions or to graphic representations, Bühler does not solve the problem that confronts him but moves it to a still earlier stage of development. In this case, it seems to us that he creates a logical circle in the definition, since the problem itself of absolute perception must be solved by means of the reverse influence of concepts on the stability of perception. We will consider this in the following chapter. But the main deficiency of Bühler's theory is that it tries to find a psychological equivalent of logical operations that lead to the development of a concept, in elementary processes that are identically proper to both perception and thinking. From this it is clear that all boundaries, all qualitative difference between elementary and higher forms, between perception and cognition are erased.

The concept seems to be simply a corrected and stable perception; it seems to be not a simple representation, but its diagram. From this it is understandable that specifically the theory of Bühler in its logical development led to the rejection of the qualitative uniqueness of the adolescent's thinking and to admitting that his thinking is, in the main, identical with the thinking of the three-year-old.

Together with the radical change in the logical point of view, the logical view of the concept, there is also a change in the direction of search for the psychological equivalent of the concept. Here again the words of K. Stumpf[51] are confirmed: what is true in logic cannot be false in psychology and vice versa. Comparison of the logical and the psychological in the study of concepts, so characteristic for neo-Kantians, must actually be replaced by the opposite point of view. Logical analysis of the concept, disclosing its essence, provides a key also to its psychological study. It is quite clear that when formal logic imagines the process of formation of a concept as a process of gradual narrowing of content and extending of scope, the process of simple loss by the object of a series of traits, the psychological study directs itself to finding similar processes equivalent to this logical abstraction in the sphere of intellectual operations.

This is the source of the famous comparison with the Galton group photograph, the source of the teaching on general representations. Together with the new understanding of the concept and its essence, psychology is confronted by new problems in its study. The concept begins to be understood not as a thing, but as a process, not as an empty abstraction, but as a thorough and penetrating reflection of an object of reality in all its complexity and diversity, in connections and relations to all the rest of reality. It is natural that psychology will begin to seek an equivalent of the concept in a completely different area.

It has long been noted that the concept in essence represents nothing other than a certain aggregate of judgments, a certain system of acts of thinking. Thus, one of the authors says that the concept considered psychologically, that is, not only from the one aspect of content as it is in logic, but also from the aspect of the form of the concept in reality, in a word, as an activity, is a certain number of judgments and, consequently, not a single act of thinking, but a series of these acts. The logical concept, that is, the simultaneous sum total of traits, different from the aggregate of traits in its form, is a fiction, among other things, completely essential for science. Regardless of its duration, the psychological concept has an internal unity.

Thus, we see that for the psychologist, the concept is an aggregate of acts of judgment, apperception, interpretation, and recognition. The concept taken in action, in movement, in reality, does not lose unity, but reflects its true nature. According to our hypothesis, we must seek the psychological equivalent of the concept not in general representations, not in absolute perceptions and orthoscopic diagrams, not even in concrete verbal images that replace the general representations—we must seek it in a system of judgments in which the concept is disclosed.

Actually since we have rejected the representation of the concept as a simple aggregate of some number of concrete traits that differs from a simple representation only in that it is poorer in content and more extensive in scope of form, seemingly a large envelope empty of content, we must assume beforehand that the psychological equivalent of the concept can only be a system of acts of thinking and some combination and processing of patterns.

The concept, as has already been said, is an objective reflection of a thing in its essence and diversity; it arises as a result of rational processing of representations, as a result of disclosing connections and relations of the given object with others and, consequently, it includes a long process of thinking and cognition that is seemingly concentrated in it. For this reason, in the definition cited above, it seems completely correct to indicate that from the psychological aspect a concept turns out to be a long activity that includes in itself a series of acts of thinking.

K. Bühler comes close to the truth when he says that an abstract word, for example, "mammal," for us adults, educated people, not only is a representation of all kinds of forms of animals associatively linked, but, what is more important, is a rich complex of judgments, more or less introduced into the system, from which, in conformity with circumstances, one judgment or another is at our service.

A great merit of Bühler is his pointing out that a concept arises not mechanically like a group photograph of the objects in our memory, that functions of judgment take part in the development of a concept, that this thesis is correct even for single forms of concept formation, and that for this reason, concepts cannot be pure products of associations, but have their place in the connections of knowledge, that is, concepts have a natural place in judgments and conclusions, acting as a component part of the latter. From our point of view, only two points are in error. First, Bühler assumes the connection of the concept with the complex of judgments introduced into the system to be an associative connection that arises outside thinking. He erroneously assumes the process of judgment to be a simple reproduction of judgment. None of the representatives of the teaching on general representations as a basis of concepts would take exception to such an associative understanding of the character of the connection between a concept and acts of thinking. Actually, there is almost nothing that a concept can be associated or connected with. The circle of various associations is, of course, absolutely unlimited, and for this reason, the presence of associative connections with judgments still says nothing about the psychological nature of the concept, nothing is changed in its traditional understanding, and it is completely compatible with identifying the concept with a general representation.

Bühler's second error is the representation that concepts have their own natural place in acts of judgment making up their organic part. This point of view seems to be erroneous to us because a concept, as we have seen, makes up not simply a part of judgment, but arises as a result of the complex activity of thinking, that is, as a result of multiple operations of judgment, and is disclosed in a series of acts of thinking. Thus, from our point of view, a concept is not a part of judgment, but a complex system of judgments combined as a certain unit and a special psychological structure in the full and true sense of the word. This means that the system of judgment in which a concept is disclosed is contained in a contracted, abbreviated form, as if in a potential state, in the structure of the concept. This system of judgment, like any structure, has its unique properties that characterize it specifically as a whole system, and only an analysis of this system can bring us to understanding the structure of a concept.

Consequently, from our point of view, the structure of a concept is disclosed in a system of judgments, in a complex of acts of thinking that represent a single whole formation which has its own principles. In this representation, we find the main idea on the unity of form and content as the basis of the concept realized.

Actually, the totality of judgments introduced in the system represents a certain content in an ordered and connected form and it is a unit of a series of points of content. Also, the totality of acts of thinking, acting as a single whole, is constructed as a special intellectual mechanism, as a special psychological structure, and is made up of a system or of a complex of judgments. Thus, the unique combination of a series of acts of thinking acting as a certain unit represents a special form of thinking, a certain intellectual method of behavior.

With this we can conclude the review of the changes that occur in the content of an adolescent's thinking. We can assert that all changes in the content, as we have pointed out repeatedly, necessarily also presuppose a change in the form of thinking. Here we come as close as possible to the general psychological law which states that a new content does not mechanically fill an empty form, but content and form are factors in a single process of intellectual development. It is impossible to pour new wine into old skins.

This applies completely also to thinking during the transitional age.

30

It remains for us to consider the important changes that the form of thinking undergoes during the transitional age. Actually, the response to this question has been determined in the preceding course of discussion. It consists in the theory of the concept that we attempted to develop briefly above. If we accept the outlined view of the concept as a certain system of judgments, then we inevitably will agree also that the unified activity in which a concept is disclosed, the unified sphere of the manifestation of the system, is logical thinking.

From our point of view, logical thinking is not composed of concepts so much as of separate elements; it is not added to concepts as something standing above them and developing after them—it is the concepts themselves in their action, in their functioning. Like a certain expression that defines function as an organ in action, we could define logical thinking as concept in action. From this point of view, in the form of a general premise, we could say that the most important revolution in forms of thinking in the adolescent is the revolution that occurs as a result of the formation of concepts, and mastery of logical thinking represents the second basic consequence of the acquisition of this function.

Only during the transitional age is mastery of logical thinking a real fact, and only owing to this fact are those deep changes in the content of thinking which we mentioned above possible. We have much evidence from investigators who place the development of logical thinking at the transitional age.

In the words of E. Meumann, for example, real logical deduction in the form in which textbooks use it, becomes easy for the child only quite late. Approximately toward the last year in a German school, that is, at 14 years of age, the child appears to be capable of seeing the connection between deductions made and to understand them. True, Meumann's opinion has been disputed many times. It developed that logical thinking appears not long before the period of sexual maturation, and the attempt to reject Meumann's position has always taken two different directions.

Some authors try simply to lower the age indicated by Meumann, and their common disagreement with Meumann was only a seeming disagreement. Thus, in a recent study, H. Ormian found that mastery of logical thinking begins at age 11. Other authors, as we shall see subsequently, also indicate age 11-12, that is, the age when primary education ends, as the period when the child's prelogical form of thinking ends and the threshold of mastery of logical thinking is crossed.

The opinion that attempts simply to lower by two years the time of appearance of logical thinking indicated by Meumann is not at variance, as we can see, with the position defended by Meumann himself, because he has in mind the final mastery of logical thinking in its developed form. Some authors, who studied the whole process of development of concepts more finely and precisely, indicate its beginning. And all agree that only after primary school age and only with the beginning of the adolescent years is the transition made to logical thinking in the real and true sense of the word.

There are authors who differ radically and decisively with this position. On the basis of serious study of the thinking of the very young child and with almost no reference to the study of the thinking of the adolescent, these authors, as we indicated many times, are inclined to reject all differences between the thinking of the three-year-old and the adolescent. On the basis of purely external data, the investigators ascribe developed logical thinking to the three-year-old, forgetting that logical thinking is impossible without concepts and concepts develop relatively late.

The controversy created by this psychological disagreement can be resolved only if we are able to answer the question, is the very young child capable of abstract thinking and concepts, and how do concepts and logical thinking differ qualitatively from generalization and the thinking of the very young child. Essentially, in all the preceding exposition, we proceeded from a desire to answer this question. Specifically for this reason we did not limit ourselves to a simple statement that the formation of concepts begins at the transitional age, but resorted to the method of genetic sections, and by comparing various stages in the development of thinking, we tried to show how a pseudoconcept differs from true concepts,[52] how complex thinking differs qualitatively from thinking in concepts and, consequently, how what is new that makes up the content of the development of thinking in the transitional age is inferred.

Now we would like to reinforce the position arrived at experimentally by a consideration of the results of the studies of other authors especially dedicated to the study of the characteristics of the thinking of the child up to the transitional age. These studies, set up with a completely different goal, seem almost specially directed to refuting the idea that the child of early, preschool, and school age is already capable of logical thinking.

The basic conclusion that can be reached from these studies is the discovery of the fact that the forms of thinking that resemble logical forms externally essentially conceal qualitatively different thinking operations. We have in mind three basic points connected with disclosing the qualitative uniqueness of the thinking of the child and the principal differences between it and logical thinking. Considering again the results of the work of others, we must resort to the method of genetic sections and try to find the uniqueness of thinking in concepts and to compare it with other genetically earlier forms of thinking.

For this reason we must obviously digress from the thinking of the adolescent and concentrate our attention on the thinking of the child. But in essence, we will always keep in mind specifically thinking in the transitional age. We only want to find the path to recognizing its characteristics through comparative-genetic study and comparison with earlier forms of thinking because, as we have already indicated, the argument about whether the formation of concepts is an achievement of the transitional age in its essentially modern formulation is reduced to the question: is a child capable of logical thinking and the formation of concepts?

31

As we have already said, we have no other means of understanding that which is new that develops in the thinking of the adolescent in comparison with the thinking of the child than through a comparative study of genetic sections of the developing intellect. Only by comparing the intellect of the adolescent with the intellect of the young child of preschool and school age, only by comparing these four sections made at early stages of development, will we be able to include the thinking of the adolescent in the genetic chain and to understand what is new, what develops in that thinking.

We also said that specifically the erroneous interpretation of early sections in the development of the intellect and interpretation based exclusively on apparent similarity, on external traits, usually led to overestimating the child's capability of logical thinking and, consequently, to an underestimation of that which is new that develops in the thinking of the adolescent.

We formulated the task that confronts us in the following way: we must consider whether the child is capable of logical thinking in the essential sense of the word, whether the child has the function of forming concepts. In order to answer this question, we must turn to a series of newer studies that leave no doubt with respect to the problem that interests us. Recently D. N. Uznadze[53] did special work on this problem; through various experiments, he undertook systematic study of the formation of concepts at the preschool age. The study (D. N. Uznadze, 1929) involved 76 children age two to seven years. The experiments required classification of various objects into groups, then followed experiments with naming a new thing with some kind of unfamiliar name and experiments of generalizing the names given and defining the new words. Thus, the experiments encompassed different functional points in the formation of concepts.

The basic task of these studies, as we have said, was to disclose what are the equivalents to our concepts at the preschool age, what makes a mutual understanding of the adult and the child possible regardless of the fact that the child has not yet mastered the development of concepts, and finally, how these equivalents are unique at the early stage of development.

We cannot consider in detail the course of the study, and will turn directly to the basic results in which we will find the answer to the question that interests us. As a general characterization of three-year-olds, Uznadze assumes that it can be said that words which they use evoke in them visual, whole undifferentiated images of objects that are also the meaning of these words.

Thus, the three-year-old does not apply true concepts, but in the best case uses only certain equivalents of these in the form of undifferentiated whole examples of an idea. The three-year-old takes a significant step forward along the path to the development of concepts, and one of the greatest achievements of Uznadze's research is that he tries to trace step by step, year by year the internal process of change in the structure of the meaning of children's words.

We cannot present the course of development year by year. We are interested only in the final conclusion. Uznadze says that finally in the seven-year-old, the developing forms of thinking attain decisive dominance. In them, 90% of sound combinations form real words in which meaning is not a whole idea, but mainly an appropriate individual trait. This is especially evident in experiments with generalizations in 84% of which the process occurs on the basis of similarity of individual traits. With respect to this, the seven-year-old attains a stage of development that makes him capable for the first time of an adequate understanding and treatment of our thinking processes. Thus, genuine school maturity occurs only with the end of the seventh year of life, only at the time that the child becomes capable of a true understanding and processing of thinking operations; before that he uses only equivalents of our concepts pertaining to the same circle of objects, but with a different meaning. The author does not analyze the uniqueness of children's meaning, but the indication of the whole concrete-like and undifferentiated character of these formations is a basis for bringing them close to the complexes we found in the experiment with complex forms of thinking.

In essence, with the help of the more penetrating research of Uznadze, we were able to show that the characteristics of thinking that former research ascribed to the young child are actually predominant by the eighth year. This is the principal merit of Uznadze's work. He succeeded in showing that where there is an obvious predominance of logical thinking there are only equivalents of our concepts that permit an exchange of thought, but not an adequate application of appropriate operations.

In application to the young child, these equivalents have long been recognized by investigators. Thus, W. Stern (1922, 1926) in a study of children's language, citing W. Ament (1899), establishes that in children's speech from the very beginning there is no differentiation of symbols for individual and generic concepts. The child is more likely to begin from certain preconcepts from which only gradually both types in which we are interested develop. But, in contrast to Ament, Stern takes a decisive step further and asserts: as long as we speak in general of concepts, we interpret the first verbal meanings logically.

Moreover, this must be decisively rejected. Only according to external form do they seem to be concepts. The process of their psychological development is completely alogical and rests on much more primitive functions than the function of concept formation. These are quasi- or pseudoconcepts. Analysis of pseudoconcepts allows Stern to reach the conclusion that the first words are simply symbols of familiarity, that is, what Groos calls a potential concept. This is the basis on which Stern interprets the change in meaning of words at an early age of which we spoke above. In subsequent analysis the author comes to the conclusion that the first individual concepts that encompass a certain concrete object develop in the child. For a child, a doll is always the same doll that is the child's favorite toy; mama is always the same person that satisfies the child's needs, etc.

It is enough to look at Stern's examples to see that that which we term an individual concept rests exclusively on recognizing the identity of one and the same object—operation, which even animals have and which in no way permits us to speak of concept in the real sense of the word.

As far as generic concepts that encompass a whole group of objects are concerned, according to Stern, they require a somewhat longer period of development. They exist at first only in a preparatory stage in which they encompass a concrete plurality of similar specimens, but not an abstract commonality of traits. Stern calls these plural concepts. As Stern maintains, the child now knows that a horse is not simply a single specimen that appeared once, but that it can be found in many specimens.

However, the statements of the child always refer to only one specimen or another that is at the time the subject of his perception or expectation. He places each new specimen among many others that he perceived previously, but he still does not subordinate all of these specimens to a general concept. On the basis of our experience, we conclude that the child approaches this only in his fourth year.

Our studies convinced us that for the child the initial function of the word is indicating a specific object, and for this reason, we understand these plural concepts as a verbal indicative gesture which he makes each time toward a concrete specimen of one thing or another. Just as with the help of a pointing gesture, attention can be called each time to only some specific, single object, using one of his first words, the child always has in mind a concrete specimen of some general group.

In this case, in what is a real concept manifested? Only in that the child recognizes the similarity or belonging of different specimens to one and the same group, but as we have seen before, this is also proper to animals at the earliest primitive stages of development. As we remember, when the situation requires it, instead of a stick, a monkey uses many very different objects which it classifies in the same group because of a similar trait. Stern's assertion that a child masters general concepts by the fourth year, completely rejected in the studies of Uznadze cited above, seems to us to be a natural consequence of inserting logic into children's speech, of intellectualism, of ascribing to the child, on the basis of external similarity, a developed and logical thinking; this is the most essential deficiency of Stern's important research.

Uznadze's achievement is that he showed how insupportable it is to ascribe the formation of general concepts to such an early age. He increased the period indicated by Stern by three to four years. But it also seems to us that he still makes a substantial error, similar to the error of Stern, which consists in his accepting as true concepts, formations that appear to be similar to concepts. It is true that a child by the age of seven takes a decisive step along the path of developing his concepts. We could say that specifically by this time, he makes a transition from syncretic ideas to complex thinking, from lower forms of complex thinking to pseudoconcepts. But, as Uznadze points out, identifying concrete common traits as the single symptom of formation of concepts in the seven-year-old is, as we have seen, nothing other than a potential concept or a pseudoconcept. Identifying a common trait by no means constitutes a concept, although it is a very important step along the path to its development. Our studies, which disclosed a complex, genetic diversity of forms in the development of concepts, are a basis for the assertion that Uznadze's analysis is also incomplete, that by the age of seven, the child has not mastered the formation of concepts, although he takes a very important step on the path to this achievement.

32

In this respect, the remarkable studies of J. Piaget[54] on speech and thinking in the child and his judgments and deductions leave no doubt. These studies (1932) undoubtedly constituted an epoch in the study of children's thinking and played the same role in the study of the thinking of the schoolchild as the studies of Stern and other authors played in their time in the study of early childhood.

By means of extremely clever and penetrating studies, Piaget succeeded in showing that the forms of thinking during early school years, regardless of their apparent similarity to logical thinking, are in fact qualitatively different from operations of logical thinking, and in them other patterns are dominant that differ substantially in structural, functional, and genetic relations from abstract logical thinking, which, in the strict sense of the word, begins only after primary school age, that is, at the age of 12.

As Piaget says, Jean Jacques Rousseau liked to repeat that "the child is not a small adult," that he has his own needs and his mind is adapted to those needs. All the studies of Piaget follow this basic line; his studies also try to show that with respect to thinking, the child is not a small adult and that the development of thinking when he makes the transition from primary school age to secondary does not consist exclusively of a quantitative growth, enrichment, and extension of the same forms that were dominant in the first stage.

Analyzing the thinking of the schoolchild and the adolescent, Piaget establishes a number of qualitative differences and shows that all of them represent a unit based on one principal, general cause.

In this respect, it seems to us that E. Claparède, in his foreword to Piaget's work, correctly evaluates its great merit: Piaget posed the problem of the child's thinking and its development as a qualitative problem. Claparède writes that we might have defined the new idea to which Piaget brings us by comparing it to the opinion generally tacitly accepted. While the problem of the child's thinking was usually treated as a quantitative problem, Piaget changed it to a qualitative problem. While in the child's development, what was usually seen was the result of a certain number of additions and subtractions, acquisition of new experience and exclusion of certain errors, we are now shown that the child's intellect changes its character gradually. If the child's mind frequently seems to be quite muddled in comparison with that of the adult, this is not because of his having somewhat more or less of some elements or because it is full of gaps and bumps, but because he depends on a different type of thinking, a type that the adult has long since left behind in his development, as Claparède emphasizes.

Thus, in the problem that interests us, Piaget's studies directly continue the work started by other authors and can be directly connected with the work of Uznadze. Piaget begins where the research of Uznadze ends and seems to reconsider the conclusion that Uznadze reached. Actually, beginning at age seven, a great upward shift occurs in the child's thinking that consists of his moving from subjective, syncretic connections to complex, objective connections that are extremely close to the concepts of the adult. For this reason there may be the impression that a child of seven thinks like an adult, that he is capable of using our thinking operations. But Piaget shows that this is just an illusion.

We cannot discuss in detail the course of his research and must limit ourselves to certain basic conclusions that may have a direct relation to our theme. Piaget's general conclusion is the following: formal thinking develops only at age 11-12. Between 7-8 and 11-12, there is syncretism; contradictions are found almost exclusively in purely verbal thinking not based on direct observations. Only at age approximately 11-12 can we actually speak of the child's logical experience. Nevertheless, age 7-8 represents a serious forward step. Forms of logical thinking appear in the area of visual thinking.

This is how we may present the basic results of Piaget's research. His data show that the thinking of the child passes through three major phases (if we put aside the thinking of the earliest age). During early and preschool age, thinking is egocentric. The child thinks in whole connected graphic impressions that are usually termed syncretic. Pre-causality dominates his thinking. By age 7-8, the child's thinking is altered significantly: the characteristics of early thinking drop off and are replaced by a structure of the child's thinking that is closer to logic. However, the features that characterized the child's thinking at the early stage do not disappear altogether. They are only transferred to a new area, specifically the area of purely verbal thinking.

The child's thinking now is seemingly divided into two large spheres. In the area of visual and effective thinking, the child no longer exhibits the characteristics that he exhibited at an earlier stage of development. But in the area of purely verbal thinking, the child still is subject to syncretism, he still has not mastered the logical forms of thought. This basic law Piaget terms the law of shift or displacement. Using this law, the investigator tries to explain the characteristics of thinking during the first years of school.

The essence of the law is that the child, perceiving his own operations, in this way transfers them from the plane of action to the plane of speech. In the transfer, when the child begins to reproduce his operations verbally, he is again confronted by the difficulties that he overcame in the plane of action. Here a shift will occur between two different methods of mastery. The dates will differ, but the rhythm will remain similar. The shift between thinking and action can be observed continually and has a major potential for understanding the child's logic. It holds the key to elucidating all the phenomena disclosed in our studies.

Thus, as a characteristic of the thinking of the schoolchild, Piaget sees in the transfer to the verbal plane, to the plane of thinking in speech patterns, the same operations that the child has already mastered in the plane of action, and for this reason the whole course of development of thinking is not subordinate to the continuity and gradualness that the associationists, H. Taine and T. Ribot, ascribed to it, but discloses a step backward, interference and transitions of various duration. All the characteristics of the very young child's thinking do not finally disappear. They only disappear from the plane of his concrete thinking, but they move, shift, to the plane of verbal thinking and are manifested there.

We might formulate the law of shift as follows: on the plane of verbal thinking, the schoolchild displays the same characteristics and the same differences from the logic of the adult as the preschooler displayed on the plane of visual and action thinking. The schoolchild thinks just as the preschooler acts and perceives.

With the law of shift, Piaget connects the law of realization established for the intellectual development of the child by E. Claparède, who in a special study attempted to elucidate the development of the child's realization of similarity and difference. It developed that realizing similarity appears much later in the child than realizing difference. In the plane of action, however, the child adapts earlier and more simply to similar than to different situations. Thus, in action, he reacts to similarity earlier than he does to difference. On the other hand, distinguishing objects creates a state of nonadaptation, and specifically this nonadaptation prevents the child from realizing the problem. On this basis, Claparède deduces a general law which states that we realize only to the extent of our unsuccessful adaptation.

The law of shift explains for us why and how the development of thinking occurs during the transition from the preschool to school age and shows that the child begins to realize his operations and his nonadaptation only when he needs to realize them. In particular, using a concrete example, Piaget shows what an enormous role social factors, to use his expression, play in the development of the structure and function of the child's thinking. He shows how logical reflection of the child develops under the direct influence of an argument that arises in the children's group, and only when an external social need arises to prove the rightness of his thinking, to argue for it, to motivate it does the child begin to use the same operations in his own thinking also. Piaget maintains that the logical reflection is a discussion with oneself that reproduces a real argument in an internal aspect. For this reason it is completely natural for the child to master his internal operations, his visual and action thinking, and he becomes capable of directing these earlier and of realizing them sooner than he masters the operations of his verbal thinking. Piaget assumes that it would be no exaggeration to say that because logical thinking does not exist before the age of seven or eight but appears at the age of seven or eight only on the plane of concrete thinking, the child continues to be at the prelogical stage of development on the plane of verbal thinking.

In order for the child to approach logical thinking, an exceptionally interesting psychological mechanism, which Piaget discovered in his studies, is needed. Logical thinking becomes possible only when the child masters his thinking operations, subjects them to himself, begins to control and direct them. According to Piaget's opinion, it is incorrect to equate all thinking without exception to logical thinking. The latter is distinguished by its substantially new character in comparison with other forms of thinking. Piaget says that this is man's experience of controlling himself as a thinking being, experience similar to what a man exercises over himself in controlling his moral behavior. Consequently, this is an effort to realize one's own operations and not just their result, and to establish whether they agree with each other or are in opposition to each other. In this respect, logical thinking is different from all other forms of thinking. Thinking in the ordinary sense is the perception of certain realities and realizing these realities, but, according to Piaget, logical thinking presumes the realization and control of the construction mechanism itself. Thus, logical thinking is characterized most of all by mastery and control. In this sense, Piaget compares mental experience with logical experience in the following way: the need of results of our mental experience is the need of facts. Need resulting from logical experience is mandatory for the operations to agree with each other. This necessity is moral, emanating from the obligation to remain true to oneself. For this reason, the thinking of the child age 8 to 12 exhibits a dual character.

Thinking is connected with actual reality, with direct observation; logical, formal-logical thinking is not yet available to the child. At approximately 11-12 years, on the other hand, the child's method of thinking comes somewhat closer to the thinking of the adult or, in any case, to that of the uneducated adult. Only by the age of 12 does logical thinking appear that assumes an unfailing realization and mastery of thinking operations as such. From the psychological aspect, this is the most essential trait that Piaget identified in the development of logical thinking. He establishes that the new realization is due directly to a social factor and that the incapacity for formal thinking is the result of the child's egocentrism.

At the age of approximately 12, life takes on a new direction, and this brings the child to completely new problems. We see here an exceptionally clear example of how the life around the child elicits ever newer problems that require mental adaptation on his part, how, in the process of solving the problems, the child masters ever newer content of his thinking and how the new content nudges him to the development of new forms.

Better and more graphic evidence of this is the dependence that exists between the development of an argument in a group of children, the need to present evidence and argue, the need to firmly ground and confirm one's own idea, and the development of formal-logical thinking. On the basis of this, Piaget says that specifically owing to the law of shift, the test of the three brothers of Binet–Simon[55] is accessible only to a child age 11, that is, at an age when formal thinking begins. Piaget believes that if this test were performed for the child instead of being told to him, if the personages were presented to him concretely, the child would make no mistakes. But as soon as he begins to consider, he makes mistakes.

Realization of his own operations has a direct and very close relation to language. Piaget notes that this is why speech is such an important factor. It indicates realization. This is why we must study the forms of verbal thinking in the child with such care.

33

It remains for us to say something about an essential factor that will explain for us what interferes from the psychological aspect with the development of abstract thinking at this time. Studies have shown that the school-age child realizes his own thinking operations inadequately still, and for this reason he cannot fully master them. He still has little ability for internal observation, for introspection. Piaget's experiments showed this extremely graphically. Only under the pressure of argument and objections does the child begin to try to confirm his idea before the eyes of others and begin to observe his own thinking, that is, look for and differentiate through introspection the motive that drives him and the direction toward which he aims. In trying to confirm his idea in the eyes of others, he begins to confirm it for himself also. In the process of adapting to others, he gets to know himself.

Piaget tries, using special methods, to establish the capacity of the schoolchild for introspection. He assigned the child small problems and when he got an answer, asked: "How did you get this?" or "What did you say to yourself in order to get this?" Most suitable for the experiments were simple arithmetic problems since they make it possible, on the one hand, to trace the path the child took to get the answer and, on the other hand, introspection becomes exceptionally accessible to the child since he can very easily establish the path and trace his thinking.

With the solving of simple arithmetic problems, Piaget studied 50 children ages 7 to 10. He was struck by the difficulty with which the children answered the question as to how they got the answer, regardless of whether it was correct or not. The child was not able to reproduce the path that his thinking took. After reaching a solution, he invents another way. All of this occurs as the child solved the problem in the same way that we solve an empirical problem by manipulation, that is, realizing every result, but not directing or controlling separate operations, and what is most important, not picking up the whole consequence of our thinking with the help of introspection.

The child seemed not to realize his own thoughts or, in any case, seemed incapable of observing them. Let us recall a single example. The child was asked: "When will it be 5 minutes sooner than 50 minutes?" He answered: "In 45 minutes." This showed that the child understood "5 minutes sooner" as "sooner by 5 minutes." When he was asked how he got this result, the child could neither describe the course of his thought, nor even say that he took 5 from 50. He answered: "I looked for it" or "I found 45." If he was asked further how he found it, if they insisted that he describe how he was thinking, the child presented another and some kind of new operation, completely arbitrary, and applied earlier to the response, "45." For example, one boy answered: "I took 10, 10, 10, and 10 and added 5."

Here we have direct evidence of the fact that the child still does not realize his internal operations and consequently, is not capable of controlling them, and this is the source of his incapacity for logical thinking. Introspection, perceiving one's own internal processes, is, therefore, a necessary factor for mastering them.

Let us remember that the whole mechanism of controlling and mastering behavior, beginning with propriocentric irritations that arise with any kind of movement and ending with introspection, is based on self-perception, on reflection on one's own processes of behavior. This is why the development of introspection is such an important step in the development of logical thinking, and logical thinking is certainly conscious and at the same time it is thinking dependent on introspection. But introspection itself develops late and mainly under the influence of social factors, under the influence of the problems that life puts before the child, under the influence of inability to solve problems of increasing complexity.

34

We must not in the least be surprised that the schoolchild, seemingly externally managing to deal with devices of logical thinking, nevertheless has not yet mastered logic in the true sense of that word. Here, we observe an extremely interesting parallel to the general law of child development: as a rule, the child always masters external forms earlier than the internal structure of any mental operation. The child begins to count long before he understands what counting is and he applies it intelligently. In speech, the child has such conjunctions as "because," "if" and "although" long before the realization of causality, conditionality, or opposition appears in his thinking. Just as grammatical development in children's speech precedes the development of logical categories corresponding to these language structures, the mastery of external forms of logical thinking, especially as applied to external concrete situations in the process of visual and action thinking, precedes internal mastery of logic. For example, Piaget established in special studies that conjunctions expressing opposition were not completely understood by children before the age of 11-12, whereas they appear in children's speech extremely early. Moreover, in some completely concrete situations, the child uses them extremely early and properly.

Special study showed that conjunctions such as "although," "regardless of," "even if," etc. are acquired by the child in their true meaning quite late. A study of sentences requiring completion after these conjunctions showed a positive result on the average in 96% of schoolgirls age 13.

Using a method corresponding to Piaget's, A. N. Leont'ev[56] also developed sentences that the child had to finish after appropriate conjunctions expressing causal relation, opposing relations, etc. The children were given 16 tasks to do.

We will present quantitative data on the study of one group of schoolchildren. The data show that only in class IV did the child finally master the logical categories and relations corresponding to the conjunctions "because" and "although." Thus, in class IV in the school studied, on the average 77.7% of the sentences that included "because" and "although" were logically correctly completed.

As is known, solving any problem is considered feasible for one age or another when 75% of the children solve the problem. True, the children in the group studied ranged in age from 11 to 15. Their average age was between 12 and 13. As we can see, only at this age does the average child[57] finally master relations of causality and opposition in completely concrete situations.

The range of these data is extremely interesting. The minimum number of solutions observed in the children in this group was 20% and the maximum, 100%. Separate examples of unsuccessful solutions show to what degree the child approaches a logical form in the guise of ideas syncretically close to the unsuccessful solutions. Thus, a child who solved 55% of the problems wrote: "Kolya decided to go to the theater because although he did not have any money"; "If an elephant is stuck with a needle it will not hurt him although it hurts all animals because they don't cry"; "The cart fell and broke although they will rebuild it"; "After the bell rang, everyone went to assembly because although there was a meeting." Another child who did 20% of the problems wrote: "If an elephant is stuck with a needle, it will not hurt him although his skin is thick"; "The cart fell and broke although not the whole thing." A child who did 25% of the problems wrote: "Kolya decided to go the theater because he had money"; "The pilot flew an airplane and fell although he did not have enough gas"; "A boy in Class III still counts poorly because he cannot count"; "When you cut your finger, it hurts because you cut it"; "The cart fell and broke although it was broken," etc. A child who did 20% of the problems wrote: "The cart fell and broke although its wheel did not break"; "If an elephant is stuck with a needle, it will not hurt him although he has a thick skin," etc.

From these examples, we see to what degree the child associatively, syncretically, according to impression, matches two ideas that are actually connected: the thick skin of the elephant and the painlessness of the prick and the broken wheel and the breakdown of the cart. But the child finds it difficult to qualify the relation of the two ideas as a logical relation. His "because" and "although" alternate. Frequently both "because" and "although" occur in the same sentence, as the examples above indicate.

35

Using a concrete example, we would like to show the characteristic of thinking during the primary school age that is a holdover of the deficiencies of the very young child's thinking which also separates his thinking from the thinking of the adolescent. We have in mind verbal syncretism, a trait that marks the thinking of the schoolchild as described by Piaget. As syncretism, Piaget understands the undifferentiated combination of the most varied impressions that the child takes in simultaneously that comprise the initial nucleus of his perception. For example, when a five-year-old is asked why the sun does not fall, the child responds: "Because it is yellow"; "Why is the sun hot?" "Because it is high" or "Because there are clouds around it." All of these impressions simultaneously perceived by the child are merged into a single syncretic image, and for the child, these initial syncretic connections take the place of developed and differentiated temporal and spatial, causal and logical connections and relations.

The child of primary school age, as we have already said, gradually overcame syncretism in the area of visual and practical thinking but transferred this characteristic to the area of abstract of verbal thinking. To study this characteristic, Piaget presented 10 proverbs and 12 sentences to schoolchildren ages 8 to 11. The child had to select a sentence for each proverb that expressed the same idea as the proverb but in other words. Two sentences of the 12 had no relation in meaning to the proverbs and the child was to remove them. It became clear that the children correlated the proverbs and sentences on the basis not of the objective connection of ideas, not according to the abstract meaning they contained, but according to the syncretic, graphic, or verbal connection. The child matched two different ideas if they had only some kind of common graphic factor, and he constructed a new syncretic pattern in which both ideas were included. Thus for the proverb, "The cat is away and mice are dancing," a child age 8 years 8 months selected the sentence, "Some people bustle a lot, but do nothing." The child understood each of these expressions if they were presented separately, but here he responded as if they meant the same thing. "Why do these sentences mean the same thing?" "Because there are almost the same words." "What does this sentence mean, 'Some people ...'?" "It means that some people bustle a lot, but then they can't do anything—they are a little tired. There are some people who bustle; and it doesn't make any difference, like cats when they chase chickens and birds. Then they rest in the shade and sleep. There are also a lot of people who run around a lot and then when they can't run any more, they lie down."

Instead of approaching and generalizing the two ideas according to the objective meaning, the child assimilates or merges them into a syncretic image misrepresenting the objective meaning of both sentences.

Under the direction of A. N. Leont'ev, our colleagues conducted a series of systematic studies involving level I schools for normal children and for mentally retarded children. The studies showed that verbal syncretism when studied under special experimental conditions actually is manifested as a characteristic of children's thinking over the whole course of school age. Leont'ev modified Piaget's test: the sentences presented in the test contained some traps—common words or common images with the proverbs to which they referred in their meaning. Because of this, in the experiment we obtained some seemingly condensed data that show extremely exaggerated expression of the verbal syncretism of the schoolchild. We succeeded in establishing an exceptionally interesting point: verbal syncretism appears in the child only because this test is especially difficult for children's thinking. Piaget indicated that the test is meant for 11- to 16-year-olds, that is, essentially it is feasible only for the adolescent. But specifically by applying it at an earlier age, we were able to produce a genetic section of the intellect in the process of solving the same problem and to consider the new element that appears in the intellect when solving similar problems. The difficulty of the proposed test is that it requires abstract thinking in a concrete form.

If we had given the schoolchild similar problems, but separately for matching sentences concrete in meaning and situations abstract in meaning, he would be able to solve both, as comparative studies have shown. But here the difficulty is that both the proverb and the sentence are constructed graphically, concretely; however, the connection or relation that must be established between the one and the other is abstract. The proverb must be understood symbolically; the symbolic attribution of an idea to another concrete content requires a complex merging of abstract and concrete thinking that is feasible only for the adolescent.

We must say that these experimental data must not be generalized, regarded as absolute and transferred to all thinking of the schoolchild. It would be absurd to maintain that a schoolchild is not capable of matching two ideas or seeing an identical meaning in two different verbal expressions except when guided by the graphic sense of the one and the other. Only under special experimental conditions, by means of a trap, only with especially difficult merging of abstract–concrete thinking does this characteristic appear as a dominant trait of thinking.

Mentally retarded children in the transitional age continue to give the same matches that the normal schoolchild gives at the earliest school age.

Let us give some examples. Thus, the child of 13 (I^*—10 years of age) who matched the proverb, "A thread from his village is a shirt to the naked" with the sentence, "Don't try to be a tailor if you never held a thread in your hands" explained this by the fact that thread appears in both. To the proverb, "Don't sit in a sleigh that isn't yours," he matched the sentence, "In the winter people ride in sleighs and in the summer, in carts" and explained it: "Because in the winter people sled and there are sleighs here."

Frequently the child in his justification explains not the process of matching but some single phrase separately. It is very typical for the child to understand correctly each sentence taken separately, but to have great difficulty in understanding the relation between them. Obviously, the graphic thinking that continues

---

*I–Mental age.—Editor's note.

to be dominant in the verbal intellect is not suited to establishing relationship. For example, for the proverb, "Not all that glitters is gold," a child of 13 years 10 months selected the sentence, "Gold is heavier than iron," explaining: "Gold glitters, but iron doesn't." For the proverb, "A thread from his village is a shirt to the naked," a child of 12 selected the sentence, "One should not postpone things," explaining: "Because if he doesn't have a shirt, he must not postpone, but must hurry and make one." For the proverb, "Strike while the iron is hot," a child of 13 years 5 months selected the sentence, "A blacksmith who works without hurrying frequently does more work than one who hurries. That's what they say about the blacksmith." The common elements of the subject, the common elements of the images are enough for matching the two sentences that differ in meaning, that state opposing ideas and are in contradiction to each other: one maintains it is necessary to hurry while the other, that it isn't necessary to hurry. The child identifies the one with the other without noticing the cryptic contradiction, being guided exclusively by the common image of the blacksmith which makes them similar.

We see that the difficulties in establishing relations, the insensitivity to contradiction, syncretic matching not according to objective, but according to subjective connections are typical of the verbal thinking of the schoolchild just as visual thinking is of the preschooler. Frequently such associative matching has a simple justification: "Because here and there we are talking about gold"; "Here and there about the sleigh." For the proverb, "The more quietly you go, the farther you'll get," the same child selected the sentence, "A job that is hard for one person to do can be easily done by group effort," explaining: "It's hard for one to do it, but a horse is one. It's hard for it—we have to ride more quietly."

For the proverb, "The more quietly you go, the farther you'll get," a child age 13 years 9 months selected the sentence, "In the winter we ride in sleighs and in the summer, in a cart," explaining: "It's easier for a horse to pull a sleigh and without hurrying, it goes fast." The same child was a good example of how thinking overcomes contradiction, combining different factors of contradictory statements. Matching the proverb we remember [Strike while the iron is hot.] to a sentence pertaining to a blacksmith, the child includes both points of the contradiction in a syncretic pattern and explains: "The blacksmith who works without hurrying and the hotter the iron, the work goes better."

For the proverb, "In for a little, in for a lot," a child of 13 years, 5 months selected the sentence on the blacksmith and explained: "Maybe the horse had a loose shoe and the blacksmith will fix it." Here we see very clearly a fact noted by Piaget that in matching ideas, a child does not distinguish logical justification from factual. Having seen the factual connection between the blacksmith, riding, and the horse, the child is satisfied with this and his thought goes no further. Frequently, the child matches ideas that seem to us to have absolutely no connection to each other. The unique relation appears that Blonsky termed syncretism of incoherent connectedness in children's thinking.

For example, for the proverb, "Don't sit in a sleigh that isn't yours," a child of 14 years 7 months selects the sentence, "If you already got somewhere, then it's too late to turn back from half-way there," explaining: "If you sit in a sleigh that isn't yours, then the owner can throw you out when you're half-way there." Frequently in such cases, the sense of the sentence is twisted to mean the opposite. The child does not feel constrained by the given premises and changes these in order to adapt them to the conclusion.

We will limit ourselves to the following two examples. To the proverb, "Not all that glitters is gold," a child of 13 years 6 months selected the sentence: "Gold is heavier than iron," explaining: "It isn't just gold that glitters, iron does too." Or for the proverb, "A thread from his village is a shirt to the naked," he selected the sentence: "Don't take up trade as a tailor if you have never held a thread in your hands," explaining: "If you didn't pick up a needle, then you must pick it up."

The examples presented, as we have already said, characterize the thinking of a retarded child. Here we see only the manifestation of those characteristics that persist in a cryptic form in the normal schoolchild also at an earlier stage of development.

In this research, A. N. Leont'ev came across a most important fact: when the child is asked to explain why he matches a given proverb with a given sentence, the child frequently reconsiders his decision. The need to justify the match, to express in words and set out the course of his judgment for another leads to completely different results.

When the child, having matched two sentences syncretically, comes to explaining it aloud, he notices his mistake and begins to give a correct response. Observations showed that the child's justification is not simply a representation in words of what he has done—it represents the whole process of the child's thinking on new bases. Speech is never simply attached as a parallel series, it always represents a process.

In order to confirm this, we undertook a special study in which the child was given two pages of tasks constructed according to the same principle, but with different material. In the first instance, the child, in matching a proverb with a sentence, thinks for himself, depending on processes of internal speech; in the second, he is required to think and reason aloud. As we might have expected, the study showed that between the two methods, thinking to oneself and thinking aloud, there is a great difference for the schoolchild. The child matching sentences syncretically while thinking to himself, begins to match similar proverbs according to an objective connection as soon as he makes the transition to explaining it aloud. We will not stop to give examples. We will only say that the whole process of solving changes its character strikingly as soon as the child makes the transition from internal to external speech (A. N. Leont'ev and A. Shein).

In school-age pedology, we tried to establish that internal speech is generally developed only at the beginning of school age. It is a young, weak, unstable form not yet fully functional. For this reason the discrepancy between internal and external speech of the schoolchild is the most characteristic feature of his thinking. In order to think, the schoolchild must speak aloud and to another. We know that external speech, serving as a means of communication, is socialized earlier in the child than internal speech, which he has not yet mastered.

We have already presented the opinion of Piaget on the fact that the child has not yet mastered his own processes of thinking and become conscious of them. A controversy, the need to justify, to prove, to argue—this is one of the basic factors in the development of logical thinking. For this reason, socialized speech is also more intellectual, more logical.

Thus, we see that internal speech does not appear during school age simply as the spoken word transferred inward, ingrown, and having lost its external part. We could not give a more false definition of internal thinking than in that certain formula: "Thought is speech minus the sound." From the fact of divergence between internal and external speech in the schoolchild, we see the degree to which internal and external speech is formed at that age on different bases, how internal speech still retains features of egocentric thinking and moves on a plane of syncretic matching of ideas, and external speech is already quite socialized, recognized, and directed in order to move along a logical plane.

This study had already been conducted when it became clear to us that, strictly speaking, we approached a fact long known in school practice from the other end. Let us recall the proven device of all schoolteachers who make pupils who solve a problem incorrectly solve it aloud. The pupil, in solving this same problem to himself, gives an absurd answer. When he is made to solve the problem aloud, the teacher teaches him to be conscious of his own operations, to follow their course, to correct it sequentially, and to control the course of his thoughts. We might say that in making the child solve the same problem aloud, the teacher transfers the child's thinking from the syncretic plane to the logical plane.

Let us recall Piaget's observation, which we cited, about the relative weakness of introspection that the child exhibits in solving arithmetic problems. We will remember that the child solving a simple arithmetic problem either correctly or incorrectly often cannot say how he solved the problem, which operations he used—up to this point he is not consciousness of the course of his own thinking and does not correct it. In the same way, it is often hard to say why it is difficult to remember one event or another.

At this stage, the child's thinking has an involuntary character. Absence of arbitrariness and of consciousness of his own thinking operations is also exactly the psychological equivalent of absence of logical thinking. As research shows, specifically with the end of the initial school age, the child begins to understand properly and be conscious of his own operations that he carries out with the help of words and the meaning of the word as a certain sign or an auxiliary means for thinking. Before this time, as Piaget's research showed, the child continues to remain at the stage of nominal realism, considering the word as one property among a number of the properties of the object.

Not understanding the arbitrariness of verbal meaning, the child does not distinguish its role in the process of thinking from that of the object, from that of the meaning that is grasped with the help of that word. To the question, "Why is the sun called the sun?" an 11-year-old boy responds: "For no reason. It's a name." "And the moon?" "For no reason too." Any kind of names can be given. Such answers appear only at age 11-12. Before that, the child does not recognize the difference between the name and the thing named and tries to base one name or another on the properties of the thing they represent.

The unconsciousness of one's own operations and the role of the word is retained in the primitive adolescent even at the stage of sexual maturity. We cite several examples from the research of Golyakhovskaya on explaining some representations and the perception of pictures in Kazakh children. A girl of 14, daughter of a poor peasant, is illiterate. The question: "What is a dog?" The answer: "It's not a man, it's unclean, not for eating. And this is why it's not a man, it's unclean and is called a dog." A girl of 14, daughter of a peasant of average means, is slightly literate. Question: "What is a sparrow?" Answer: "Something that flies, with wings. Because it's small, we call it a sparrow. In Kazakh language, it's called an animal." Question: "What is a rabbit?" Answer: "An animal. Since it's white and small, we call it a rabbit." Question: "What is a dog?" Answer: "It's an animal too. Since it's unclean, and not for eating, we call it a dog.".

A boy of 12, son of a rich landowner, semi-literate. Question: "What is a rock?" Answer: "It comes out of the ground as a rock by nature. That's what we call a rock." Question: "What is the steppe?" Answer: "What was created in the beginning. Of course, the steppe was created. Then we called it the steppe." Question: "What is sand?" Answer: "From the very beginning sand was formed from under the earth. Then we called it sand." Question: "What is a dog?" Answer: "From the very beginning there was a dog and now we call it a dog." Question: "What is a marmot?" Answer: "It's a special animal. From the very beginning it was made a marmot. Then he started to dig a den and began to live there. How do I know this? There was some kind of single marmot and he had children. I concluded that he was created a marmot."

Here the characteristic of thinking that the word is considered as an attribute of the thing, as one of the properties of the thing, is clearly evident. Only with progressing socialization of the child's thinking does intellectualization occur. Being conscious of his own and others' thoughts in the process of verbal communication, the child begins to be conscious of his own thoughts and to direct their course. Progressing socialization of internal speech and progressing socialization of thinking are the basic factors in the development of logical thinking during the transitional age, the basic and central fact of all changes that occur in the adolescent's intellect.

36

Thus, we see that only concrete thinking of the schoolchild is logical thinking in the true sense of the word, but on the plane of verbal thinking, abstract thinking, the schoolchild is still susceptible to syncretism, is insensitive to contradictions, is not capable of perceiving relations and uses transduction, that is, conclusion from the particular to the particular, as a basic device of thought.

Piaget maintains that the whole structure of children's thinking up to age 7 or 8, and even to a certain extent until deduction in the true sense of the word appears at the age of 11 or 12, can be explained by the fact that the child thinks of particular or special cases and does not establish common relations among them. Piaget demonstrated that this characteristic of children's thinking, which Stern termed transduction when applied to an early age, was retained on the plane of abstract thinking by the schoolchild who had not yet finally mastered the relation of the general to the particular.

As we have said, underdevelopment of logical thinking consists of the child not being conscious of his own process of thinking, not having mastered it. Piaget says that introspection is actually one of the types of consciousness or more precisely, it is consciousness to the second degree. If the thought of the child did not meet with the thoughts of others and did not elicit adaptation of his own thoughts to the thoughts of others, the child would never become conscious of himself. Logical confirmation of any judgment occurs on a completely different plane than the formulation of that judgment. While judgment may be unconscious and may arise from preceding experience, logical confirmation arises from contemplation and searching, in short—it requires a certain constructive self-observation of one's own thoughts and it requires thinking which alone is capable of meeting logical requirements as Piaget assumes.

Applying the conclusions of his research to the formation of concepts, Piaget establishes that up to the age of 11 or 12, a child is not capable of giving an exhaustive definition of concepts. He always makes judgments from some concrete, direct, and egocentric point of view, not yet having mastered the relation of the general to the particular. The concepts of the school-age child include a certain generalization and uniting of various traits, but the generalization is still not realized by the child himself and he does not know the basis for his concept. The absence of a logical hierarchy and synthesis between various elements of one and the same concept is what characterizes the child's concept.

In these equivalents, children's concepts still retain a trace of what Piaget calls serial position, that is, an insufficient synthesis of a number of traits. In his opinion, children's concepts are a serial position, but not a synthesis, that is, a unity related to the unity in which various elements merge in the syncretic image—a subjective unity. From this, in the process of being developed and used, children's concepts display serious contradictions. These are concepts-aggregates, as Piaget terms them. They continue to dominate in the determinations of the child and are evidence that the child has not yet mastered the hierarchy and synthesis of elements contained in the concepts and does not maintain in the field of his attention all of the traits in their entirety, operating with one, then with another of these traits. According to Piaget, the child's concepts resemble a metallic ball that attaches sequentially and randomly to five or six electromagnets and jumps randomly from one to another.

More simply, synthesis and hierarchy of elements that are dominant in a complex concept and the relations between elements comprising the essence of the concept are still inaccessible to the child regardless of the fact that these elements and their combination are already accessible to him. This is manifested in operations with concepts. Piaget shows that the child is not capable of systematic logical addition and logical multiplication. As the research of Piaget shows, the child is not capable of simultaneously fixing his attention on a series of traits that are part of a complex single concept.

In the field of his attention, these traits alternate, and each time his concept is diminished from some one aspect. The hierarchy of concepts is not accessible to him, and for this reason, although his concepts externally resemble our concepts, in essence they are only pseudoconcepts. This is the main goal of all of our research in which we are trying to show that the thinking of the child of school age is at a different genetic stage than the thinking of the adolescent and that the formation of concepts appears only during the transitional age.

Subsequently we will return to this central point, but now we must note one of the ideas that Piaget expressed in passing, an idea that, in our opinion, contains the key to understanding all the characteristics of children's thinking that Piaget established. He said that the child never enters into genuine contact with things because he does not work.[58] This connection of the development of higher forms of thinking, particularly thinking in concepts, with work seems to us to be central and basic, capable of disclosing the characteristics of children's thinking and that which is new, which appears in the thinking of the adolescent.

We will be able to return to this problem in one of the following chapters of our course. Now we would like to consider the problem that seems to us to be closely linked to the forms of merging of abstract and concrete thinking in the adolescent.

37

In a special study, Graucob considers the formal characteristics of thinking and language during the transitional age. He bases his study on the correct position that not only the scope and content, but also the formal character of thinking at this age is closely connected with the general structure of the personality of the adolescent. This work draws our attention along two lines. First, it shows the same idea that we tried to defend above, but from a different aspect. We tried to show that neither the preschoolchild nor the schoolchild is capable of thinking in concepts and that, consequently, it appears no earlier than during the transitional age. But a number of studies show that during the transitional age, this form of logical, abstract thinking in concepts is still not the dominant form, but is fresh and young and only just developed and not yet secure.

Wholly conscious and verbally formulated thinking is not at all the dominant form of thinking in the adolescent. As Graucob correctly notes, most often we find forms of thought in which only the results are distinctly formulated in concepts while the processes leading to those results are not consciously realized. In his graphic expression, the thinking of the adolescent at this time resembles a mountain chain, the peaks of which sparkle in the morning light while everything else is hidden in darkness. The thinking is stepwise and if it is reproduced precisely, it sometimes leaves the impression of being disconnected and without an adequate basis.

It is understood that we are speaking only of spontaneous thinking of the adolescent. His thinking connected with school is in a much more systematized and deliberate form.

Second, the new form of thinking during the transitional age is a merging of abstract and concrete thinking—the appearance of metaphors, words used with a figurative meaning. Graucob correctly notes that the thinking of the adolescent still flows partially in a pre-speech form. True, this pre-speech thinking is not directed mainly toward single, visually present objects and toward external, evoked, eidetic, visual images as it is in the child. It differs from the visual thinking of the child, but it seems to us that the author does not formulate the problem quite correctly when he considers this thinking as a type of metaphysical thinking that in the formal respect is similar to the contemplation of mystics and metaphysicians.

We think that pre-speech and some post-speech thinking frequently does not occur entirely with the participation of speech; nevertheless, as we will try to show in a subsequent chapter, it is done on the basis of speech. A. A. Potebnya compares thought without words to a chess game without looking at the board. He says that in a similar way it is possible to think without words, being limited only to more or less clear pointing to them or directly at the content of what is being thought, and such thinking is found much more frequently (for example, in sciences that partially replace words with formulas) specifically as a result of its greater importance and in relation to many aspects of human life. Potebnya adds that we must not, however, forget that knowing how to think humanly but without words is possible only through words and that deaf-mutes without speaking teachers (or trained speakers) would remain almost animals forever.

This reasoning seems to us just about right. To know how to think like a human, but without words is possible only through words.

In the next chapter, we will try to consider in detail the influence that verbal thinking has on visual and concrete thinking, radically restructuring these functions on new bases. For this reason, we think the author correctly indicates that the combination of speech and thinking during the transitional age is much more firm than in the child; this is apparent in the increasing mastery of speech, in enrichment with new concepts, but most of all in the formation of abstract thinking and in the accompanying elimination of eidetic tendencies.

Graucob believes that, except for early childhood, at no stage in human life can one observe with such clarity as in the transitional age that the development of thinking moves forward together with the development of speech; together with verbal formulation of thinking, making newer and sharper distinctions becomes possible. In the expression of Goethe, language in itself is creative.

Investigating the appearance of metaphors and words used in a figurative sense during adolescence, the author quite justifiably indicates that this unique combination of concrete and abstract thinking must be considered as a new achievement of the adolescent. The verbal tissue of the adolescent exhibits a much more complex structure. Connections of coordination and subordination come forward, and this more complex verbal structure is an expression, on the one hand, of increasingly complex but still not fully clarified thinking, and on the other, a means for further development of the intellect.

How does the metaphor or figurative sense of the word differ qualitatively in childhood and in the transitional age? Even in a child's language, there are graphic comparisons that reinforce the tendency of children toward eidetism. But these comparisons do not involve anything abstract. Metaphors in the true sense of the word do not exist for the child. For him, metaphors are an actual matching of impressions. It is not the same for the adolescent. Typical here is a unique relation of the concrete and abstract that is possible only on the basis of highly developed speech.

We see to what degree the usual comparison of the abstract and the concrete is incorrect and how these two forms of thinking actually are not in contradiction but are mutually connected. Graucob says that during adolescence, the abstract is assimilated more easily when it is reflected in some concrete example of a concrete situation. Thus, he says, we come to a seemingly contradictory result that indicates that, regardless of the development of abstract thinking and the gradual disappearance of eidetic contemplation that parallels it, concrete, graphic comparisons in the language of the adolescent increase and reach a peak, after which they begin to decrease, approaching the language of the adult.

The metaphors of the child, the author continues, leave the impression of something objective, natural. In the adolescent, they are the fruit of subjective processing. In the metaphor, objects are matched not organically, but with the aid of the intellect, and metaphors develop not on the basis of synthetic contemplation, but on the basis of a combining introspection. For this reason, the rapprochement of abstract and concrete thinking is the distinguishing trait of the transitional age. Even in lyric poetry, the adolescent is not free of reflection. His fate consists of the fact that where he must be a thinker, he poetizes, and where he performs as a poet, he philosophizes.

Illustrating metaphors in the speech and thinking of the adolescent, Graucob establishes a series of exceptionally unique metaphors in which their original meaning appears as if in inverted form. Remote, abstract concepts must elucidate what is simple, concrete, and close. In these metaphors, the abstract is not elucidated with the help of the concrete, but the concrete is frequently elucidated with the help the abstract.

In the next chapter, we will consider in detail the unique merging of abstract and concrete thinking that is typical for the transitional age. Now we are interested in the fact that factors of the abstract and concrete are contained in the thinking of the adolescent in proportions and qualitative relations that are different from those in the thinking of the schoolchild.

Kroh, noting correctly that the development of thinking is usually underestimated in theories of the transitional age, establishes the fact, decisive for elucidating the development of intellect, that with the end of [primary] school begins the process of differentiation in thinking influenced by external causes.

Never does the influence of the environment on the development of thinking acquire such great significance as specifically at the transitional age. Then as the intellect develops, the city and the village, the boy and the girl, children of various social and class levels are distinguished more and more. Obviously, the process of development of thinking at this age is directly affected by social factors. In this we see the direct confirmation of the fact that the adolescent's main successes in the development of thinking are in the form of cultural development of thinking.

Not biological development of the intellect, but mastery of historically developed synthetic forms of thinking comprises the principal content at this age. This is why the series of monographs that Kroh cites show that the process of intellectual maturation in different social strata presents a very different picture. External factors that form intellectual development assume a decisive significance in the transitional age: the intellect acquires methods of action that are the product of socialization of thinking and not of its biological evolution. Kroh, as we shall see, establishes that subjective and visual images begin to fall away at approximately age 15-16. In the author's opinion, the main reason for this is the adolescent's development of language, socialization of his speech, and development of abstract thinking. The visual bases for speech diminish. Conceptions that are the basis for words lose their specific meaning. In the child, the visual experience determines the content and frequently also the form of the child's expression. In the adult, speech depends much more on its own bases. In words-concepts, it has its material in grammar and syntax, its normal rules of formulation. Language more and more separates from visual conceptions and becomes more autonomous to a significant degree. This process of automatization of speech occurs predominantly during the transitional age, as Kroh assumes.

E. Jaensch, the author of studies on eidetism, correctly indicates that during historical human development also, in the transition from primitive to developed thinking, speech played a decisive role as a means of liberation from visual images.

Remarkable in this respect is the fact, pointed out by Kroh, that in deaf-mute children eidetic images can be found even when they have almost disappeared in their peers. This is indisputable evidence that elimination of eidetic images is influenced by the development of speech.

Connected with this is another trait of thinking during the transitional age—the transfer of attention of the adolescent to his own internal life and transition from the concrete to the abstract. Gradual introduction of abstraction into the thinking of the adolescent is the central factor in the development of the intellect during the transitional age. However, as Kroh points out correctly, isolating separate properties in a complex of things is already available to the young child. While we usually understand attention that isolates as abstraction, we must mention abstraction that isolates, which is also available to animals; to say that this kind of abstraction is an acquisition of the transitional age is not correct.

Abstraction that generalizes must be distinguished from abstraction that isolates. It arises when the child subordinates a number of concrete objects to one general concept. But the child forms and uses even this kind of concept extremely early. Obviously this does not comprise what is new, what engages the thinking of the adolescent. Abstraction that generalizes leads the child to thinking of contents that are not accessible to visual perception. When people say that the adolescent first involves the abstract world for himself, then the statement, in the words of Kroh, must not be understood in the sense that this form of abstraction becomes accessible only at this age.

It is much more important to emphasize something else: as a rule, comprehended mutual relations of similar abstract concepts become accessible to the adolescent. Not so much do separate abstract traits in themselves become accessible at this age as do connections, relations, and interdependencies of traits. The adolescent establishes relations between concepts. By means of judgments, he finds new concepts.

It seems to us that Kroh's mistake was his opinion that the use of proverbs and abstract expressions presented in a visual form is a transitional stage from concrete to abstract thinking. Kroh believes that this form usually was not noted by investigators and, moreover, that it is an end stage of the development of abstract thinking for many people.

As we have said and as we will try to explain in detail subsequently, merging of the abstract and the concrete is not accessible to the child and is not at all a transition from concrete to abstract thinking, but a unique form of changing concrete thinking, a form that already appears on a base of the abstract similarly, as Potebnya says, to knowing how to think without words is determined in the last analysis by the word. The same thing pertains also to logical conclusions.

Although, as Deuchler pointed out, these conclusions are evident as early as in the four-year-old, they are still based completely on a visual or graphic combination of premises and their content. The logical requirement for the result obtained, like the whole path of logical consideration, is still not accessible to the child. The normal child becomes capable of these operations only during the period of sexual maturation. Such an intelligent understanding of logical-grammatical thinking occurs only at that time. In the child, mastery of grammar is based mainly on the feeling for language, on the habits of speech, on the formation of analogies. Kroh justifiably connects these successes in the adolescent's thinking with his successes in the area of mathematics. He asserts that the comprehended course of evidence and independent discovery of mathematical laws and conditions are actually possible only during the transitional age. A serious change in the content of thinking of the adolescent is coupled with these features of formal thinking. The task of self-knowledge, prepared by understanding other people and mastering mental categories, brings the adolescent to directing his attention more and more toward the aspect of external life. For the adolescent, separating the internal from the external world is a necessity related to the needs and the tasks with which development confronts him. Kroh believes that the task of creating a life plan requires greater separation of the essential from the nonessential as time goes on. Without a logical evaluation, this cannot be done. For this reason, it is understandable that development of higher forms of intellectual activity is so very important during the transitional age. Genuine, correlated, abstract thinking becomes all the more crucial.

It does not arise at once of course. The child knew previously how to perceive data visually and the relatively complex connection of things, meanings, actions. He was in a state to understand and apply abstractions of various kinds. The transitional age brings with it only the capability of an intelligent correlation of abstract concepts and general content. Real logical capabilities develop together with this. Kroh repeats that the child's environment has a decisive influence over this thinking. According to the author's observations, in a peasant environment, we frequently encounter adults who have not gone beyond the intellectual level of a schoolchild. Over their whole life, their thinking has not moved beyond the sphere of the visual, never made the transition from specifically logical thinking to its abstract forms.

Since soon after finishing school, the adolescent enters the kind of environment in which higher forms of thinking have not been mastered, it is natural that he himself does not reach a higher degree of development, although he displays great ability. It cannot be more decisively confirmed that the formation of concepts is the product of the cultural development of the intellect and depends in the last analysis on the environment.

In various spheres of practical life there are completely different methods of applying intellectual activity which, on the one hand, are determined by the prevailing structure of that sphere of life and on the other, by characteristics of the individual himself.

Kroh's most important conclusion, it seems to us, is the conclusion regarding the central significance of intellectual development for the whole transitional age.

The intellect plays a decisive role for the adolescent. Even in selecting one profession or another, processes of a typical intellectual nature are applied to a large degree. Together with E. Lau (1925), Kroh maintains that specifically in the adolescent, the influence of the intellect on will is exceptionally strong. Considered and conscious decisions play a much greater role in his whole development than does the influence of the usually overrated increasing emotionality.

In the next chapter, we will try to elucidate in detail the central significance of intellectual development and its leading role.

Using the method of genetic sections and their comparative study, we were able to establish not only what is lacking during the initial school age, but also a number of mechanisms that aid in developing the central function of the whole age, the formation of concepts.

We saw what a decisive role in this process is played by introspection, realizing one's own processes of behavior and controlling them, transfer of forms of behavior arising in the group life of the adolescent to the internal sphere of the personality, and the gradual growing into new methods of behavior, transferring inward a number of external mechanisms and socialization of internal speech and, finally, work as a central factor of all intellectual development.

Further, we can establish the significance the acquisition of a new function—the formation of concepts—has for all the thinking of the adolescent. We have shown that if objects are represented in thinking in an immovable and isolated form, then a concept actually combines the content of the thinking. However, if we assume that an object is disclosed in connections and mediations, in relations with the rest of reality and in motion, we must conclude that thinking that has concepts at its disposal begins to master the essence of the object and discloses its connections and relations with the other object and begins for the first time to combine and correlate various elements of experience, and then the complicated and comprehended picture of the world as a whole is disclosed.

The concept of number may serve as a simpler example of the changes that concept introduces into the thinking of the adolescent.

38

We would like to use a graphic example to show what new material thinking in concepts introduces into the recognition of reality in comparison with concrete or visual thinking. To do this, we need only compare the concept of number that the educated person usually has with the idea of number based on direct perception of number that prevails among primitive peoples. Just as in a very young child, the perception of number is based on number images, on concrete perception of form and size of a given group of objects. With transition to thinking in concepts, the child is liberated from purely concrete numerical thinking. In place of a number image, a number concept appears. If we compare the concept of number with a number image, at first glance it may seem to justify premises of formal logic relative to the extreme poverty in content of the concept in comparison with the riches of the concrete content contained in the image.

Actually, this is not so. The concept not only excludes from its content a number of points proper to the concrete perception, but for the first time, it also discloses in the concrete perception a number of such points that are completely inaccessible to direct perception or contemplation, points that are introduced by thinking and are identified through processing the data of experience and synthesized into a single whole with elements of direct perception.

Thus, all number concepts, for example, the concept "7," are included in a complex number system, occupy a certain place in it, and when this concept is found and processed, then all the complex connections and relations that exist between this concept and the rest of the system of concepts in which it is included are given. The concept not only reflects reality, but also systematizes it, includes data of concrete perception into a complex system of connections and relations, and discloses the connections and relations that are inaccessible to simple comprehension. For this reason many properties of size become clear and perceptible only when we begin to think of them in concepts.*

As a rule, it is pointed out that even a number has some qualitative characteristics. Nine is a square of three, it can be divided by three, it occupies a definite place and can be placed in a definite relation to any other number. All of these are properties of number: its divisibility, its relation to other numbers, its construction from simpler numbers—all this is disclosed only in the concept of number.

Investigators, for example, H. Werner, turn very frequently to number concepts to elucidate the characteristics of primitive thinking; these concepts disclose these characteristics most graphically. M. Wertheimer,[59] when he tries to penetrate primitive thinking using analysis of number images, proceeds in the same way. We have the same, completely satisfactory device available to disclose the reverse qualitative uniqueness of thinking in concepts and to show how concept is infinitely enriched by elements of mediated knowledge of the subject, raising its very content to a new height.

We shall limit ourselves to an analysis of an example that clearly shows what a systematizing and ordering function thinking in concepts fulfills in recognizing reality. If for the school-age child, the word represents a family of things, then for the adolescent, the word represents a concept of things, that is, its essence, laws of its structure, its connection with all other things, and its place in the system of already recognized and ordered reality.

39

A number of investigators who use the method of describing a picture to determine the nature of children's visual thinking note the transition to a systematic development of experiment and realization. Piaget indicates the nature of the thinking of the school-age child by the term "serial position," which indicates the weakness of synthesis or combination in the thinking of the child. Just as the child does not simultaneously combine all the traits included in a concept, but thinks alternately of one then another trait as being equivalent to the content of the concept as a whole, precisely so does he not order, not bring into the system the structure of his thoughts, but places them as if in a row, one after another, without combining them.

As Piaget says, in the thinking of the child, logic of action dominates, but not logic of thought. One thought is connected with another, as one movement of the hand elicits another and is connected with it, but not as thoughts are constructed hierarchically subordinate to one main thought. Piaget and R. Rosselo[60] recently

---

*In opposition to Kant, Hegel was *essentially* completely correct. Thinking going from the concrete to the abstract does not deviate—if it is *correct . . . from* truth, but approaches it. The abstraction of *material, a law* of nature, abstraction of *value*, etc., in a word, *all* scientific (correct, serious, not foolish) abstractions reflect nature more deeply, more reliably, more *fully*. From a living contemplation to abstract thinking *and from it to practice*—such is the dialectical path of recognizing *truth*, recognizing objective reality (V. I. Lenin, *Complete Works*, Vol. 29, pp. 152–153).

TABLE 3

Age, years	Purpose-directed and functional definition of concept, %
6	79
7	63
8	67
9	64
10	57
11	44
12	34
13	38
14	38
15	31

applied the method of describing pictures to the study of the development of thinking in the child and adolescent. These studies show that only with the beginning of adolescence does the child make the transition from the stage of enumerating separate traits to the stage of interpretation, that is, combining visually perceived material with elements of thinking that the child introduces into the picture on his own.

Forms of logical thinking are the basic means for describing pictures. Forms of logical thinking seem to order the material of perceptions. Perceiving, the adolescent begins to think; his perception is turned into concrete thinking and is intellectualized. C. Burns studied concepts in 2000 children, age six to fifteen, using the method of definition. The results of his research are presented in Table 3, which indicates that during this period, the number of purpose-directed and functional definitions decreases by a factor of more than 2.5, yielding to logical definition of concept.

M. Vogel (1911) established that the relations the adolescent finds through thinking increase as he approaches the transitional age. Specifically, judgments pertinent to causes and effects increase by more than 11 times with the transition from school age to adolescence. These data are particularly interesting in connection with the pre-causal thinking that Piaget established as a characteristic of the initial school age.

The basis for pre-causal thinking is the egocentric character of the child's intellect, which leads to confusing mechanical causality with psychological causality. According to Piaget, pre-causality is a transitional stage between motivation, the purposeful basis of phenomena, and causal thinking in the true sense of the word. The child frequently confuses the causes of a phenomenon with purpose and, in Piaget's words, it is as if nature were the product or, more accurately, a duplicate of thoughts in which the child tried to find sense and purpose at every moment.

The studies of H. Roloff show that the function of defining a concept increases markedly in the child between ages 10 and 12, the time of the beginning of the transitional age. This is observed in conjunction with the development of logical thinking of the adolescent. We have already cited the opinion of Meumann regarding the late appearance of deduction in the child (approximately age 14). H. Schüssler, disputing the opinion of Meumann, sets the intensification of this process at age 11-12 and 16-17. H. Ormian puts the beginning of formal thinking at about age 11.

No matter what we think of these studies, one thing remains completely clear: in agreement with all of this data, somewhat inconsistent from the external aspect, thinking in concepts and logical thinking develop in the child relatively late: only at the beginning of the transitional age does this development take its principal steps.

E. Monchamps and E. Moritz recently again studied the thinking of the child and the adolescent using description of pictures. In contrast to the usual experiments, which were limited to describing simple pictures accessible to a very young child's understanding, the new studies establish, as the last stage of visual thinking, the stage of precise synthesis that is accessible only to half of adult educated people and which assumes not an average, but a superior intellectual giftedness.

According to these data, the time of sexual maturation was marked by the fact that a typical form of children's thinking at the age that interests us seems to be a partial synthesis, that is, elucidation of the general sense of the picture accessible usually at the sixth stage of development. The same data show to what extent the child's development and his movement along the stages is determined by social-cultural conditions. A comparison between those studying in public schools and those studying in privileged schools discloses substantial differences: whereas 78% of the children from privileged schools reached the sixth stage at the age of 11, approximately the same percentage was reached by those studying in the public schools at the age of 13-14.

The studies of H. Eng (1914), who tried to elucidate the development of concepts using the method of definition, also show that this development has significant success beginning at age 12. By age 14, the number of correct responses increases by a factor of almost four in comparison with the age of ten.

Recently, G. Müller studied the logical capabilities of adolescents using two tests. The adolescents were required to establish the relation between concepts and to find new concepts that are in a certain relation to the given concept. The distribution of the solutions of these problems according to age shows that logical thinking becomes the dominant form in boys at the age of 13 and in girls at the age of 12.

40

In conclusion, it remains to be said that we have spent so much time on the development of thinking because, for the transitional age, we cannot consider it as one of the partial processes of development in a series of other such partial processes. Thinking at this age is not one function in a series of other functions. Development of thinking has a central, key, decisive significance for all the other functions and processes. We cannot express more clearly or tersely the leading role of intellectual development in relation to the whole personality of the adolescent and to all of his mental functions other than to say that acquiring the function of forming concepts is the principal and central link in all the changes that occur in the psychology of the adolescent. All other links in this chain, all other special functions, are intellectualized, reformed, and reconstructed under the influence of these crucial successes that the thinking of the adolescent achieves.

In the following chapter, we will try to show how the lower or elementary functions, being processes that are more primitive, earlier, simpler, and independent of concepts in genetic, functional, and structural relations, are reconstructed on a new basis when influenced by thinking in concepts and how they are included as component parts, as subordinate stages, into new, complex combinations created by thinking on the basis of concepts, and, finally, how, under the influence of thinking, foundations of the personality and world view of the adolescent are laid down.

Chapter 3
DEVELOPMENT OF HIGHER MENTAL FUNCTIONS DURING THE TRANSITIONAL AGE

1

The development of higher mental functions during the transitional age reveals most clearly the patterns that characterize the process of development of the nervous system and behavior.

One of the basic laws of development of the nervous system and behavior is that as higher centers or higher formations develop, lower centers or lower formations yield a substantial part of their former functions to the new formations, transferring these functions upward so that the tasks of adaptation that are done by lower centers or lower formations at lower stages of development begin to be done by higher functions at higher stages.

In this case, however, in the words of E. Kretschmer,[62] the lower centers do not simply move aside as the higher centers gradually develop but continue to work in a common union as a subordinate unit directed by the higher centers (younger in the history of development) so that in an undamaged nervous system, they usually cannot be considered separately.

Kretschmer maintains that only in a pathological state, when the higher centers are functionally weak or separated from the subordinate centers, does the general function of the nervous apparatus not simply stop, but the subordinate unit becomes independent and exhibits elements of its old type of functioning which had remained in it. Kretschmer formulates this general neurobiological law as follows: if within the psychomotor sphere, the action of the higher unit becomes functionally weak, then the closest lower unit becomes independent and operates within its own primitive laws.

The three basic patterns, observed in the development of the nervous system, specifically—preservation of lower centers in the form of separate stages, transition of functions upward, and emancipation of lower centers in pathology—conform perfectly to the history of development of mental functions. Specifically, all mental development during the transitional age is an example of the concrete expression of these three basic patterns.

As we have said, the principal content of development during this age is a change in psychological structures of the adolescent's personality, a change consisting in the transition from elementary and lower processes to a maturation of the higher processes. Higher functions develop according to completely different laws than the elementary or lower functions. Their development does not occur in parallel with the development of the brain and the appearance in it of new sections or growth of older sections. They are a different type of development, a different type of mental evolution. These higher functions that are the product of the historical development of behavior arise and are shaped during the transitional age in direct dependence on the environment that develops during the process of social-cultural development of the adolescent. They usually are not constructed together with the elementary functions as new members in the same series nor above them as an upper story of the brain above the lower; they are constructed according to the pattern of development of new complex combinations of elementary functions through the development of complex syntheses.

We know that every complex mental process that is at the base of higher functions is, in Kretschmer's expression, more than the sum of the elements from which it developed. In Kretschmer's words, it is basically something new, a completely independent psychological formation, a firm unit that cannot be reduced to its elements. This law of independence of higher syntheses is the basic neurobiological law that can be traced from the simplest reflex processes to the formation of abstraction in thinking and speech.

Only by considering the higher mental functions as a product of such syntheses will we learn to recognize correctly their relation to lower or elementary processes that have already been quite well developed when sexual maturation begins. This connection is twofold. On the one hand, the higher functions arise in no other way than on the basis of the lower: in the last analysis, they are not physiological processes of a new kind, but a certain complex combination, a complex synthesis of the same elementary processes. In this sense, the attempts of many contemporary psychologists to ignore the connection between the higher processes and the lower and to remove from psychology the patterns that characterize the fate and development of elementary functions seem fallacious to us. According to the sound observation of Kretschmer, there is a clear need to understand association in analyzing many problems of higher psychology, for example, the psychology of children's thinking, of the primary intellect, and of the flow of ideas. The theory of the structure of higher mental life without an associative understructure is absolutely unthinkable.

Also unjustified is the attempt to reduce higher functions, as does E. Thorndike, to simple associations that are only quantitatively increased. It is just as wrong to ignore the law of independence of the higher syntheses. All mental neo-formations that we can determine in the adolescent have at their base the complex and essentially dual relation between the elementary processes and the higher processes.

In essence, this relation, empirically established by modern psychoneurology and prompted by the study of the development of the nervous system, does not represent anything new from the point of view of dialectical logic. Hegel points to the double meaning of the German word, "to remove." He says that it can mean, first, "to remove," "to reject," and in keeping with this, we say: "the law, the institution, is abolished, eliminated." But it also means "to preserve," and in this sense, we say that something was put away. This duality in word usage must not be considered as accidental. It reflects the real, objective relation that is at the base of the process of development in which each higher step rejects the lower step, but rejecting it, it does not destroy it, but keeps it within itself as a preserved category, as its integral part.

The whole history of mental development during the transitional age consists of this transition of functions upward and the formation of independent higher syntheses. In this sense, in the history of the adolescent's mental development, a strict hierarchy is dominant. Various functions (attention, memory, perception, will, thinking) do not develop side by side like a bundle of branches placed into a single vessel; they even do not develop like various branches of a single tree that are connected by a main trunk. In the process of development, all of these functions form a complex hierarchic system where the central or leading function is the development of thinking, the function of forming concepts. All the other functions enter into a complex synthesis with this new formation; they are intellectualized and restructured on the basis of thinking in concepts.

In essence, completely new functions appear before us that have patterns different from their elementary precursors; only the circumstance that the lower functions yielded part of their activity to the upper, higher functions frequently brings about a situation in which the higher, logical memory is compared to the elementary, mechanical memory, the logical memory being seen as a direct continuation of the mechanical memory and both being considered as part of one and the same genetic line. Precisely in this way, the transition of functions upward leads to the fact that higher or voluntary attention is merged with elementary, involuntary attention and considered as a direct continuation of the latter.

We shall try to show how a series of new, higher syntheses, new higher functions occurs, which includes corresponding elementary functions as subordinate units, as a sequestered category, the higher functions having obtained from these subordinate units a part of their activity that was transferred upward.

2

We shall begin with the function of perception. In a certain sense, this function is usually considered as the earliest in the history of the child's mental development. The child begins to perceive earlier than he can direct his attention, remember, or think. For this reason, this earliest function is considered as an elementary function and its processes are hidden from direct observation. Moreover, the new psychology destroys the legend that perception does not develop at all, that it functions in the infant from the very beginning just as it does subsequently in the adult, that in the process of a universal change in mental functions, perception has the privilege of not developing, not changing but remaining as it is. Actually, perception in the infant resembles the perception of the adult as little as do memory or thinking at these two stages of development.

At each new age level, perception changes qualitatively and in the transitional age, scientific analysis discloses the complex changes and the complex restructuring that occur then. We cannot at this time even sketchily outline the history of the development of perception in its main points. For our purpose, it is enough to indicate in a very few words the two basic types of changes that occur in this function in the process of its development. We might call the first type of change the primary revision or primary syntheses of perception. Among these is the development of such properties of perception as relative constancy of size of perceived objects, their form and color. All these points vary depending on a number of accidental conditions of our perception, and constancy of perception that is due to a complex fusion of processes of perception with processes of memory develops only gradually.

If we look at a pencil, placing it close to our eyes and then move it ten times farther away, the image on the retina also decreases by a factor of ten. It will equal the image that a pencil ten times smaller would make when looked at if placed at the first distance. However, a pencil moved ten times farther away from the eyes does not seem to us to be ten times smaller. We know how to distinguish its size from the size of a pencil that is ten times smaller placed right in front of our eyes.

Precisely so, as E. Hering[63] has noted, a piece of coal at noon reflects three times more light than a piece of chalk at dawn. Regardless of this, even at dawn chalk seems white and coal at noon remains black. Precisely so, in the perception of one and the same object from very different sides, from different angles of sight, its form always seems to us to be constant although the real reflection of this form on the retina varies endlessly.

What is the source of the constancy of our perception, its independence of accidental changeable conditions? H. Helmholtz[64] expressed the hypothesis that unconscious deductions are working in this case. Later studies showed that what operates here are complex processes of combination, fusion of present stimulation and stimulation produced from memory and that the real process of perception always includes certain correctives introduced into it by memory. Looking at an object, we not only perceive it, but also remember it. Behind the process of perception there is, in essence, a complex process of uniting present sensations and eidetic images.

We will not stop now to consider in detail the mechanism of developing the constancy of our perception, since these processes are more characteristic for childhood than for the transitional age. In general, they end before the onset of sexual maturation, and the psychology of the adolescent may proceed from them as from ready data. Compared with these processes, other processes that perception undergoes might be called a secondary processing or processes of secondary syntheses in the area of perception. Here a merging occurs of perception and thinking, a connection of perception with speech.

A study was made only recently of the complex effect of processes of speech on the child's visual perception. It developed that the processes of development of speech and of thinking in words reprocess the child's visual perception in a complex way, restructuring it on a new base; particularly during the transitional age, together with the formation of concepts, a change occurs in the old proportions, in the old relation of visual and nonvisual, concrete and abstract factors in the sphere of perception.

In order to elucidate the role of speech and thinking in words in perception, we will refer to our own experiments using the method of describing pictures, a method which is closely linked with the studies of perception of the adolescent referred to above. As we know, this method was introduced into psychology a long time ago and is usually used to establish the development of a child's perception of reality. In the picture, the child sees one bit or another of reality familiar to him. After the child perceives and describes this picture, we can develop some concept of how he perceives reality as a whole, what kind of patterns are dominant in his perception. As we know, W. Stern and other authors established four basic stages through which the development of the child's perception passes, if we can judge by the child's descriptions of the pictures. At first, the child simply enumerates separate objects in the picture, then he names actions carried out by these objects, later his descriptions begin to produce traits that he interprets and on the basis of these he merges what he sees with what he knows relative to what is in the pictures and finally this process ends with describing the picture as a whole and with establishing the relations between its various parts. Corresponding to this, there are four stages in the development of the child's perception: objects, actions, qualities, and relations. According to this hypothesis, a child of three perceives the world as an aggregate of separate objects; later he perceives reality as an aggregate of acting objects and people and still later, he makes the transition to correlated thinking and perceives reality as a united whole. This is how the course of the child's perception is described by many other contemporary psychologists.

If we had used the method of describing pictures as our basis, we would have been led to precisely the same conclusions. However, these conclusions are in serious contradiction with what we know from other sources about the development of the child's perception. Thus, we know that the child very early perceives activity, actions that become isolated for him from the whole other mass of perceptions. A moving object is isolated in the child's perception extremely early. For this reason there is little probability that the child perceives reality first as an aggregate of objects and then begins to turn his attention to actions and their perception.

Further, in the psychology of perception, the idea has long been drifting about that the development of perception proceeds from the part to the whole and is composed of separate elements as a house is built of separate bricks. Primitive perception of animals discloses an opposite path of development. Initial, diffuse, complete perception of a whole given situation precedes distinct perception of its separate parts. In precisely the same way, new experiments of H. Volkelt[65] and others showed that in the child at a very early age, perception of the whole precedes the perception of parts: the whole is not composed of separate sensations, but separate sensations are differentiated and isolated from an initial whole perception. Once again the pattern just presented according to which the child's perception moves from separate objects to discerning the whole is strongly contradicted.

Finally, the special studies of W. Eliasberg and others showed that the child is capable at a very early age of establishing a number of connections, dependencies, and relations. A study of syncretism in children's thinking also showed that there is not a separation of elements, but an incoherent cohesiveness of thought, a global intertwining of impressions, like a cluster; syncretic images complex in composition characterize children's thinking at the very earliest stages. All of this as a whole, makes us doubt that the path of development of children's perception established by traditional psychology corresponds to reality.

We tried to confirm this pattern experimentally in the following way. In experiments, we asked children to tell first what was in a picture then next not to say anything about the picture, but to act out what was in the picture. Comparing the spoken description with the acted version of the content of the picture by one and the same child, we were able to establish that children at the object stage of perception who simply enumerated separate parts of the picture, in acting out, conveyed the content of the picture as a whole. In this way, we established that perception of a picture is not an exception to the general rule according to which development of perception proceeds from the whole to the parts.

Moreover, another, extremely interesting and complex question confronted us, whose solution is the key to a correct understanding of the alterations in perception of the adolescent. The question is: why does the child perceiving a picture as a whole and reproducing it as a whole in play take the path of analysis and enumeration of parts when speech is coupled to perception of a picture? The answer can be reduced to the fact that speech, being involved in the processes of visual perception by the child, does not proceed in parallel to these processes as a peripheral series of reactions, as an accompaniment that goes along with a basic melody. On the contrary, speech is interwoven with processes of visual perception and forms new and complex syntheses, restructuring these processes on a new base.

A cursory analysis is sufficient to show that speech modifies perception. It directs attention to a certain aspect, extremely curtails the situation perceived, giving a kind of stenographic record of what is perceived. It automatically analyzes what is perceived, breaking it down to objects and actions. Also, it synthesizes what is perceived, reflecting apparent connections in the form of spoken judgments. When a child, looking at a picture of a running boy, says: "The boy is running," he condenses the apparent situation extremely, he analyzes it because he perceives the boy and the fact that he is running separately, but expresses both the one and the other using words. Combining these words into judgments, he introduces a certain meaning into the perception.

This is how the processes of thinking and processes of perception merge, how perception is intellectualized, how it is converted into visual thinking. In this sense, K. Bühler is completely justified in insisting on the close tie between speech and thinking, and he shows how a certain spoken pattern also becomes a pattern of thinking. Bühler maintains that we may with complete justification say that speech thinks for man.

Isolated objects of perception became connected because of thinking; they became ordered and acquired sense—a past and a future. Thus, speech leads to thinking about perception, to analysis of reality, to the formation of a higher function in place of an elementary function.

If we turn to the perception of an adult, we will see that it represents not only a complex synthesis of present impressions and images in memory, but its basis is a complex synthesis of processes of thinking and processes of perception. That which we see and that which we know, that which we perceive and that which we think merges into one, and when it seems to me that I see a number of objects that fill my room, identifying that which I perceive with that which I actually see is a simple illusion. I can see dimensions, form, color of these objects, but I cannot see that this is a *cabinet*, this is a *table*, this is a *person*.

Ordered and comprehended perception, connected with thinking in words, is the complex product of a new synthesis in which visual impressions and processes of thinking are merged in a single alloy that can justifiably be called visual thinking. In contrast to the developed thinking of an adult, a child's thinking unites, orders, and comprehends what is perceived entirely differently. For this reason, the hypothesis of E. Claparède,[66] who says that the child sees differently than the adult, and the statement of K. Koffka[67] that the child lives in another world than we adults do are true in a certain respect. The developed perception of an adult places a net of ordering, logical categories over reality. His is always a comprehended perception. The transition from perception to visual thinking is a special case of the transition of a function upward of which we spoke earlier.

The transition of a function upward is not done instantly in a leap. The transition begins very early in childhood. Bühler, analyzing children's drawing, states on a firm basis that from the moment that things acquire names in the consciousness of the child, the formation of concepts begins, and then in place of concrete images, concepts appear and verbally formulated knowledge in concepts begins to dominate in the memory of the child. As the child's drawings show, he begins very early to reflect and to convey not that which he sees, but that which he knows. His memory is no longer a store for single images, but is an archive of knowledge. Specifically this explains the graphic and sometimes "x-ray" drawings of the child, which frequently appear without the child's referring at all to a visual image. Specifically this is what distinguishes the thinking of the young child from the thinking of animals.

Modern logicians and psychologists, in Bühler's opinion, are inclined to believe that higher vertebrates use concepts, indicating, for example, the fact that a dog recognizes his master in various clothing and in various situations and chases any rabbit as a rabbit regardless of its different external appearance. But at best, Bühler believes that here we must speak only of precursors of human concepts because animals lack the most important thing, specifically the ability to name things.

Thus, we see that under the influence of speech, the perception of the child undergoes a complex restructuring comparatively early. What that is new does the transitional age bring that distinguishes the perception of the adolescent from the perception of the child in this respect? We have F. Berger's extremely interesting studies (1929). They deal with the problem of perception of categories and its pedagogical significance. The most important conclusion of the study is the conclusion that the perceiving and ordering function of psychological categories appears quite distinctly in the experiences and memories of the child only with the onset of sexual maturation. Berger set a goal of elucidating how, in the process of perception, ordering and correlation of the whole multitude of things and internal impressions develops.

Children age 10 to 17 were shown a film with no explanation. How children of different ages perceived its content was studied. Berger succeeded in establishing that in a 10-year-old, the content of another's internal life is perceived in an external way, as undifferentiated, and only at the age of 12 or 13 does the child take serious steps on the path to understanding another's psychology. In the words of Kroh, this shows that categories needed to perceive another's internal life begin to function only after primary school age.

It is interesting to note that one of the results of this research is the fact that long before he enters school, the child is capable of observing not only separate objects, but also their properties and changes. There is little evidence of this when the child is given only one picture of some kind to describe. Sometimes the impression is that the child perceives only the substantially concrete and gradually involves in his perception the sphere of actions, qualities, or relations. This is specifically the kind of conclusions that Stern reached when he ascribed dominance of the object stage to the preschool age. As new research shows, the child at the earliest age level perceives quality, relation, and action. Nevertheless Kroh tried to find confirmation for Stern's hypothesis: at certain periods indicated by Stern, the forms of perception move to the foreground especially markedly which could, in essence, be observed significantly earlier and which are manifested especially in the practical behavior of the child. Here we have the possibility of seeing how verbal mastery of the categorical tissue of reality develops.

Thus, we see that a systematic, ordered, categorical picture of reality develops only during the period of sexual maturation. Together with this, we can establish that the child has mastered the perception of quality, relation, and action long before he entered school. Again we are confronted by the same question: what distinguishes the perception or visual thinking of the child from the perception of the adolescent? What is new is not that perception meets speech for the first time and is converted into visual thinking. As we have seen, this occurs relatively quite early. What is new is that the adolescent's verbal thinking itself makes a transition from the complex type to thinking in concepts, and together with this, the nature of the participation of verbal thinking in the adolescent's perceptions also changes radically. Speaking of thinking, we have already seen that the words of the child and the adolescent pertain to one and the same circle of objects. Their object reference coincides. But behind them lies a completely different meaning. The child realizes the meaning of a word as a complex of concrete objects connected by a factual tie; the adolescent realizes the meaning of a word as a concept, that is, as a complex image of the object, reflecting its ties and relations with the reality of its essence.

Thus, the visual thinking of the adolescent includes abstract thinking, thinking in concepts. The adolescent not only is conscious of and comprehends the reality that he perceives, but also comprehends it in concepts, that is, for him, in the act of visual perception, abstract and concrete thinking are complexly synthesized. He orders apparent reality without referring it to formerly established complexes, but through concepts developed in thinking. Categorical perception develops only during the transitional age. We could say that both the child and the adolescent relate *in the same way* to what is perceived with a system of connections hidden behind words, but the system of connections itself in which what is perceived is included is *seriously different* for the child and the adolescent, just as the complex and the concept are different; broadly speaking, the child, in perceiving, remembers more, the adolescent thinks more.

In this sense, A. Gelb very graphically contrasts the perception of man and the perception of an animal. He says that for an animal, what exists is not a world of objects, but a world of objects of his action. In different situations the connections with various actions of objects must appear to the animal as being completely different. A container from which he drinks and a container which is rolling in a field are for him two different objects since in each case, the container is a part of two different situations.

In the experiments of W. Köhler, we find a clear confirmation of this change in the meaning of an object depending on different concrete situations. A monkey that repeatedly reached fruit hung high by using a box as a base carefully tried one day to get the hanging fruit directly from the ground without using the box on which another monkey was lying. It would be wrong to assume that the monkey did not notice this box because, tired by its fruitless efforts, it approached the box several times and even sat on it, but left again. It would also be wrong to assume that for some reason it forgot its usual method of using the box. As soon as its friend got off the box, the monkey immediately grabbed it, put it in the right place, and reached the fruit. K. Koffka maintains that the behavior of the monkey gives the impression that if the thing is removed from its usual situation, only with utmost effort can it be transferred to another whole. The box on which the monkey was lying is a thing for lying, not a thing for getting fruit.

Experimental studies of animals are full of such examples. The object has no meaning outside a concrete situation. In different situations, one and same object has different meanings determined by its function in action. The same thing is apparent for a long time in the determinations of a child when he names objects according to the actions that are carried out with it. Only a concept, creating a concept of an object, allows freedom from an immediate situation. As we shall see later, when thinking in concepts becomes dysfunctional, the world of object consciousness is also disturbed. We might say that only with the help of the word can a child recognize things and only with the help of a concept does he come to a realistic and intelligent perception of the object.

And what about the animal, what about the child, what about the deaf-mute child? Can they know reality? In the first years of life, the child sees the situation, but does not have a conception of it, does not analyze it, does not register it; he does not have a conception of it, but experiences the situation. His conception is an integral part of direct adaptation; it is not separated from action, from appetite. Later we will speak of a patient who knew the purpose of objects and carried out intelligent actions with them when prompted by hunger or thirst, but did not recognize the objects outside these situations.

Conception in the sense of an ordered, categorical perception is not possible without speech. The word takes a thing wholly out of the process of adaptation, out of the situation, and makes it the object of a conception. Of course, animals have rudiments of a conception, roots of a conception. There are rudiments of conception even before the appearance of concepts in syncretic images, in complexes of thinking. But intelligent conception becomes accessible only to one who has mastered concepts. Gelb summarizes this role of concepts for intelligent perception of reality in the following statement: "For an animal there is only what surrounds it (*Umwelt*), for man—the world (*Welt*)."

3

The adolescent's memory exhibits a similar change during the transitional age. The question of the development of memory is one of the most intricate and complex questions in psychology. Psychology that does not differentiate between the development of lower and higher functions is full of contradictory statements about the development of memory. Some authors assume that development of memory is intensified during the transitional age; others maintain that it experiences a certain decrease; finally, a third group places the peak of its development significantly earlier and assumes that memory remains at approximately the same level during the whole transitional age.

M. M. Rubinstein maintains that the question of memory development during youth is debatable. Many, like J. Sully (1901), maintain that memory crosses its highest point at 12 years. Others apply to it the general law of development and believe that it is not an exception to the general rule and attains a higher level during mature years. This means that even during youth, it increases.

M. M. Rubinstein speaks in favor of the second point of view. If memory in itself were actually at the zenith of its development at 12 years of age, he believes that taken as it is in life, it finds so much support in extended interest, in associative enrichment, in great stability of will and emotional stability, in more consistent logic, etc. (in the process of life, all of this has a fundamental significance), that this is clear: without special causes, memory in youth cannot become weaker, but on the contrary, it becomes stronger.

We see that psychology is forced to limit itself to general descriptions instead of a factual answer to the question of the development of memory during the transitional age, but the formulation of the question itself seems to be correct. The organic bases of memory and its elementary functions scarcely develop at all noticeably during the transitional age. They evidently reach apogee significantly earlier than at the age of 12 and do not exhibit any substantial movement forward during the time that interests us. But higher or logical memory developed on the basis of synthesis of intellect and memory is a true achievement of the transitional age. Here we are dealing with a phenomenon similar to the development of perception.

There is no doubt about one thing: the key to understanding the development of memory in the adolescent must be sought not in the changes that occur within memory itself, but in those that encompass the relation of memory to other functions that alter its place in the general structure of mental processes. In order to determine the existence of changes in the adolescent's memory, using the method of comparative genetic sections, we can examine the relation between memory and thinking during primary school age. The comparative study shows us that the relation of these two basic processes is inverted during the transition from the primary school age to adolescence.

During primary school age, as in early years, the intellect depends to a large degree on memory. Thinking is done mainly through remembering. Analysis of thinking operations discloses patterns that do not characterize thinking as much as they characterize the activity of memory. In recent times, a series of beautiful experimental studies have disclosed the essential role of memory in the processes of thinking.

Without exaggerating, we can say that primitive thinking at early stages of development in onto- and phylogenesis is essentially only the function of memory. Moreover, at primitive stages, memory contains three different functions in an undifferentiated form: remembering, imagining, and thinking.

In a special study of visual thinking, Schmitz set up the task of elucidating the relation between intellect and eidetic tendency,[68] that most clear form of concrete memory in the visual thinking of the child. She proceeded from the data of M. Zillig (1917), who established that there are definite relations between a clearly expressed eidetic tendency and a low intellect, and even between a strong eidetic tendency and retardation. Other studies showed that high intellectual giftedness is also combined with eidetic rudiments. O. Kroh (1922) was the first to point out that, in general, there is little probability that a simple correlation can exist between intellect and eidetism. Actually, Schmitz' study showed that there is no simple connection between the one and the other and that eidetism may be combined with various degrees of intellectual giftedness.

For elucidating the question of the relation of visual and nonvisual thinking, the problem of the relations between intellect and memory is of great interest. If it is impossible to establish a connection between intellectual giftedness and eidetic tendencies, then the following question becomes much more interesting: is there not a definite relation between visual images of clearly distinct eidetics and their thinking?

The studies of Schmitz, which we mentioned, dealt with this problem. It encompassed a large number of schoolchildren in various stages in school and found interesting relations between memory and intellect. In general, from our point of view, this study confirmed the idea we expressed that eidetic images contain elements of three future independent functions in an undifferentiated form: memory, imagination, and thinking. In schoolchildren, all of this operates as a unit, so that no precise boundary can be made between the three processes which later separate into independent functions. The connection of eidetic tendency and activity of fantasy, which Zillig established, is also confirmed in the studies of Schmitz. But it seems that even the intellectual activity of eidetics casts light on the origin of intellect and its primitive stages.

Let us consider the studies of one of the school classes of children age 10-11, 53% of whom were eidetics. The children were given tests intended for 10-year-olds on the Binet–Bobertag scale.[69] Qualitative analysis of the responses and errors of the children showed a close tie between thinking and memory at this level; in all cases, in the expression of Schmitz, the child answered questions having in mind a concrete case. He remembered some kind of story, tale, picture, experience. What Schmitz was able to study by means of the test was a complex of recollections from which the child drew some component appropriate to the answer. For example, to the test question, what must you do if you are late for a train, the child answered: "You have to spend the night at the station." This kind of an answer seems wrong if it is considered from the point of view of thinking, but it is based on the following recollection. The child and his parents at one time took a trip to Kassel. Since the last train to Marburg had already left, they had to spend the night at the station waiting for the first morning train. From the example, it is clear to what degree the child's thinking is directed by recollection and to what degree the solving of the intellectual problem is for him a matter of selecting from recollections components that correspond to the new situation.

The study brought Schmitz to an incontrovertible result: children age 10-11 answer a question posed in a general form, as is usually done in testing, not by judging the general character, but almost always with a concrete judgment. The question elicits in them some kind of definite experience with which the question has only external or verbal similarity. Schmitz assumes that the child brings up this recollection and uses it as a basis for his answer, which frequently does not at all convey what is most essential in the experience, but only isolates some component that is dominant because it was colored with emotion or connected with other elements.

Thus, what is, in the final analysis, in the forefront in this kind of intellectual activity is actually the activity of memory that elicits some experience. For this reason, in Schmitz' opinion, we cannot reach a conclusion regarding children's intellect by means of tests; the conclusion will more likely pertain to the activity of their memory.

Confirmation of these data was obtained in a study of eidetics meant to elucidate whether visual images serve as a support in their responses or whether these images are the primary element that is the basis of their answers. The study was done with 28 eidetics using tests for 10- to 11-year-olds and 12-year-olds. They were required to define the concepts "sympathy," "dependence," and "justice" and form sentences with the three words: gold, misfortune, saving, etc.

Even in their looks and posture while they thought before arriving at an answer, it was possible to see whether visual images were participating in the child's thinking. In a positive case, the bright look of the child wandered over the wall, along the surface of the table, over the cover of his notebook. In the opposite case, the look wandered about the room with no definite direction. Many children got the answer without any participation of an image and only when they answered when being questioned did the children produce a corresponding image. Such cases were excluded from the general count. In other children, on the other hand, all solutions to the intellectual problem were elicited by a concrete, visual image.

In explaining the concept, "sympathy," the schoolchild thinks of having to stay at the bedside of an ill person yesterday and today and visually represents his bed. Another child, in explaining this word, sees two images: his mother giving a piece of bread to a beggar and himself giving bread to his younger brother on the playground. As an explanation, he adds: "Because bigger boys can stand hunger more easily than small children." His explanation of sympathy develops from these images: if someone does not have bread, people give him something. Another example shows quite graphically that defining a concept is based on concrete images and that a verbal definition of a concept is a translation of image concepts.

The general count shows that 28 of 109 answers (25%) were arrived at by the children on the basis of visual images. For this reason, we must ascribe a greater significance to sensible memory in their answers to the questions. Of these same 109 answers, 33 (30%) were influenced by an idea and only in the remaining cases could we establish neither a visual image nor an idea as the basis for the answer. The children said that they only thought about it. A new study confirmed these results. It developed that in only 20 answers (18%) did the children reveal that they did not think of anything definite. Of 89 answers that referred to a concrete case, 65 were connected with a definite experience of the child, 24 with reading, and only 5 with what they had learned in school.

Schmitz came to the conclusion that the close tie between memory and intellect in schoolchildren makes tests for giftedness which test memory and not intellect completely unacceptable. However, we might reach a broader conclusion from this study, seeing in it a clear confirmation of the great dependence of the primitive

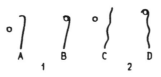

Fig. 1

intellect of the child on his memory. The thinking of the child is not yet separated from remembering. His intellect is based mainly on memory. The basic question on the correlation of image memory (eidetism) and giftedness cannot *for this reason* have an unambiguous solution; in the process of development, the relation of the memory and the intellect changes, and this *change* of the interfunctional connection and relation of two types of processes forms the basic content of the development of memory during the transitional age. The same question set up in the light of the general hypotheses we developed gets a clear and fully definite answer, not statistically but dynamically, about the evolution of *interfunctional connections* that are the basis for the change with age of the higher mental functions.

In this respect, of interest is the participation in the visual thinking of the child of dynamic, practical components which the author indicates. Visual thinking, as the study shows, is very closely linked with the dynamic, active, and motor factors and forms a single complex with them. The visual-dynamic processes represent equivalents of eidetic phenomena, as Metz demonstrated, and, according to the accurate observation of Schmitz, concepts at the early stage of the child's development predominantly approximate the motor, dynamic form and, because of this, evoke a readiness to react and represent an essentially special form of practical behavior.

The basis of primitive thinking based on memory is an unbreakable combination of visual-contemplative and practical-dynamic elements which support each other. This observation led Schmitz to say that, among the civilized people of Europe, we should turn attention to the presence of so-called manual concepts that Cushing observed in primitive peoples.

Here we cannot help but recall the interesting studies of E. Jaensch. He demonstrated experimentally that eidetics think with the help of images in which the dynamic, practical, and visual elements are merged into one. This author asked 14 eidetics to visualize the image of a target (apple, rock, ball, piece of chocolate) and a stick with a bent end. The stick and the target were a distance away from each other. When the eidetic got the instruction to think that he wants to capture the target, for 10 of the 14 subjects, the visual images shifted in space in such a way that they gave a solution to the problem as shown in Fig. 1. The tool and the target unite, and what he later would carry out with his hands took place in the child's visual field.

It is easy to see that these experiments present a perfect analogy to the well-known experiments of Köhler with monkeys, and provide a key to a correct understanding of experiments with animals. Jaensch believes that Köhler's experiments are concerned with the fact that the animal with the help of some kind of spatial shifts in the visual field moves the stick toward the target at first in perception and then in fact. Spatial displacement of the object with a glance at some target represents this kind of union of the visual and dynamic elements. In this form, we evidently have the most primitive intellectual acts of animals.

It seems to us that, on the basis of this experiment, Jaensch needlessly reaches a negative conclusion on the presence of intelligence in the chimpanzee. The fact that the animals do not act blindly, but are directed by visual perception and approximation, in his opinion, need not lead to the conclusion that they act intelligently. Jaensch assumes that something resembling our geometric-optical illusion develops in the monkey, a direction of attention, a sensing of a seeming movement of the object, etc. We believe that we are actually dealing here with a very primitive optoid form of intellect that is still not separated from perception and in which visual and actual moments are locked into a single synthesis. It is interesting that other studies of children's concepts indicate that, during childhood, the development of a concept is in essence a function of memory. As we have seen, K. Groos considered the child's potential concept as a function of habit, as a device for similar general impressions. He termed these formations pre-intellectual concepts, indicating that they do not yet have anything inherently in common with the intellect. These potential concepts, which are based on a device of a purely operative character, include a practical factor and are to a certain degree "manual concepts." The so-called functional definition of the concepts of the child is also nothing other than a "manual concept" translated into words, a common, practical mind-set. In this respect, children's concepts, which are more general at the beginning and become more concrete at the end, undergo an interesting evolution. Groos provides the following example: a girl, age $8^1/_2$, when asked what a chair is, answered: "It's furniture on which people sit." This definition of the concept is somewhat broad since it also includes a bench.

Much more typical is the answer of a 12-year-old, mature girl asked what is a table: "It is a four-angled board with four legs." A few years ago, this same child would have accepted as a table any oval or round or three-legged table. But if at a more mature age, the girl gave this unsatisfactory answer, this indicates that her former judgment depended in no way on a clear concept, but only on the mind-set for a certain general impression.

This example also shows us a feature of many children's definitions. Obviously, the girl applies this definition to all tables without much thought, satisfied that she indicated a recollection that appeared in her consciousness.

For the school-age child, the definition of a concept, as we can see, is still to a large degree a product of recollection. Groos believes that the girl gave only a factual description of one example although she meant to produce a real definition.

In school-age children, we frequently see definitions of concepts in which this method is very clear. We will borrow a few examples of children's definitions from Grünewald: "What is a thing?" "It's a table." "What is a sheet?" "It's a sheet of blotting paper." We have already given A. Messer's example of a definition of reason given by a class I pupil: "Reason is when I am hot and I don't drink water." The basis for this kind of definition is some kind of concrete impression. Groos believes that this impression is not a concept broken down into separate traits, but only a mind-set associated with a word. When the child hears that someone wants to tell him a story of some kind of reasonable action, he experiences a simply pre-intellectual mind-set for similar impression, and this is quite enough for a logical solution by means of judgment.

K. Groos is correct in saying that such examples also cast some light on the behavior of adults when an image is more effective than definition.

This latter feature of children's definitions consists of the fact that in this case a preference is disclosed for actions in general and voluntary actions in particular. Thus, an active "manual concept" is found to be the basis for children's definitions.

In Binet's experiments, a child explains that a knife is what we cut meat with, a cap is what we put on our head, etc.

K. Bühler also considers the connection between children's concepts and memory. He believes that our definitions consist of our defining something by its natural connection with other concepts. In principle, a small child proceeds exactly the same way, but his connections of things assume a somewhat different imprint. Connections according to purpose, according to practical use are for the most part the basis of these "manual concepts" translated into words. From Binet's experiments, we see that to the question, "What is a snail?" the child answers, "It's—so we can crush it, so they won't eat the lettuce. That's all." "It eats lettuce, they crush it so that it won't eat in the garden" (age 15); "It means that it shows its horns, it means that it should be crushed." It seems that the child is in a garden making observations and practical disposal, and showing his knowledge. But the child abandons the formula, "this is for" or "in order to," which is the usual pattern for translating a "manual concept" into a verbal definition when little stories are brought to the forefront or once the child makes observations. "What is a carriage?" "Men sit in it, they strike a horse with a whip and then the horse runs"; "And what is a bus?" "So that many ladies could sit there. There are soft seats. Three horses. They sound a 'ding,' and they run."

Again we see that the basis for a child's concept is remembering or a general motor mind-set. A concrete situation that arises in the process of defining a concept affects the child in such a way that he establishes not a natural connection of a given concept with others, as an adult would, and not a concrete connection according to a recollection, as we saw in the examples just given, but a connection that is completely accidental, encouraged by the order of the words presented to him. K. Bühler gives examples of this kind of perseveration: first comes the horse, it bites, then comes the lamp, it does not bite, then comes the house, it does not bite, etc.

Summarizing the features of children's concepts, Bühler says that, in general, the idea of purpose is dominant. It is typical to designate this whole age as the age of practical, purposeful orientation. The sphere of things and events that the child manages with this category is not very large, of course, and the merging of purposeful connections, being broken at every nearest member, still remains without stable ordering threads. However, in this small kingdom, there is clarity and order.

We might add that the clarity and order that rule in the thinking of the child at this stage are created by the fact that his thinking is still wholly dependent on his practical, active habitual mind-set and on his concrete, visual, graphic recollection. Intellect appears here as a function of habit and memory. Concepts are based on translating the motor mind-set and visual image into words.

A digression into the study of the features of the thinking of the school-age child and its connection to memory was necessary in order to establish precisely what kind of changes occur in the memory of the adolescent. To do this, we again must resort to a comparative study of two genetic sections. We anticipated the basic conclusion of this study in a hypothetical form when we expressed the idea that the principal change that occurs in the development of the memory of the adolescent consists of an inversion of the relations between memory and intellect that exists during primary school age.

If in the child, intellect is a function of memory, then in the adolescent, memory is a function of intellect. Just as the primitive thinking of the child depends on memory, the memory of the adolescent depends on thinking; while in the child a concrete-graphic and practical content is hidden behind an evident verbal form, in the adolescent, real concepts are hidden behind the outward appearance of images in the memory. This central factor in the history of the development of memory has not been adequately studied thus far.

Developmental psychology has thus far studied changes with age of the functions taken in isolation and separately, one after another, and usually approached the development of mental functions as if they formed a series composed of relatively self-sufficient and independent elements moving in parallel. The basis for this, in a cryptic form, is the assumption that evolution of mental functions resembles a bundle of cut branches placed in one vessel. Too little attention has been paid to the functional and structural relations between separate processes according to the order of separate functions that develop with each age situation, and in connection with this, inadequate consideration was given to the complex combinations, those higher syntheses, whose development so enriches the transitional age. Even the trends in psychology that noted the self-sufficiency of thinking and the fact that it cannot be reduced to associations do not deal with the problem in its full depth and do not disclose the basic fact that, in the process of development, an essentially new function, a new combination of processes, a new self-sufficient synthesis occurs that might be termed logical memory.

The old experiments of K. Bühler (1912)[70] showed that memory of ideas and memory for words and other images exhibit different patterns. O. Külpe says that if ideas do not differ from images, then ideas must be remembered with the same difficulty as images. Associations between ideas are formed incomparably more rapidly and firmly than between words. Who can learn sets of 20-30 words having heard them once so well that he could quickly respond with the correct word when one member of a set is given? If anyone were in a state to do that, we would consider the person with such a phenomenal memory very extraordinary. However, as experimental studies have shown, such a result can be easily achieved when paired ideas are memorized.

K. Bühler gave a subject a series of paired ideas among which a connection had to be established. He established how easily this was done and how long both ideas were retained. Even after a day this kind of series can be reproduced without error. In another series of experiments, the same author presented 15 phrases or fragments of ideas, and after a break gave a second series of sentences related in sense to the first series or their parts with partial sense.[71] Thus, one and the same idea was presented in a different form: the first parts in the first series and the second parts, in the second. The order of the first and second parts did not coincide. The subject, hearing the second parts, was asked to complete them mentally with corresponding parts from the first series. All the subjects did this. In the series, corresponding parts were separated from each other by several clauses, but a mental review of all the material was possible, and this undoubtedly contradicts the law of association which operates in the sphere of images.

These experiments demonstrated that separate ideas not only are exceptionally easily retained and preserved, but also that they unite with one another, seemingly upsetting all laws of memory.

Thus, it was experimentally established that remembering ideas is subject to completely different laws than remembering images. One such fact is enough to understand what kind of radical qualitative transformation in the activity of memory occurs in the adolescent during the transition from visual to abstract thinking. We have seen that the child's thinking depends specifically on concrete images, on visual representations. When the adolescent makes the transition to thinking in concepts, his remembering what he perceived and logically comprehended must disclose completely different laws than those that characterized remembering during primary school age.

Intellectual mnema, that is, gradual drawing together of memory and intellect, in the expression of F. Geise, is the basis of memory development at this age. We can understand what kind of progress in memory, what kind of rise to a higher stage is achieved here. Continuing the graphic comparison of Külpe, we could say that in making the transition to remembering in concepts, the adolescent achieves results that would undoubtedly be evidence of an outstanding, phenomenal memory if he were remembering in images.

But the growth of logical memory occurs not only quantitatively, not only from the aspect of content—memory is filled not so much by images of concrete objects as by their concepts, connections, relations. There is also a growth of the qualitative character of the function of remembering itself from the aspect of its composition, structure, and method of action. The subsequent course of its development changes radically.

In "Primary School Pedology," we elucidated the basic traits that make up the transition from the development of direct, eidetic, natural memory to mediated, cultural, mnemotechnical memory. We saw that in this case the child follows the same course to mastering his memory using artificial signs, going from using memory to managing it, from mnema to mnemotechnique, the same course that all of humanity once followed in the process of the historical development of memory.

It is understood that the transition is not instantaneous. It is prepared for in the process of childhood development, and we face the problem of using genetic sections and their comparative study to find what is new in this area that occurs during the transitional age and to develop a solid basis for it. We have already said: the process of formation of concepts begins in the child at the moment the first words appear; at an early age, the child's drawings indicate that his memory is an archive of knowledge and not a storehouse of images. Even at an early age, the participation of speech in processes of memory, verbalization of memory, is very appreciable. The child frequently remembers not a direct, concrete situation, not one event or another, but a seemingly verbal record of that event. Remembering in signs, remembering in words is characteristic even in early childhood.

Some psychologists, reducing thinking to speech habits, are inclined to see in the functioning of the speech aspect of our habits the most concrete expression of the activity of memory. J. Watson, for example, considers memory as a reproduction of speech records of concrete experiences and actions. However, we know that the very meaning of the word, the very method of using the word as a sign for a number of objects, the very type of intellectual operations that are the basis of generalization achieved through words, are substantially different in the schoolchild and in the adolescent. From this it is clear that verbalization of memory and remembering with the help of speech records also change substantially from primary school age to the transitional age.

We can formulate the central points of all of these changes in the following way: the memory of the adolescent is liberated from eidetic visual images, and verbal memory, remembering in concepts, directly connected with comprehension, analysis, and systematization of material, are brought to the forefront; with the transition from image to concept, the character of the processing of material in verbal remembering undergoes the same changes as thinking in general. Finally, in connection with the powerful development of internal speech and definitive elimination of the break between internal and external speech, the adolescent's verbal memory itself, being converted into one of the intellectual functions, depends mainly on internal speech. Thus, a relation develops that is completely the opposite of what we established for a much earlier stage in the development of memory and thinking. If there, the definition of a concept is, in essence, a translation of a concrete image into words or a motor situation, then here remembering of concrete images and motor situations is replaced by assimilation of corresponding concepts. If there to think meant to remember, then here, remembering means to think.

To state it briefly, we can say that the child, in becoming an adolescent, makes a transition to an internal mnemotechnique, which is usually termed logical memory or an internal form of mediated remembering. This transition from outward to inward is connected with the powerful development of internal speech, but it requires a more detailed explanation, since it makes up the common trait in the development of all intellectual functions of the transitional age and pertains in equal measure to attention and to memory. For this reason, we shall postpone elucidating the law of the transition of functions from the external to the internal until we have considered the more important changes that occur in the development of attention in the adolescent.

4

The changes in attention that occur during the time of sexual maturation have attracted extremely little attention from investigators thus far. Most authors bypass this problem in silence or devote several lines to it, limiting themselves to a cursory and summary indication of the quantitative increase in stability and activity of attention noted in the adolescent. It seems that not one of the authors discloses the radical and major change in the processes of attention during the transitional age. Moreover, this change is no less important and essential than similar changes in perception and memory.

In a word, we have before us the problem of the origin of a higher synthesis and simultaneous action of a number of more elementary functions, a new, complex combination, a new and complex structure characterized by its own special laws. For this reason, we must again seek the key to understanding the problem in the mutual relations and mutual dependencies of attention and other functions, and primarily, of thinking. We would expect that the development of attention during this period will exhibit laws similar to those that we established with respect to perception and memory. An essential difference in these laws is the fact that the changes pertain not to the internal structure itself of the elementary function of attention and not even to the appearance of certain new properties within this function, but to the relations of the given function to other functions.

The elementary function of attention as it appears in its purest form in early childhood appears as a subordinate factor in a new, complex synthesis with intellectual processes. Attention is intellectualized just as memory, is and if for childhood, a dependence of thinking on attention is characteristic, then, according to P. P. Blonsky's valid point, with the onset of dominance of voluntary attention, these relations are inverted. Voluntary attention is characterized primarily by its connection with thinking. Again, it would be a mistake to assume that this change appears suddenly. It is, of course, prepared for by the preceding development of attention.

When we speak of active attention, Blonsky assumes that we have in mind that the attitude of sense organs is determined by thought. The most developed attention is determined principally by thought (voluntary attention). This active, voluntary attention is undoubtedly a late product of development. Blonsky cites T. Ribot,[72] who expressed the idea that voluntary attention is the product of civilization. Actually, Ribot's theory of attention was the first to develop the idea that voluntary attention is the product of cultural development of mental functions. Voluntary attention is characteristic of neither animals nor infants.

Ribot terms this form of attention artificial (1897) in contrast to natural, involuntary attention and sees the difference in that art uses natural powers to accomplish its tasks. In this sense, in the words of Ribot, this form of attention is also called artificial. Ribot showed how attention opens up the complex process of change; it is only a link in the chain of cultural development of humanity that led from a primitive wild state to a state of organized society. He indicates that this progress in the area of mental development forced man to make the transition from the dominance of involuntary attention to the dominance of voluntary attention. The latter serves simultaneously as the result of and the reason for civilization.

Specifically, Ribot points to the psychological relationship between work and voluntary attention. His opinion is that as soon as the need to work appeared, voluntary attention became a factor of primary importance in the new form of the struggle for life. As soon as the capacity developed in man to devote himself to work that was not attractive but necessary, voluntary attention also came to be. It is easy to prove that before the appearance of civilization, voluntary attention did not exist or was only momentary. Ribot maintains that work is the most pronounced concrete form of attention. Finally, as a summary of his thinking, Ribot formulates the idea that voluntary attention is a sociological phenomenon. Considering it as such, we will better understand its genesis and instability. Voluntary attention is adaptation to conditions of higher social life.

With this thesis, Ribot discloses the origin of voluntary attention in the phylogenetic plan. In ontogenesis, we cannot, of course, rightly expect a full repetition of the same path of development. We know that there is no parallel between the one process of development and the other and that in development, the individual masters the same forms that in their time arose in the development of the species by means of quite different paths. But the psychological nature of voluntary attention is fully disclosed in Ribot's analysis, and this nature already hands us the key to understanding the development of voluntary attention in the child. Even here, we must approach voluntary attention as a product of the cultural development of the child; we must see in voluntary attention a form of adaptation to higher social life and we should expect it to display patterns typical for the whole course of the cultural development of behavior.

And actually, this expectation does not disappoint us. How does the traditional view usually characterize the development of attention during the transitional age?

M. M. Rubinstein maintains that with all individual variety, at this time attention in its living form cannot but acquire a greater range and stability not only because interests are extended and become more stable, but also because its basic element, the will, becomes more enduring and stronger. Because of this, the attention of the youth becomes longer and more active. In addition to this, it acquires greater capacity for stably considering an abstract content and for being controlled by the internal logic of the material and has less need for support from external impressions—stimuli in all their variety.

This is all that traditional psychology of adolescence has to say about the problem in which we are interested. In different variants and versions, it repeats one and the same idea on the extension of the range of attention, on increase in its stability, on increase in arbitrariness, activity, and, finally, on the change in its direction and on its connection with interests and abstract thinking. But to combine all of these different symptoms, to present them as a part of a whole, deliberate picture and to show the need for these changes at specifically this age and their development from one source, one cause, and, finally, to establish the connection of these changes to the general changes in intellectual development of the adolescent—none of this could traditional psychology do. However, in one thing it is undoubtedly correct: it seeks specific changes in the adolescent's attention in the area of its relations to other functions, specifically in its closer relations to thinking.

Following the path we selected, we actually discover the close connection that exists between the development of attention during the transitional age and the function of formation of concepts. Let us recall that this connection has a dual character: on the one hand, a certain degree in the development of attention, just as of other intellectual functions, is a necessary precursor to the development of thinking in concepts, and, on the other hand, the transition to thinking in concepts also represents a rise of attention to a higher level and its transition to a new, higher and complex form of internal voluntary attention.

We will consider the internal functional connection between the character of childhood concepts at a different stage of their development and attention. It seems that Piaget was the first to voice the idea that we must look for the cause of the child's incapacity for logical concepts in the underdevelopment of the child's attention. We recall that N. Ach indicated the role of the word as an active means of directing attention during the transitional age and ascribed to the word an important role in the formation of concepts in the adolescent.

As we have said, Piaget encountered the fact that the child's thinking is marked by the absence of a logical hierarchy and synthesis between different elements of one and the same concept. Where we simultaneously, synthetically think of all the component elements of a concept, a child, on the contrary, thinks not simultaneously, but alternatively, one trait after another. According to Piaget's determinations, children's concepts are the product of serial position, but not of synthesis of a certain number of elements, still various and not perceived in their interrelations. These concepts-conglomerates differ from our concepts mainly, as Piaget says, in that various traits entering into the composition of the concept penetrate into the field of consciousness at different moments, and for this reason, the child comprehends each trait separately, not synthesizing it with the other traits. The child takes each trait in isolation; in the adult, the basis of a concept is synthesis, a hierarchy of elements.

The same narrowness of children's attention that does not allow simultaneous thinking of a number of traits is also apparent when we study the logical thinking of the child. The child does not comprehend all the data that he must take into account simultaneously, but considers one condition then another alternately, and for this reason his conclusion is correct always in one specific relation. Where it is necessary to consider two or more conditions simultaneously, his idea meets with insurmountable difficulties. For this reason, the basic form of children's thinking is the form that W. Stern called transduction in very young children and that Piaget extended to verbal thinking of the schoolchild. Comprehension in the child does not move either from the general to the particular or from the particular to the general, but always from the particular to the particular or from unit to unit. We see that the unique character of the child's concept and the unique character of thinking is related to this kind of structure of the concept and depends directly on the narrowness of the child's attention.

Considered from the psychological aspect, this kind of concept-conglomerate, as Piaget terms it, is nothing other than a transitional form from complex thinking to thinking in concepts. Actually it is not a concept, but a complex of certain traits connected with each other on the basis of actual closeness, but still not representing the unity that characterizes a true concept. The concept-conglomerate is, essentially speaking, a pseudoconcept or a complex, since the child attaches to the given concept any object that coincides with any of the traits of this concept. Thus, the most varied objects coinciding with the given concept in various traits may appear in actual relation to it without there being any kind of internal relationship between them. But is this the same characteristic feature of thinking in complexes that we described above?

In order to elucidate the unique character of children's thinking, Piaget, as we have said, refers to the child's narrowness of field of attention. He maintains that in order to form a judgment of relations, a broader field of attention is necessary than for predicative judgments or, in any case, as G. Revault d'Allones (1923) said, more complex patterns of attention are required. Any relation assumes consciousness of two objects at once. P. Janet frequently stressed this idea. The field of the child's attention is narrower than ours and it is less synthetic. The child cannot encompass in one process of thinking all the data of a test; he perceives objects one after the other and not simultaneously. Because of this, the child converts judgments on relations into a series of simple predicative judgments.

Piaget continues: here we must still explain why the child has a narrower field of attention than we do. The fact that in the child, consciousness of his own thinking and conclusions is much weaker than in us does not yet mean that attention directed toward the external world (connected with perception, with understanding another's speech, etc.) must be subject to the same law. On the contrary, children's attention may be more plastic than ours, as frequently happens with children's memory or even with that of mildly retarded persons. The difference is due to the degree of organization and the structure of schematism of attention.

This structure or organization of children's attention is characterized primarily by its connection with the child's egocentric thinking; the processes of his thinking determine the character of his attention. For this reason, for the child, there are strict differences between direct, concrete perception and abstract thinking. He considers things not in their internal relations to each other but always in those relations that he can perceive directly. He considers them not sequentially one after the other, but fragmented, without synthesis or in a vague amalgam (syncretism).

It is Piaget's idea that this is what constitutes the narrowness of the child's attention. He sees many things, frequently more than we do. He is especially observant with respect to a large number of details that we do not notice, but he does not organize his observations and he is not capable of thinking of more than one thing at a time. His multiple attention is not proportional to his apperceptive attention, just as the organization of his recollection is not proportional to the plasticity of his memory. In this sense, we may say that it is not the egocentrism of thinking that results in the narrowness of the field of attention, but that these are related phenomena. They both arise from the primitive methods of thinking that assume a directly personal perception for the absolute point of view, and both lead in the same way to the incapacity for logically thinking of relations.

Thus, Piaget discloses this aspect of the matter; he shows the undoubted connection between the child's syncretic thinking and the character of his attention. This connection finds complete confirmation in what we know in general about the development of children's attention. The most elementary function of attention, involuntary attention, like memory is more plastic and richer in the child than in us. The narrowness of the child's field of attention does not consist of the fact that the child perceives few things; he perceives more of them than the adult and with a greater number of details, but this attention is organized completely differently. He does not have what might be called control itself of the mechanisms of attention that would control this process and subject it to his will.

In this sense, Piaget is right in referring to the studies of Revault d'Allones, who distinguishes two basic forms of attention: direct attention and indirect, instrumental attention. The latter is characterized by the fact that between the object of attention and the thinking person, another factor intervenes—it is the means by which a person actively directs his attention to an object which does not interest him directly and does not directly attract his action, but to which he wants nevertheless to direct his attention. We cannot now consider in detail what it is that plays the role of this means, only that signs, words, and certain patterns evidently play that role. As Revault d'Allones noted, because of this, the whole operation takes on an indirect, instrumental character and the whole process of attention assumes a completely new structure, a new organization. We can speak of voluntary attention when we consider anything to which our attention is directed through symbols, whatever they might mean, for example, a concept.

We can summarize the results of our discussion in the following way. The child's thinking is marked by primitive organization of attention. His attention has a direct character, it is involuntary, it is controlled from outside. Objects attract or repel his attention. In the adolescent, together with maturation of thinking and the transition to thinking in concepts, higher forms of attention also develop: mediated attention, which has the same relation to involuntary attention as mnemotechnique has to mechanical memory. We could see this role of attention when we spoke of perceptions and their change during the transitional age.

W. Köhler in his new work (1929) on the problem of human perception indicates that in situations that allow a person to fix easily on an object which he must isolate from a given structure, animals lose their orientation and their reaction becomes confused. Köhler observed this many times in monkeys. These animals also appeared to be incapable of changing this sensory organization by force of will. They, much more than humans, are slaves of their sensory field.

This means that the attention of an animal is determined by the organization of his visual field. Because of this, the animal is a slave of his visual field, the animal does not know how to control his attention, and for this reason, cannot free himself from the controlling influence of the structure of his visual field. With certain caution, we might say that a child also to a much greater degree than the adolescent is slave to his sensory field. Just as in the area of memory, he *remembers* more than he *memorizes,* in the area of attention, things control his attention much more than he himself controls it.

To conclude our discussion of attention, we will consider the extremely important genetic law that characterizes the development of all higher mental functions—of logical memory, voluntary attention, and thinking in concepts. This law has a much broader significance than in the area of attention alone. For this reason, we will consider it in detail in the closing chapter of our course in discussing the structure and dynamics of the personality of the adolescent. But even now, unless we know this law, we will notice a substantial gap in the general picture of the development of the functions under consideration, including attention. The essence of the law is that it identifies four basic stages through which every mental function of a higher order passes in development. We have already said repeatedly that higher forms of memory, attention, and other functions appear not suddenly and not in a prepared form. They do not drop at a certain moment from above; they have a long history of formation. This is precisely the case with voluntary attention. In essence, its development begins with the first pointing gesture with which adults try to direct the attention of the child and from the first independent pointing gesture with which the child himself begins to direct the attention of others. Later, in an infinitely more developed form, the child masters a whole system of these means for directing the attention of others. Sensible speech is such a system of means. Still later, the child begins to apply to himself the same methods of behavior that others applied to him and that he applied with respect to others. In this way, he learns to control his own attention and to transfer his attention to the voluntary level.

Of all the stages of which the process of development of attention as a whole is made up, we will consider only two basic stages: the first encompasses school age and the second, the transitional age. These two genetic sections are of interest to us now for establishing the features of attention during the transitional age. In a general form, we might say that the first stage is the stage of external mastery of one's own mental functions—memory and attention, and the second, the stage of internal mastery of these processes. The transition from external to internal mastery makes up the most essential trait that distinguishes the adolescent from the child.

We have seen that external mnemotechnique is characteristic for the school-child, and internal, for the adolescent. In precisely the same way, external voluntary attention is characteristic for the child and internal, for the adolescent. This transition from outward to inward, which was graphically termed the process of revolution, consists of the fact that the higher form of behavior is formed in the process of social-cultural development of the child and is assimilated by him from the people around him. As Ribot points out, the higher form of behavior develops in the process of adaptation to higher social life. For this reason, of necessity, it is at first an external operation and occurs through external means. Other people, using words, direct the child's attention, turning it from some elements in the visual field toward others or even directing it to internal processes of thinking. The means in this case remain outside, and the operation itself is still divided between two different people.

Attention directed in this way is objectively voluntarily directed attention, but involuntary from the point of view of the child himself. Assimilating this form of mastering attention, the child at first masters a purely external operation and transfers it into the sphere of his own behavior in the form in which it is developed among people. He just unites in one person the two parts of the operation that were earlier divided between him and the adults around him. For this reason, the initial stage in the development of any higher function is the stage of external operation accomplished through external means. Then gradually, to the extent that the operation is assimilated by the child, to the extent that it is firmly established in the circle of basic operations of his behavior, to the extent that it grows into the general structure of his thinking, it loses its external character and is transferred from outside inward and begins to operate mainly through internal means. This process of transition of the operation from outside inward we call the law of revolution.

Our colleague, A. N. Leont'ev,[73] made a special study of the development of mediated attention at different ages (1931, pp. 154-180). The children were presented with a problem to solve in which they had to maintain in their field of attention a series of factors stipulated by the instruction, but had to direct their attention not along the habitual path of associative thinking, but along the indirect path of circumstantial thinking.

The child was asked questions. For some of them, he had to answer by naming some color. There were two colors that the child was not to mention, as in the game, "Don't buy the white or black." Also, the child was not to use the same color twice; at the same time, the child had to respond correctly to questions. For example, in a series in which red and blue could not be named, the child was asked:

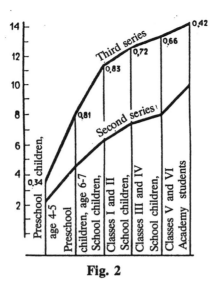

Fig. 2

"What color are tomatoes?" He answered: "They're green when they're not ripe." Solving this problem is possible only with an active control of attention and with an ability to maintain a number of factors in the field of attention simultaneously.

This kind of problem, as the study demonstrated, cannot be solved even by a school-age child if he is not given auxiliary means in the form of colored cards that the child spreads before him and uses to support his attention. We know that the child can simultaneously perceive a number of external objects, but the internal organization of his attention is still extremely weak.

The experiments succeeded in tracing how the solution of this same problem changes for children at various stages of development and for adults with the help of the same external means. Quantitative results of this study are presented in Fig. 2. As we can easily see, the difference between two paths of solving the same problem, using and not using external means, measured by the number of correct responses that the child gives, discloses a definite pattern in development.[74]

This pattern is expressed in the fact that the difference between involuntary and voluntary attention in preschoolchildren is extremely insignificant. In schoolchildren, it becomes more significant, reaching a maximum toward the end of the primary school age and increasing by almost 10 times in comparison with preschool age. Finally, it drops again in adults, nearly approaching preschool age in corresponding indexes.

This quantitative characterization shows three basic stages in the development of mediated attention. First of all, the stage of natural involuntary acts is characteristic for preschool age. At this stage of development, the child is not capable of controlling his attention with the help of the organization of special stimuli-means. Introducing a number of cards into the operation does not increase success in solving the problem; the child is not capable of using them functionally. The next stage of development is characterized by a sharp difference in the indexes in both basic series. Introducing the cards that the child uses as a system of auxiliary external stimuli significantly increases his capacity for the operation. This is the stage of predominant significance of the external sign. Finally, we see that in adult subjects

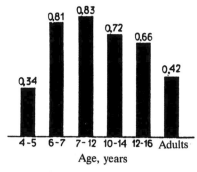

Age, years

Fig. 3

the difference between indexes of both series again levels off and their coefficients become level, but at a new and higher point.

This does not mean that the behavior of the adult reverts to involuntary, natural behavior. At the higher stage of development, behavior remains complex, but it also becomes emancipated from external signs. What occurs is what we arbitrarily designate as a process of revolution of external means. The external sign is converted into an internal sign.

The pattern established experimentally initially for the selection reaction was later confirmed in the study of attention and memory that involved more than 1000 subjects (A. N. Leont'ev, 1931, p. 94). These data can be easily presented in the form of coefficients expressing the dynamics of relations between nonmediated and mediated remembering. If we were to present graphically the pattern of change in separate stages in the course of cultural development and formation of any higher mechanism of behavior, we would obtain two curves with concave sides turned toward each other and drawn together in the lower and upper regions. This pattern, presented in Fig. 2, which expresses visually the course of development of higher intellectual processes, we term the parallelogram of development (A. N. Leont'ev).[75] Let us recall that we have already mentioned the parallelogram of development in connection with nonverbal thinking of man when we attempted to establish that knowing how to think in a human fashion, without words, can only be done with words.

Here too in the behavior of the preschoolchild, the same independence from mediating signs is exhibited externally as in the voluntary attention of the adult. But according to internal structure, we have before us two completely different processes.

We must note that the problem of external similarity of the higher form of voluntary attention and the elementary form of involuntary attention was disclosed in psychology in all its clarity by E. Titchener.[76] In his theory, we see not only a confirmation of the patterns we found, established on a completely different path of research, but also a precursor of this theory of voluntary attention that develops before our eyes, which can fully justifiably be termed the genetic or historical theory of attention.

Titchener differentiates the two forms of attention: it can be passive and involuntary or active and voluntary. These forms of attention, in Titchener's words, are characteristic for different stages of mental development. They differ from each other only in complexity as earlier and later forms and manifest the same type of consciousness, but in different periods of mental development. Passive or involun-

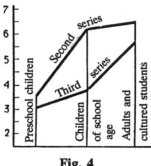

Fig. 4

tary attention can, for this reason, be termed primary attention because it represents the earliest stage of the development of attention. However, the development of attention does not stop at this stage. If it is characteristic that at this stage, impression alone attracts and retains our attention, the reverse relation is characteristic for the second stage, in which we pay attention to an impression by our own effort.

Titchener states that a problem in geometry does not make as strong an impression on us as a clap of thunder. The clap of thunder captures our attention completely independently of us. In solving a problem, we also continue to be attentive, but we ourselves must maintain our attention. Attention to such an object is usually termed active or voluntary. Titchener calls it secondary attention and believes that it is the inevitable result of the complexity of the neural organism. It develops from conflict between primary attentions, from their collision, and from the fact that we become winners in this struggle, in this conflict. Secondary attention, in Titchener's opinion, originates with the conflict of primary attentions, from competing external perceptions and the struggle of incompatible motor positions. As long as even some traces of this conflict remain, our attention will be secondary or active.

However, there is still a third stage in the development of attention. It consists in nothing other than in returning to the first stage. When we solve a problem in geometry, we gradually become interested in it and devote ourselves completely to it, and shortly, the problem acquires the same power over our attention as the clap of thunder had when it appeared in our consciousness. Difficulties are overcome, competitors are eliminated, and distractedness disappears. It would scarcely be possible to cite weightier evidence for the derivation of secondary from primary attention than the fact of conversion of secondary attention into primary.

Titchener's analysis is not limited to establishing three stages in the development of the process of attention. He tries to match the process of the relations of these three stages to the development through time of a person. He maintains that the psychological process of attention is simple at first and then becomes complex; specifically where there is indecision and comprehension, it attains a very high degree of complexity. Finally it becomes simple again. Considering life as a whole, we might say that the period of study and questioning is the period of secondary attention, and the following period of mature and independent activity is the period of derived, primary attention.

Titchener's definition is not sufficiently precise. It would be more correct to say that at the last stage of development, attention is simplified only externally and again returns to the form that was dominant during the primary stage. According to internal structure, at the third stage, it is much more complex than at the second, but the conflict is transferred within and the means with which this conflict is overcome also become ingrown into the personality.

A second point consists of the fact that it sharply separates the mature life of the adult from the time of studying and education, forgetting the transitional age as a uniting link between the one and the other. If we introduce these correctives into Titchener's discussion, we will see that it is specifically the adolescent age that is the transition from the second to the third stage in the development of attention or the transition from external to internal attention. We term this transition the process of revolution. An elegant picture of a gradual interiorization opens before us, that is, a gradual transition inward of higher mental functions at this age. We have seen that specifically here the process of development of internal speech is finally finished, and the break between external and internal speech that was so clearly evident during early years[77] is eliminated.

We have seen that internal mnemotechnique or logical memory becomes the basic form of accumulating experience during the transitional age. Finally, we have seen that the most typical feature of the evolution of this function is contained in the revolution of voluntary attention during the time in which we are interested. This cannot be the result of an accidental coincidence, but has causes in the deeper and common laws of formation of the personality of the adolescent, of which we shall speak in greater detail in the closing chapter of the course.

We will not stop now to bring these partial patterns that we found, which characterize the development of separate functions, to their common and deep roots. We shall be satisfied with establishing the internal, functional, and structural connection that exists between separate factors. Actually, we have already indicated that the drawing together of memory and attention with intellect is the most essential and distinctive trait of the transitional age. These functions make a transition from the system of perception to the system of thinking. We have seen that there is a close connection between the primitive concept of the schoolchild, a concept-conglomerate or a complex, and the narrowness of the field of attention. We have seen further that the transition to thinking in concepts in the true sense of the word presumes not a simple quantitative extension of the field of attention, but a transition to a new form of organization of this field. In the child, multiple attention frequently is not less rich, but richer than in the adult. The child can include a greater number of objects in his field of attention and a much greater number of details. The attention of the adult is characterized by a different structure and a different type of activity. We have found that this change consists in a transition from nonmediated, elementary attention at early stages of development to mediated attention, the activity of which is accomplished with a number of auxiliary internal means.

Now, without going into disclosing the deep causes of the connections between thinking in concepts and the higher form of attention, we would like to indicate that both these forms of activity again reveal a close genetic and functional dependence and connection. Just as involuntary attention showed a relationship to complex thinking, thinking in concepts and internal voluntary attention mutually support each other. This connection, like the connection between thinking and memory, has a dual character. On the one hand, a certain stage in the development of attention is a required precursor for the development of concepts. Specifically the narrowness of the field of attention is responsible for the inability of the child to think of all the traits in a hierarchic synthesis. On the other hand, the development of attention itself, its transition to a higher form, is possible only because the function of attention, like memory, is intellectualized, connected with thinking, and enters as a subordinate factor into a new, higher, complex formation that in essence represents a qualitatively new function.

If we continue to call this function attention also, then we will do so exclusively on the basis of external traits, on the basis of the fact that the result of this activity appears to be identical with the result of the activity of elementary attention, that in functional respects, the lower and higher forms of attention are equivalent, that is, the higher form assumes the function of the lower and begins to carry it out. We have before us no more than a partial case of the general law of transition of a function upward about which we have already spoken. For this reason, strictly speaking, psychological terminology and classification of function may sometimes refuse to admit to being one on the basis of function in the lower and upper levels of development owing exclusively to their transition upward.

Just as a transfer of some functions to a higher, newly constructed center is not a basis for considering this center as identical with the lower center which had thus far carried out the same functions, the higher mental function, not destroying but removing the function that was active before, is not simply its continuation, its higher form. The new center that arises in the history of the development of the brain is not simply a perfected old system, although it would have certain functions in common with it and would operate with them in a complex unit. Precisely so, the new function of attention is not simply a perfected and developed old form of this activity, but a qualitatively new formation that includes lower processes of attention in itself as a factor removed in a complex synthesis, as a peripheral form.

Piaget's merit was that he knew how to find the internal connection between the type of activity of attention and the type of thinking. However, Piaget himself considers the connection he found to be a static and purely descriptive definition of the phenomenon. He establishes the relationship of the two mental functions that develop together, but does not disclose the mechanism of this connection. Moreover, he assumes that here we do not need to note the causal connection, that both factors are derived from one common source.

Disclosing the process of the development of attention, we have tried to show that the connection here is more complex and more general, characteristic not only for attention, but also for other functions such as perception, memory, etc. A reciprocal dependence of one function on the other is present here. Here causes and effects change places. That which serves as a precursor of development of higher forms of thinking is itself transformed and raised to a higher level under the influence of the new type of thinking. For the purposes of our discussion, it is important to note that there is a close connection between thinking in concepts and internal voluntary attention. This connection is that attention controlled by thinking in concepts is directed by this unique method to one object or another.

Just as a concept itself is not direct, but mediated thinking, so precisely attention controlled by a concept in a different way than this is done at the primitive stage of development is an aggregate of traits that make up the concept in their complex structural unity. In internal voluntary attention, our intellect thus acquires a new function, a new method of activity, a new form of behavior, since a new complex mechanism, a new *modus operandi* of our attention appears.

5

We must still consider the evolution of this function during the transitional age in order to conclude the history of the development of higher mental functions of the adolescent as well as the history of his cultural development considered from the functional point of view. We have in mind practical activity, practical thinking, or operative intellect, as it is sometimes called.

The old psychology, in considering the development of the forms of thinking of the adult cultured person, usually ignored the historical approach to the problem of thinking. Because of this, psychology presented the actual course of the historical development of thinking in a grossly distorted way and sometimes in a directly inverted form. It placed the initial and earliest forms of thinking at the end of development and the latest, at its beginning. This is also how the matter stood regarding the problem of practical thinking. Based mainly on self-observation, the old psychology took as primary the development of internal thinking connected with speech and with representations but in practical, reasonable action, saw only the realization or continuation of processes of internal thinking. The cultured adult usually thinks first and then acts; from this, psychology concluded that this is also what happened in the history of the development of thinking: thinking came first and then action. In connection with this, the old psychology placed the end of childhood and the beginning of the transitional age, the maturing of reasonable goal-directed, practical activity of the child at a comparatively late time.

Like the base of many fallacies, this too contains a grain of truth corresponding to reality. We shall try to disclose this grain of truth hidden under a false interpretation. During the transitional age, an extremely important leap is made in the development of practical, goal-directed human activity; here for the first time possibilities open up for actually mastering professional work, the concrete realization of practical thinking. Newer research has also confirmed that in the area of practical thinking, the transitional age represents a crucial point.

The study of practical intellect has shown that the end of the primary school years (10-11) corresponds to the transition from mechanical play to mechanical intellect, and only after this does the period of mechanical thinking in the true sense of the word begin. Zagorovskii says (1929, p. 53) that a number of German investigators (H. Meyer and G. Pfahler, O. Lipmann and V. Neubauer)[78] note that during the first school years mechanical giftedness is lower than general giftedness, but between the third and fifth years of training, a reversal occurs in the development of mechanical abilities, and at age 13-15, the adolescent leaves the stage of naive physics behind. The experiments of Meyer and Pfahler showed that at age 12-14, children are capable of solving mechanical problems independently.

The studies of V. E. Neubauer (1928)[79] basically confirmed these conclusions. Neubauer gave children of different ages construction material of which they were to build different things and draw them. The author studied what and how a child builds and draws. Of all Neubauer's conclusions, we shall consider what interests us, the basic pattern of development of the mechanical thinking of the adolescent. From the age of 5 to 9, pattern predominates in the child's drawing. The age of 9 to 12 is the transitional period, which is characterized by a dominance of perspective images. At age 12-13, the development of the child's own technical drawing begins. From the point of view of the relation that exists between the building and the drawing, Neubauer distinguishes three different methods of thinking.

The first is characterized by the child's indicating in the drawing the basic distinguishing trait of the object he built, for example, the wing in a wind mill. The drawing seems to serve an identifying purpose and is an allusion to the external form of the object. The second stage is a detailed presentation of the form or external appearance of the object. The child is usually not satisfied with presenting one characteristic trait; he tries more or less faithfully to present a general description, the general external form of the object built. Finally, the drawing acquires a

Table 4

| Age | Features of the drawings, % | | | | | |
| | Typical traits | | Form | | Functioning | |
	Boys	Girls	Boys	Girls	Boys	Girls
5	100	100	—	—	—	—
6	100	100	—	—	—	—
7	100	100	—	—	—	—
8	63	82	25	18	12	—
9	65	70	20	15	15	15
10	47	70	10	17	43	13
11	50	67	12	4	38	29
12	35	36	6	12	59	32
13	38	69	7	12	55	19
14	35	37	5	30	60	33
15	34	40	—	—	66	60

completely new function: the child makes the transition to presenting the internal dynamism, the method of functioning, the reason for building the object. Table 4 indicates the results of Neubauer's study. From the table it is easy to see that only with the beginning of the transitional age does the third form of drawing begin to dominate in the picture.

Neubauer, generalizing the data of the study, notes three basic stages in the development of the mechanical thinking of the child. At the first stage (age 5-9), mechanical understanding is in an embryonic state. The child's drawing is still directly connected with play and presents the characteristic traits of the object in a graphic form. Drawing several objects at the same time is nothing other than a purely mechanical combination, a purely external uniting. At the second stage, the circle of the objects the child draws is extended and machines are included in the drawing. The child draws the external form in greater detail; the combination of separate objects has a more connected, complex character. Finally at the third stage, the child draws machines mainly, and his attention is directed toward presenting the external connections of the parts, toward functioning. The combination of parts and elements acquires a predominantly mechanical character. The third stage, according to V. E. Smirnov (1929), coincides with the beginning of maturation of the functional reorganization of the organism when the person experiences especially keenly the changes in his organism.[80] Thus, we can see that in the practical thinking of the adolescent serious changes actually occur during the time of sexual maturation. We shall define more precisely what these changes are and what causes them. We shall begin with negative definitions.

First, we can scarcely take the connection with the change in functioning of the organism itself as a real explanation of these changes. This kind of explanation seems to us to be extremely strained and improbable. Assuming that the adolescent makes the transition to drawing the principle of the working of some mechanism on the basis that the functioning of his own body has changed and that because of this, his attention is drawn toward these changes, seems to us to be a direct reduction into a single unit of the most disparate points between which there are actually many connecting links.

Second, it seems to us that such a purely descriptive study of facts empirically established without genetic analysis, without disclosing the causal-dynamic connections that are the basis of the phenomenon, leads to the false conclusion that practical thinking in the real sense of the word seems to appear only during the transitional age.

We can find an allusion to correct understanding of this question in the studies of Pfahler, who, in Kroh's words, indicates that the ability to understand and adequately reproduce the internal connections of word and action, the internal complex of action, becomes possible only on the basis of psychological consideration, only during the transitional period. We are again approaching the device we have tested, to which we resorted repeatedly in explaining a change in one function or another during the transitional age. We might expect that in the area of practical activity, during the transitional age, we will not find any kind of new elementary forms of behavior that would not be known to the child.

In addition, we cannot expect to find any kind of substantial changes and substantially new formations within the function of practical thinking itself. We must anticipate that changes characteristic of the adolescent will appear in the area of interrelations, interconnections between this function and other functions, in particular, between this function and the central function that controls all mental development—thinking in concepts.

Actually, the study shows that it is not only this function that undergoes changes of one kind or another, but its relations with other functions change, its moving toward thinking in concepts occurs, and again there is a dual dependence between each special function and the central function. The special function enters into a new and complex synthesis. It is simultaneously a precursor of the development of thinking in concepts and itself is elevated to a higher level under its influence. The formation of a new independent synthesis that has its own special laws, the appearance of an essentially new form of activity, a new function, a new *modus operandi* is the true content of the genetic process. We shall consider in greater detail how this actually occurs.

The problem of practical thinking in modern psychology has been turned into one of the central and basic problems of all of science, and the well-known experiments of Köhler with monkeys have shown that higher primates are capable of devising and using tools intelligently. Thus, the forms of thinking earliest in the genetic respect were studied. They were forms of practical effective thinking completely independent of speech.

The experiments of Köhler give us every basis for assuming that practical, effective thinking is the most primary form of thinking in the history of mental development, which in early manifestations does not depend on more complex kinds of activity but contains this potentially, in an undeveloped form. Köhler's studies were transferred to the child and disclosed that in the child at the age of approximately 10-12 months, actions were first observed that, in the expressions of K. Bühler, completely resembled actions of the chimpanzee.

For this reason, Bühler called this the chimpanzee-like age, wishing to stress that here for the first time practical thinking of the child was evident, completely independent of speech, in the most primitive forms that are natural to monkeys. Experiments were then done with an older child, and they also showed that practical thinking develops before verbal thinking and to a large degree independently of it.

All the studies that transferred experiments with monkeys to the children's room were carried out basically in the old ways. They all looked for factors in the child that would compare his thinking with the thinking of the monkey. The authors completely lost sight of the basic difference in the structure of experience and in the development of practical thinking between man and the animal. But since modern child psychology, in Bühler's correct expression, widely uses the methods of zoopsychology, this basic difference went unnoticed.

If the basic tendency, which permeates Köhler's whole book, is a striving to show the similarity between the chimpanzee intellect and that of the human, then the tendency of child psychology is the opposite: to show the similarity of the child's intellect to that of the chimpanzee. Köhler says that his experiments disclosed the intellect of the chimpanzee to be of the same type and kind as in man. Bühler, studying the child, confirms that his actions completely resemble the actions of the chimpanzee, and for this reason the investigator termed this phase of the child's life the chimpanzee-like age.

Many authors have tried to detect specific differences in the child in various ways. Without going into a detailed analysis of all attempts, we shall note, however, that some of the authors, for example, O. Lipmann, tried to find a specific difference in the more developed biological potentials of the child as compared with the monkey. If the monkey actions are influenced mainly by the visual, structural situation, then in the child, as Lipmann showed (O. Lipmann and H. Bogen, 1923),[81] naive physics takes the foreground relatively early, something that is extremely undeveloped in the chimpanzee. Lipmann understands these words to mean the whole naive, unconscious experience relative to physical properties of his own body and surrounding objects which is formed in the child in the first years of life. Specifically this naive experience relative to the physical properties of his body and other objects and not the visual structure of the field determines the practical intellect of the child. In this way, Lipmann approaches the child as a chimpanzee that has human biology.

Other authors go much further, but according to their own expression, and try to humanize it, as S. Shapiro and E. Gerke[82] have done in introducing the methodology of Köhler into pedology. This humanizing consists of their trying to take into account as a basic factor that controls the practical thinking of the child, not naive physics, not a more complete knowledge of the physical properties of an object, but the social experience of the child.

All the past experience of the child, as these authors correctly note, is constructed along a completely different type than the past experience of the chimpanzee, and for this reason identical experiences in the monkey cage and in the kindergarten can preserve the identity of the psychological structure, can correspond in the same way to the motor apparatus of the one object and the other. But if the past experience of the child is lost from sight, the perspective of the result obtained will be radically distorted. The past experience of the child, apparent in his practical intellect, can be seen primarily in the fact that the environment in early years teaches the child to seek help in the process of adaptation not only from the means at hand in his present situation, but also from resources of past experience. For this reason, as the child grows, a generalized pattern of action develops that is applied independently of definite concrete conditions of adaptation using a similar reaction.

The behavior of the child is full of such crystallized patterns of social experience. Used in later life in play with a number of objects, the child works out certain patterns of behavior and guided by these, masters the principle itself of the given activity. For example, using strings, ribbons, or cords leads to assimilating the principle of connection. As a result, the child is wholly immersed in means of adaptation copied from the social environment.

We shall not touch on all the changes that the authors mentioned above introduce into experiments. We are interested in this case in the main approach to the child's practical intellect. The experiments showed the direct dependence of the child's practical thinking on an available store of social patterns. In addition, the authors say that the adaptive process in the child occurs mainly because of ready patterns appropriated from the social environment. Thus, we see that the search for unique human practical intellect moved along the path of attracting new factors and showed the actual complexity, and the multilevel quality of the construction of this function in man. Naive physics and a store of social patterns, as experiments have shown, are undoubtedly powerful factors that determine the uniqueness of these processes in man.

But we think that these studies still do not show what is most important, what distinguishes the practical thinking of the child from the same kind of thinking in the monkey, specifically, the connections that exist between this form of behavior and all the other functions. In the monkey, practical intellect exists in a completely different system, in a completely different structure of behavior than in the child. Only the intellect of the monkey, as the highest peak, is elevated above the other, more elementary functions. This is not the way it is in the child. From a very early age, the child assimilates a number of higher forms of behavior completely inaccessible to the monkey, specifically, an immeasurably more complete form of verbal thinking. It is impossible to assume that including chimpanzee-like reactions in a completely new structure of human intellect will leave these reactions in an unchanged form. On the contrary, we might justifiably expect that a complex interweaving occurs here, a drawing together, a synthesizing of a number of functions connected with a qualitative transformation of the practical intellect.

In our studies,[83] we turned our attention to the essential difference in the behavior of the child in such a chimpanzee-like situation. It developed that the child, confronted by the problem of mastering some goal with a tool, not only acts with it, but also talks. Experiments showed that the child in this situation exhibits active syncretism of a special type: he reacts to things and to the experimenter syncretically, combining and uniting words, which he uses in trying to affect the experimenter and himself, and the actions that he uses to affect the thing. Both reactions—action and speech—merge into one syncretic whole. We observed how, in similar situations, the child resorted to the same form of talking to himself, to conversation with himself, which Piaget called egocentric speech. If we measure the coefficient of egocentric speech for a situation rich in intellectual points, for example, in working with or using tools, it will be on average twice as high as for a neutral situation such as drawing, and what is most important, it will have a different character. Egocentric speech will syncretically merge with the actions of the child. This syncretic merging of social and egocentric speech and action in situations that include using tools has an important significance for all further development of the child's practical thinking.

Speech is not a by-product of a child's activity; speech is not a parallel function that occurs together with action. Speech and action merge, and this has a decisive significance for both action and speech. Initially, speech merges with intellectual action, accompanies it, reflecting the results of activity and its principal points. But specifically because of the fact that speech reflects and fixes separate points of practical thinking, it is converted from the reflecting, accompanying function into a planning function, shifting to the beginning of the process, transferring from one operation to another the formulaic structure of action. The initial, objective connection between speech and thinking arises in this way. Speech becomes the means for thinking mainly because it reflects an objectively occurring intellectual operation. This is a moment of major importance in the development of speech and thinking, which discloses the secret of the development of verbal thinking as a whole.

The initial syncretic merging of speech and thinking is realized gradually by the child.

It is important to note two points from the very beginning. First, the merging of speech and thinking is not invented by the child; it is not constructed by him with the help of logical operations. The child does not devise one method or another of practical behavior with the help speech. On the contrary, speech itself assumes certain logical forms, is intellectualized only because it reflects and accompanies practical intellectual operations of the child. Verbal thinking at first must arise objectively and only later subjectively. At first, it arises in oneself, then for oneself.

Speech and action, merging, themselves begin to determine the behavior of the child before the child begins to determine his own reaction with their help. Whoever actually seriously studies the connections that arise between speech and intellectual action of the child will find the central link in the whole chain of development of speech and thinking that will experimentally-genetically disclose the nature of that formation. The child relates to a situation that requires the use of tools through another person, the experimenter. Talking with him, then talking in his presence to himself, the child relates to the situation through instruction, through speech, that is, socially. Here the road is laid through speech to the intellect, first objectively through another, then for himself. Later, the experimenter is left out. Talking to oneself in his presence, that is, egocentric speech, makes a transition to talking to oneself without him, that is, to internal speech, when the child relates to the situation through his own instruction, through his own speech.

Here we reconstruct verbal thinking experimentally in its true genetic nature.

Second, practical thinking, leading to intellectualization of speech, itself becomes verbal. It is verbalized. Because of this, its potentials are infinitely extended. We have seen that initially speech becomes comprehensible because it reflects action. But when the child, using speech, begins to fix the formulaic structure of the operation, when he then begins to apply the formula to future actions, making a plan and intention in his own behavior, his practical thinking rises to a new level: the child's behavior begins to be determined not by the structure of the visual field, not by naive physics, and not even by social patterns of experience, but by a new form of activity—verbal thinking.

From the story of the drawing, we know, for example, how the replacement of the child's word with respect to the child's own action occurs. At the first stage, the child draws, then names what he drew. He does not even know what he is drawing when he is asked. He still does not have a plan, he does not have an intention with respect to his own action. Gradually, the word begins to shift, to be displaced from the end of the process of drawing to the action itself.

Not too long before the picture is finished, the child names what he has drawn, and thus the end of a process that is not yet finished is anticipated. Frequently, in the middle and sometimes even sooner, after the beginning of the process, the child tells what it will be, fixes it in words and thus subordinates all of the subsequent process to the plan and intention.

Finally, at the third stage, the word is moved to the very beginning of the process. The child determines beforehand what he will draw, and the whole process of drawing is subjected to this verbal formulation of the intention and plan itself. This shift from the end point to the beginning also characterizes the relation between practical action and its verbal formula in the child. At first the verbal formula consists of and fixes the result of the action; later it begins to reflect separate points in the abrupt change of the process of solving the problem, and, finally, it becomes a formula of a plan and intention that precedes the development of the further course of the effective operation and transfers the child's behavior to a completely different course.

It is not the laws of the visual field that enslave animals, in Köhler's expression, but laws of voluntary self-determination of one's own behavior, laws of the verbal field that become the basic factors that control the child's behavior. The monkey *sees* a situation and *experiences* it. The child, whose perception is directed by speech, *comprehends* the situation. But in addition to the situation, he comprehends, but does not experience his own actions. Just as he solves the given problem with the help of mediated activity, with the help of using tools, he begins to determine, to construct and connect his own processes of behavior into a single whole with the help of mediated activity, with the help of the word, with the help of verbal thinking.

Of course, the transition to higher forms of synthesis of practical and verbal thinking is not instantly achieved. It begins in early childhood and, as before, a basic problem arises: establishing what is new in the processes of the merging of verbal and practical thinking that is achieved specifically in the transitional age. To answer this question, we must note that, of course, even former investigators observed the great importance of speech in the practical, effective thinking child. This simply could not but be noticed no matter from which point of view the investigator approached the process. Whether the attention of the investigator was directed to naive physics or to the pattern of social experience, everywhere and always he would run across speech to which he would ascribe a secondary, although a respected place.

It would be complete blindness on the part of the investigator, a direct distortion of facts, if the role of speech in the process of behavior was not noted at least in the factual part of the study. For this reason, all authors consider speech reactions as playing a unique role in the adaptive process of the child. Thus, in experiments that required the use of tools, Shapiro and Gerke observed that speech very often served the function of noting the action. In especially difficult cases or with inadequate pressure of adaptive energy, the children were limited to establishing the facts of their inadaptability or began to dream aloud, maintaining that their wish would be granted by itself. "It will climb down now and drop down to us, it will come to us on the floor," says Borya (age 3). In general, Shapiro and Gerke noted that the number of speech manifestations was inversely proportional to the number of effective acts.

It is understandable from the point of view of the authors that speech replaces unsuccessful action, that with the help of speech, the child begins to dream aloud, wherever he cannot effectively master the situation.

These authors note that in certain cases, speech has an anticipatory and corrective significance. The child first solves the problem verbally and only then puts his solution into action, or he critiques his action, introducing appropriate corrections into the action. Speech, by virtue of specific features, significantly facilitates the subject's transition from the present situation to past experience. It very often diverts the child from the need to use the resources he has directly, diverting his adaptation in other directions. On the one hand, speech makes passive adaptation possible through verbal requests for help from the experimenter. On the other hand, speech sometimes carries the child off into an area of recollections or conversation with the experimenter not directly connected with the problem placed before him as a test subject.

All of this once again points to the significance of social experience in adaptive reactions of the child, since even a cursory analysis of the role of the child's speech displays almost in relief that he uses speech as a universal social pattern. Summarizing, the authors state that speech plays a unique role in the practical, effective adaptation of the child. It replaces and compensates for subordinate adaptation or serves as a bridge for transition from direct trials to past experience and a purely social type of adaptation through the experimenter.

Even in this description of the child's behavior during action using tools, connections between practical action and speech are very clear. However, the investigators, not giving these connections any substantial significance, consider them as a special case of patterns of social experience and ascribe a subordinate, secondary significance to the synthesis of speech and action, and sometimes do not even note this synthesis. Such authors are inclined to think that the child's speech and action are inversely proportional, thinking of it as not only a purely quantitative relation of these and other reactions, but also thinking that the substantial connection between them consists of speech replacing unsuccessful action. In any case, in all of these observations, speech is taken to be something that accompanies the process of action, but that does not lead to a radical change in its nature and to the development of a new and essentially qualitatively unique form of practical activity specific to man. Lipmann in the logs of his experiments also repeatedly reports the unique combination of social and egocentric speech of the child and his practical activity.

It is incomprehensible that the authors who take the structural point of view and reject the possibility of a mechanical, purely associative combination of the two types of activity do not note this completely new structure which develops on the basis of the union of practical and verbal thinking into a single whole. Lipmann, studying the capacity for rational action, draws a detailed parallel between children's actions and the behavior of monkeys in Köhler's experiments. Lipmann finds many similarities, but also establishes a radical difference which, as we have indicated, consists of the absence of naive physics in the monkeys and naive optics in the children.

Comparing the actions of children and anthropoids, Lipmann summarizes: as long as physical action depends mainly on visual components of the structure of the situation, the difference between the child and the monkey is only one of degree. If the situation requires comprehending relations of physical, structural properties of the things, the difference between the monkey and the child becomes apparent: the actions of the monkey depend mainly on optics, but the actions of the child depend mainly on physical relations of the things.

Again we see indications of an extremely important new biological factor that determines the practical thinking of the child in comparison with that of the monkey, but we do not see even the smallest shift toward understanding the main and radical difference between human practical activity and the activity of the animal. We say directly that if the boundary between the activity of the child and the monkey is drawn where Lipmann draws it, we will never be able to understand the development of the work activity of man.

In our studies, we were able to note that a purely verbal operation pertaining to subsequent, practical action, but separated from real action is the product of later development. For the most part, the initial verbal operation enters into an external operation as an auxiliary device. The character of its combination with the external operation is different at different stages of development. Each age has its own genetic center that is characterized by the synthesis of speech and practical thinking that is dominant at the given age. A line of development of practical activity of the child goes from center to center. As we have said, the basic changes in this process consist of speech shifting in time from the end to the beginning of the whole operation, that it makes a transition from the function of fixing and reflecting action to the function of planning it. In the correct expression of M. V.

O'Shea (1910), the child at first acts then thinks, but the adult first thinks then acts.

Our studies provide a basis for us to develop a very general sketch of the basic pattern of development of the child's practical activity. We will consider this pattern briefly. If we think of the experiments with the use of tools in genetic section, we see approximately the following course of development of this activity. At the youngest age, at 6 months, as investigators noted, there is an embryonic form of future use of tools. The child, using one object, affects another, an operation specific to human hands and not observed in animals. This is still not a purposeful operation since the action of the child is not directed toward anything, but it is a tool in itself, in its objective significance, since some middle member is present between the child and the object of his action. At 10-12 months, a true use of tools, primarily of the type that occurs in monkeys, can be observed.

A characteristic trait of this whole age is the independence of practical action from speech (chimpanzee-like age). However, we believe that the child's prattle which accompanies the activity and, in this case, actually has the character of emotional accompaniment, is of substantial significance.

Early childhood is characterized by the syncretic combination of the child's socialized speech and his action. Instead of acting directly on the object, the child turns to the experimenter with requests, or tries to affect the object with words, or, finally, changing the problem, replaces real success with words. The essential trait of the whole age is syncretic combination of the social situation and the physical situation into one nonsystematized whole. The syncretic combination should be understood as a most important genetic center which first results in the establishment of a connection, still indefinite and confused, between speech and practical thinking.

During preschool age, the child's speech has already assumed a new form and has become speech for himself, and the whole age is characterized by a syncretic combination of egocentric speech and practical action. In the true sense of the word, verbal thinking in the process of solving a problem is rarely observed. Words control and direct behavior although the child does not pronounce them for this purpose. Here we have what seems to be a less than complete point-to-point coincidence of the two operations of thinking, still not consciously and not purposefully connected with each other, but already objectively connected.

During school age, as we have seen, in the area of abstract verbal thinking, the child is still influenced by verbal syncretism, and because of this, when he is confronted by a problem of uniting into a single whole processes of internal speech and processes of practical action, a syncretic combination of these develops without dominance of internal speech over the whole practical operation.

Only during the transitional age, in connection with the development of verbal thinking in concepts, does it become possible to solve a problem verbally and subsequently implement it in action, implementation that is subject to plan, controlled by a single purpose, directed by the will which, like a law, determines the method and character of the action.[84]

Thus, gradually, the road is laid for thinking verbally, and during the transitional age, we note at a glance a dual situation: on the one hand, the adolescent masters thinking in concepts for the first time, thinking that is completely separate from concrete actions, and on the other hand, specifically because of thinking in concepts, the specifically human higher forms of relations between thinking and action, characterized by a complex hierarchic synthesis of the two forms, are created for the first time.

We have an extremely interesting similar situation in the history of development of human thinking in the phylogenetic plan. As is known, Hegel repeatedly tried to consider human practical activity, and specifically the use of tools, as putting logical inferences into action. V. I. Lenin in a note on Hegel's *Logic*, said the following with respect to the category of logic and human practice: "When Hegel tries—sometimes even tries very hard—to classify purposeful human activity in the category of logic, saying that this activity is a 'conclusion' (*Schluss*), that the subject (man) plays the role of a certain 'member' in a logical 'figure' of the 'conclusion', etc.—**This is not only stretching the point, not only a game, it is a very serious content, purely materialistic, that should be turned inside out: human practical activity must have brought human consciousness to repeating various logical figures billions of times in order for these figures to acquire the significance of axioms**" (*Complete Collected Works*, Vol. 29, p. 172). And another time, Lenin expresses the same idea about the connection of logical forms of thinking with human practice thus: "The conclusion of acting... For Hegel *acting*, practice, is a *logical 'conclusion,'* a figure of logic. And this is true! Of course, not in the sense that a figure of logic in its otherness has the experience of man (=absolute idealism) but vice versa: human experience, repeated billions of times, is fixed in the consciousness of man by figures of logic. These figures have the stability of a prejudice, an axiomatic character specifically (and only) by virtue of those billions of repetitions" (ibid., p. 198).

Action forms a judgment in speech, transforms it into an intellectual process. We have seen this in experiments with the child. What the child thinks in action, using tools being thinking in action, while using speech, changes not only the form of his thinking, introducing into it a road through speech and new forms of using experience, but he changes speech itself, forming it according to an intellectual principle, giving it an intellectual function. In the phylogenetic plan, of which V. I. Lenin speaks, speech evidently played a decisive role in the process of fixing in the human consciousness logical figures repeated billions of times in human experience.

Up to this time, the significance of speech for thinking was presented one-sidedly, but not how speech out of the amorphous mass that carries out the most various functions under the influence of practical intellect, accompanying its operations and fixing them after the fact, forges for itself an intellectual form (judgment), takes a picture, a cast of practical intellect which only later—during the transitional age—itself begins to control thinking. Thus, during the transitional age, the change in roles and interactions of speech and action thinking, which begins very early, is completed.

If at the early age, the leading, dominant function is the practical intellect and the speech of the child is intelligent only to the extent that it is not a thing separate from his action, now the action of the child takes a subordinate position with respect to thinking. In this process, we can trace not only how thinking becomes verbal, but also how speech becomes intellectual through practical action.

How does the relation of the two forms of thinking during the transitional age differ from the school age immediately preceding it? During school age, solving a problem that requires a complex use of tools is possible without external speech, by way of internal speech, but with checking it with perception, with the real situation and real action. Otherwise, without a visual situation and without visual action in thoughts, this solving leads to verbal syncretism. Only during the transitional age does internal speech, thinking in concepts, lead to the possibility of a new synthesis, a new type of connection of two forms of intellect. Only the adolescent can solve a problem of practical thinking without a visual situation, in concepts, and then transfer it to a plan of action.

As a general formula, we could say that in the process of our studies, we are in a position to trace how the road is laid to the intellect through speech. But for speech to become a road to the intellect, it must itself experience the forming influence of intellect. However, the process of the development of the planning function of speech from being a reflecting function is only a partial case of the general law of the development of regulating and comprehending processes from processes of perception. Reflection with the help of speech (a mold in speech of one's action), the development of speech formulas for successive actions, is the basis for the development of consciousness of self and higher voluntary controlling mechanisms. We have already indicated that all the controlling mechanisms of the organism are constructed on the principle of self-perception of one's own movements.

When reflection is approached without taking it in motion, investigators frequently say that if one operation or another, for example, speech or consciousness, reflects some kind of objectively occurring process, then by the same token, speech cannot carry any substantial function because reflection in a mirror cannot change the fate of the object reflected. Moreover, if we take the phenomenon as it develops, we shall see that specifically because of reflection of objective connections and especially because of self-reflection of human experience in human verbal thinking, both man's consciousness of self and his potential for consciously controlling his actions develop. "Consciousness in general *reflects* life. This is the general position of all of materialism" (V. I. Lenin, *Complete Collected Works*, Vol. 18, p. 343). "And management of nature manifested in human experience is the result of an objectively true reflection in the head of man of the phenomena and processes of nature, it is evidence of the fact that this reflection (within the limits of what experience demonstrates to us) is the objective, absolute, eternal truth" (ibid., p. 198).

We considered the development of practical activity in such detail because it is connected with the three main points of all of the psychology of the transitional age.

As Piaget demonstrated, the first point is the following: the whole school age is filled with what the child transfers from the sphere of action to the sphere of verbal thinking of the operations which he mastered at the preceding stages. We saw that this is done with the help of introspection, reflection of his own processes in consciousness. Piaget says that to be conscious of one's own operation is to move it from the sphere of action into the sphere of speech. Assimilating any kind of operation in a verbal relation, in Piaget's opinion, reproduces the abrupt changes that took place in assimilating the same operation in the sphere of action. Only the dates will be different; the rhythm remains analogous.

Thus, we see that the child's reflection of his own experience in the sphere of verbal thinking leads to a serious disproportion between experience and thinking in the schoolchild. In the sphere of practical action, he has already overcome syncretism and the features of egocentric thinking. In the verbal sphere, he is still under the influence of the factors that characterize primitive forms of thinking. The disproportion is leveled and not only leveled, but has become disproportional again in the reverse direction during the transitional age: together with the formation of concepts, thinking and its control of action increase and thereby raise the practical action of the adolescent to a higher level.

The second point consists of the fact that we are confronted here by an extremely interesting problem of the connections between the use of tools and the development of mediated processes of behavior. We have seen that the child's and adolescent's practical activity itself becomes more and more mediated by speech and that introducing speech into the processes of practical activity essentially signifies a transition of this activity from a direct, practical operation, controlled only by perception of the situation, to a process of practical thinking mediated by words. Man controls his behavior and subordinates it to a certain plan through speech and with the help of speech.

Thus, the practical activity of man is converted into a doubly mediated activity: on the one hand, it is mediated by tools in the literal sense of the word, and on the other hand, it is mediated by tools in the figurative sense of the word, the tools of thinking, means that facilitate carrying on an intellectual operation; it is mediated by words.

Finally, the third point that interests us, the most important point, is the close connection that exists between the genetic, synthetic centers of thinking and practical activity that are developing and replacing one another and the development of the work activity of the adolescent who is maturing toward mastery of higher forms of human work. We shall speak of work separately in Chapter 15, "The Working Adolescent."*

6

We began our discussion with perception, moved on to memory and attention, and concluded with practical activity. In the evolution of these processes during the transitional age, we found something in common. We saw that these processes evolve not separately and not side by side and that the history of their development resembles less than anything the sum of separate changes of each function. The evolution of the intellectual life of the adolescent stood before us as a single integral picture in which all the parts were subordinate to the connection with the center.

From this single center, from the function of the formation of concepts, we attempted to draw all peripheral changes in the psychology of the adolescent. During the transitional age, perception, memory, attention, and action are not a cluster of functions dropped into a vessel with water, not an uncoordinated number of processes, but an internally connected special system subjected in its evolution to a single law derived from the central, leading function, the function of forming concepts.

In this sense, we might note many common traits among the various functions. We succeeded in showing that laws of the development of voluntary attention are essentially the same as the laws of the development of logical memory. We would be completely justified in transposing the customary, traditional definition and speak on the same basis of voluntary memory and logical attention because the basis of the one and the other is the same. On the basis of the formation of concepts, both functions acquire an intellectual character and begin to be controlled by thinking in concepts. This makes them logical on the one hand, and, on the other hand, free, independent of more elementary patterns that form their base, freely directed by conscious, that is, voluntary thought.

We were able to show the substantial difference of the transitional age, which is expressed in the fact that relations existing between memory and intellect are inverted. If during childhood, thinking is a function of memory, then in the transitional age, memory becomes the function of thinking. We could show with an equal basis that the same thing happens with respect to perception and action of the child. At an early age, and in general, at primitive stages of development, thinking is the function of perception of the visual field. To think means to analyze one's

---

*Editor's note: See Note 1 in the present volume.

perceptions. During the transitional age, to perceive means to think of the visual in concepts, to synthesize the concrete and the general. Perception becomes a function of thinking.

Thus, with full justification, we could speak of logical and even of voluntary perception, having in mind the definitions of Köhler presented above which state that animals are slaves to the sensory field to a much greater degree than adult humans. It is precisely the same with action, controlled initially specifically by the sensory field and being the primary form of human thinking, which then becomes free, voluntary, and logical action only during the transitional age, when it is controlled by thinking in concepts.

It remains for us to take the final step. In order to find real evidence and be firmly convinced that the systematic picture of evolution of all the functions connected into a single system that we have drawn is actually true, that the development represents a single process, the center of which is the function of forming concepts, we must turn to the comparative study of data of a pathological character, data on the disintegration and disturbance of that complex unity, the development and structure of which we have just studied. E. K. Sepp[85] formulates the idea of a comparative study of any complex function in its development and disintegration in the following way. Just as geology uses every damage to the Earth's crust, its shifts, faults, and outcroppings exposed by erosion, to study the laws of formation of strata, to study the history of the Earth's development, so too the neuropathologist, using disturbances in the nervous system that result from catastrophic causes or those persistent and long-term changes, similar to erosion, that are caused by intoxication and other systemic damage to the brain, has the opportunity to judge the structure and development of the nervous system of man and the structure and development of his behavior.

Studying the exceptionally rich area of speech functions, Sepp continues, the neuropathologist has the opportunity to establish by comparison not only definite localization of the speech centers and the conditional nature of this localization, which depends on the order of formation of speech, but also the interconnectedness of speech functions and other functions of the cerebral cortex. This is possible specifically because in damage to the nervous system, we can see exposed the mechanisms that are so merged in a healthy state that they cannot be separated from the single function in which they participate.

Many such mechanisms, disclosed as a result of disturbance of the connection between them, appear to be species mechanisms, and in the newborn infant in whom behavior is not yet based on personal experience, they are the only effective mechanisms. In the adult, we find them in isolated action only in case of a disturbance of a connection in the central nervous system. Not only in the area of innate species mechanisms, but also in the area of mechanisms constructed on the basis of individual experience, on the basis of functioning activity of the cerebral cortex, in pathology, do we observe the exposure that makes it possible to study the separate mechanisms in isolated activity. Here, according to Sepp, the speech function must be brought to the forefront.

As an example of what made it possible to penetrate into the history of the development of these mechanisms that were at one time connected and into the history of the structure of the now disintegrated but formerly single functions, Sepp cites motor aphasia in polyglots, stressing that with disruption of a certain part of the cerebral cortex, the ability to speak in the native language is lost while ability to speak in the language that was used less, and is sometimes quite forgotten, is not only not lost, but is much freer and better than it was before the illness. It is obvious that engrams of the speech function depending on the order of their formation are localized in different places each time. By erasing some engrams in the cerebral cortex, pathology makes it possible for the neuropathologist to examine according to parts the history of the given personality and its formation.

Thus, we see that the brain preserves in itself in a spatial form the documented temporal sequence of development of behavior, and a disintegration of complex single functions allows us to penetrate into the history of their development. This idea has now become one of the basic methodological principles of all of psychoneurology as a whole. Development is the key to understanding pathological processes, processes of disintegration of syntheses, higher unities, and pathology is the key to the history of the development and structure of the higher synthetic functions.

We have already indicated one of the basic neurobiological laws, cited by Kretschmer, which states: if a higher center is functionally weak or separated from subordinate centers, then the general function of the nervous apparatus does not simply stop, but the subordinate one becomes independent and displays for us the elements of its old type of functioning that remain in it. The emancipation of lower centers finds a complete analogy in the emancipation of lower functions. The lower or elementary function, entering into the composition of a complex single function, when the latter is damaged, when its unity is disrupted, is separated and begins to act according to its own primitive laws. Specifically for this reason, disease is frequently expressed in the form of regression. This is as if a reverse movement of the process of development, a return to points long since passed, and consequently, a disclosure of the very secret of the structure of that complex unity, the disintegration of which we can observe and study. This emancipation contains not a parallel, but an important neurobiological law, which, as we have said, can justifiably be applied also to the history of development and disintegration of functions.

In this respect, three diseases are of exceptional interest for understanding the history of the structure of higher mental functions during the transitional age. What we have in mind are hysteria, aphasia, and schizophrenia; from our point of view, they are as if experiments, specially organized by nature, on the disintegration of the unity, the structure of which makes up the main content of the transitional age. In all three diseases, we can observe from different aspects the reverse movement of the same process of development that we study in the psychology of the adolescent from the genetic point of view.

Thus, it seems to us that a scientific understanding of this psychology would be impossible without serious study of the history of the structure of higher functions of the adolescent as compared with the history of the disintegration of the unities, the syntheses in the disease processes we have mentioned. Of these, two disease forms were usually compared to and converged with the transitional age. Psychology of the adolescent was frequently considered in the light of teaching on hysteria and schizophrenia. In that case, however, what was under consideration were relations directly opposite to those of which we are now speaking.

In pedology, a comparative study of processes of development and processes of pathological disintegration of any forms most often does not pursue the purposes that we now set ourselves. Based on the completely correct position that between disease and the normal state there is a series of fine transitions, there are no sharp boundaries that separate one state from the other, pedologists usually are inclined to understand pathology as an exaggerated norm, and for this reason consider each age in the light of diseases proper to it, trying intensely to find the basic patterns of the age reflected in the disease.

We come from a directly opposite assumption: in disease, we have the possibility of observing processes of reverse development. For this reason, we cannot in advance expect that the history of the disintegration of higher forms of behavior, as it is observed in one mental or nervous illness or another, represents simply in an exaggerated and emphasized form the history of their structure. More likely, one process is the opposite of the other rather than its condensed expression. But specifically because the disintegration of the higher forms of behavior is the reverse movement of the process of development, its study is the key to understanding the history of the development of these forms. In particular, the law of emancipation of lower functions presented above speaks specifically in favor of this kind of understanding and no other of the relation of processes of pathological disintegration and processes of development. Disease frequently is a regression, a return to the past, to already passed points of development, and it makes possible, by comparative study, finding and establishing that which is substantially new, that which is specific, the construction of which is exposed in disease as old geological strata are exposed by erosion of their surfaces.

7

Hysteria has long been considered as a disease closely linked to the characteristics of the transitional age. E. Kretschmer (1928) states that many of the symptoms of the so-called hysterical character are nothing other than solidified residue of the mind in early sexual maturation or its unfavorable changes in character under the influence of a later change in conditions of life. Further, Kretschmer enumerates a number of symptoms among which we must note a characteristic contrast between indifference and excessive pressure of amorous feeling, a contrast between devotion and childish egoism and particularly, a mixture of the playful and the tragic in the image of life.

For this reason, in Kretschmer's words, if former investigators readily defined hysterics as big children, then we prefer to say, "adult adolescents." This will correspond exactly to the period when a delay occurred in biological development: the period of early sexual maturity. The immature mind has a great tendency toward impulsive affective release and in particular, to hypobulic mechanisms. In general we might say that the period of sexual maturation is a favored soil for hysterical reactions.

Hoche assumes that every man is predisposed toward hysteria. Elucidating his position, Kretschmer adds: specifically because everyone carries in himself old instinctive forms, hidden more or less firmly by newer characterological layers of culture.* What does this mean? We can understand only what has been said in the light of two laws that pertain equally to development and to disintegration of higher forms of behavior. Let us recall that one of them speaks of the preservation of functions lower in the history of development as being subordinate factors within the higher, complex, new formations.

Thus, the mechanisms that control our behavior at earlier stages of development, and especially during the early period of sexual maturation, do not disappear entirely in the adult; they are included as an auxiliary, implementing mechanism in the composition of the more complex synthetic function. Within it, they act according to other laws than those that control their independent life. But when the

---

*In this sense, we might graphically say in connection with the future that everyone carries in himself not only his own hysteria, but also his aphasia and his schizophrenia, that is, those stages of development passed, but preserved in a cryptic form, that are exposed by diseases.

higher function disintegrates for any reason, the subordinate factors preserved within it are emancipated and begin again to act according to the laws of their primitive life. This is the source of regression in disease. Break-up of the higher function also means, in a conditional sense of course, a kind of return to a genetically prior stage of development.

Kretschmer states that this is not an accidental parallel, but an important neurobiological, basic law that in the area of the lower motor sphere has long been recognized but has not yet been applied in the area of the psychiatry of neuroses. When in the mental motor-expressive sphere, the higher factor becomes incapable of control, then the lower factor underlying it begins to work independently following its own primitive laws. This is the second of the laws we have mentioned.

What kind of subordinate factors begin to work independently in hysteria and, consequently, return us to the beginning of sexual maturation? Kretschmer calls this mechanism hypobulic and says that in primitive mental life, the will and affect are identical. Every affect is at the same time a tendency, and every tendency assumes the traits of an affect. The direct, impulsive organization of the life of the will proper to the child and especially to the adolescent at the beginning of sexual maturation, are emancipated from the higher superstructure of the will in hysteria. It is most essential that hypobulia assumes a qualitatively characteristic will form that under some circumstances may function independently and be disposed between a purposeful apparatus and a reflexive apparatus so that it can act in union both with the first and with the second, as Kretschmer assumes.

In this sense, hypobulia is not a new creation of hysteria; it is not specific to hysteria alone. In the words of Kretschmer, what we consider in the hysteric as a kind of disease of a foreign body is a demon and double of the purposeful will that we find in higher animals and in small children. For them this is will in general; at that stage of development, it is a normal and more or less the only existing method of wanting. The hypobulic type of will represents an ontogenetically and phylogenetically lower stage of a purposeful apparatus. Specifically for this reason, we call it hypobulic. Study shows that the most varied diseases are accompanied by the emancipation of the hypobulic mechanism. Kretschmer believes that the disease takes something that is an important normal component part of the psychophysical expressive apparatus in higher living beings and separates it from the normal connection, isolates it, displaces it, and compels it to function too forcefully and purposelessly, tyrannically.

From the fact that such varied types of diseases as war neurosis or endogenic catatonia have the same hypobulic roots, it follows that hypobulia is not only an important transitional stage in the history of the development of higher living beings that disappears subsequently or is simply replaced by a purposeful apparatus. We see that hypobulia has greater resemblance to a vestigial organ, the imprint of which is retained to a greater or lesser degree also in the psychological life of adult man. It is not just an atavism, a dead adjunct. On the contrary, we see that even in a healthy adult man, hypobulia as an important component part, united with purposeful function, forms what we call will. However, here it is not dissociated as it is in hysteria or catatonia, it does not present itself as an independent function, but is merged with the purposeful apparatus into a firm, single function.

The process of development during the transitional age is as if separated into parts and repeated in reverse order in hysterical illness.

That which is emancipated as an independent lower function in hysteria is, at the beginning of the transitional age, a normal stage in the development of the will. The process of its further development consists in the construction and formation of that complex unity from which the lower function is separated and isolated in illness. Kretschmer says that the question is frequently raised as to whether hysterics are weak willed. He says that when the question is posed in this way, it cannot be answered. Hysterics are not weak in will, but weak in purpose. Weakness of goal is the mental essence of the state as we see it in most chronic hysterics. Only by separating one factor of will from the other will we be able to understand the mystery; man, not knowing how to control himself, uses a great force of will, not at all without purpose, to present a picture of the most pathetic weak will. Kretschmer assumes that weakness of purpose is not weakness of will.

We could summarize the comparative study of will functions in the hysteric and the adolescent. We could say that the content of development during the transitional age is specifically the disintegration of what makes up the content of hysterical disease. If, in hysteria, hypobulia is emancipated from the control of purposeful will and begins to act according to its primitive laws, then during the transitional age, hypobulia is included as a component of an inseparable part of the purposeful will that appears for the first time at this age and is an expression of the function that makes it possible for man to control himself and his behavior and places before him certain goals, controlling his processes in such a way that they lead to the attainment of those goals.

Thus, purposeful will which manages affect, controls one's own behavior, directs one, knows how to set goals for one's behavior and attain them—this is what is new, what is the basis for the development of all mental functions at this age. But knowing how to set goals and control one's behavior requires, as we have seen, a number of prerequisites of which the main one is thinking in concepts. Only on the basis of thinking in concepts does purposeful will develop, and for this reason we cannot be surprised by the fact that in hysteria, we observed disturbance in intellectual activity, which usually escaped investigators. A decreased development of intellect or emotional disturbance of thinking were usually considered either as conditions accompanying development of the hysterical reaction or as accompanying basic emotional disturbance and its side effects.

Our studies demonstrated that disturbances of intellectual activity in hysteria have a much more complicated quality: it is a disturbance of the purposeful apparatus of thinking. The characteristic relation in the normal man between the activity of thinking and affective life is inverted. Thinking loses all independence, hypobulia begins to lead its own separate life, it no longer takes part in complex purposeful decision-making formations, but acts according to the simplest, primitive formulas.

This lack of purpose pertains also to the thinking of the hysteric; it loses its willful character. The hysteric stops controlling it, just as he is incapable of controlling his behavior as a whole.

It is understood of itself that loss of purpose leads to disorientation, to confusion, and in the sphere of the content of our thinking, to a change in feelings themselves. Kretschmer correctly states that, as a defense against the external world, the hysteric surrounds himself with a wall consisting of instinctive reactions—flight and fight. He pretends, he becomes bitter, strengthens his reflexes. In this way, he succeeds in deceiving the oppressive external world, frightening it, tiring it, and making it tractable. The internal defense against feelings corresponds to this kind of instinctive tactic with respect to the external world. Kretschmer believes that it is characteristic for the essence of the hysterical mind to avoid deep feelings rather than to confront them face to face.

We will not stop now to consider in detail the complex changes in feelings that are observed in hysteria and that essentially make up the psychological content of hysterical neurosis. We will only say that two traits characterize the changes. First, regression to childhood, which is expressed in excessively childish imitation of the mental level of a small child. This state, called puerilism and frequently evoked artificially in hypnosis, is undoubtedly related to regression in the sphere of the life of the will. The second feature is that there is a direct causal connection between the function of disruption of concepts and the change in feelings.

We have already mentioned the great significance for our internal life that the function of concept formation acquires. We are conscious of all external reality and the whole system of internal experiences in a system of concepts. We need only make the transition from thinking in concepts to thinking in complexes—and this is precisely what we observe in hysteria—to drop directly into another, genetically earlier method of orientation toward reality and ourselves. This is why the confused picture in perception and comprehension of external reality, the picture of one's own feelings and self consciousness of the personality, are the direct result of disturbance of the function of concept formation.

How is this disturbance expressed? In that the function of forming concepts, unique and complex in structure, disintegrates owing to the well-known law and exposes complex forms of intellectual activity preserved in it as a stable foundation of thinking. With the transition to an earlier function, thinking changes from the aspect of content and experience of both the external world and internal world.

We can conclude the comparative consideration of the disintegration of will and thinking in concepts in hysteria and the structure of these functions during the transitional age. Summarizing what was said, we come to a general conclusion: in hysteria, we observe the process of reverse development of specifically those functions whose structure makes up the most characteristic feature of the transitional age. The disappearance of hypobulia as an independent factor in the development of purposeful will and the disappearance of complex thinking and the appearance of thinking in concepts make up the most characteristic feature of the psychology of the adolescent. Reverse processes are the basis of hysterical illness.

This comparison returns us to the questions, considered before, on the cultural processing of tendencies and the appearance of willful mastery of one's affective life during the transitional age. Weisenberg and other biologists note the empirically established fact that sexual maturation coincides with the end of general organic maturation.[86] In this fact, the investigator is inclined to see objectively seemingly purposeful striving of nature to unite general bodily maturity and sexual maturation at one temporal point. This connection, the biological significance of which we have already considered, has an essential psychological significance. The sexual instinct of the adolescent grows and matures late and finds, when it matures, an already formed personality with a complex system of functions and an apparatus of factors and processes with which it enters into a complex interaction; on the one hand, it induces their restructuring on a new basis and on the other hand, it begins to be manifested in no other way than as complexly refracted, restructured, and included in the far from simple system of these relations.

The extreme uniqueness of human sexual maturation consists in that the three stages in the development of behavior—instinct, tempering, and intellect—do not appear in chronological order so that all instincts mature first, then everything that pertains to tempering, and finally, only then would intellect appear. On the contrary, there is an extreme genetic overlapping in the manifestation of these three stages. The development of intellect and tempering begins long before the maturing of sexual instinct and the maturing instinct finds in a ready form a complex structure of personality that changes the properties and method of action of the manifested instinct depending on the fact that it is being included as a part into a new structure. Including sexual instinct into the system of personality does not resemble the inclusion of other instincts that mature earlier, for example, sucking, because the whole into the composition of which the new, maturing function is included is essentially different.

It remains for us to compare the appearance of instinct in the mind of the idiot and in the mind of a normal 14- to 15-year-old adolescent in order to see the difference in the maturing of this instinct in the one case and in the other. In the adolescent at the moment of maturing of the sexual instinct, there are a number of fine and complex functions established by the intellect and by habits. In this whole, instinct develops in a different way: everything is reflected in consciousness, everything is controlled by will, and sexual maturation proceeds as if from two ends—from above and from below—so that, as we have seen in a preceding chapter, E. Spranger[87] accepts both processes as two independent processes—to the degree that they are independent of each other. Actually, it is essentially a single process reflected in higher forms of consciousness and behavior of the individual.

Owing to the fact that the new system of tendencies that arises together with sexual maturation is complexly refracted and reflected in the thinking of the adolescent and acts in a complex connection with purposeful actions, it acquires a completely different character and enters, as a subordinate factor, into the function that we have called will. The decisive transition from complex thinking and the function of forming concepts, which we have discussed above, is a required precursor of this process.

8

If hysteria elucidates for us very clearly the process of will construction during the transitional age, then disintegration of the function of forming concepts, observed in hysteria in a somewhat less clear form, finds an extreme expression in another disease which is characterized by disturbance of the speech function and, for this reason, is called aphasia. In the expression of Sepp, the study of aphasia is the key to understanding the intellectual work of the cerebral cortex. From the point of view of psychology of the transitional age, of all the forms of this illness, of greatest interest is so-called amnesic aphasia, which is manifested in the patient's forgetting words that pertain to a number of objects and actions and producing the words with difficulty. Losing words may assume a quantitative expression; nevertheless the basic type of impairment of speech activity as observed in aphasia usually remains the same.

The essence of changes in amnesic aphasia may be expressed in one hypothesis: the pathological disturbance results in a disintegration of the complex unity that we call the function of forming concepts. The complex connection that exists at the base of this function evidently disintegrates, and because of this, the word drops to an earlier genetic level which the normal person has left behind before the period of sexual maturation. The aphasic makes a transition from thinking in concepts to complex thinking. Here, the most characteristic and essential trait of this disease is the trait that brings it close to the mental development of the adolescent according to the law of opposites and the reverse flow of processes.

Studies of amnesic aphasia done recently show that all of the various disturbances that are observed in this case are internally connected with each other and are parts of a single picture; at its base is one principal disturbance which causes disruption of thinking in concepts. Current studies show that the disturbance does not involve an isolated speech sphere or the sphere of concepts, but, in the expression of A. Gelb and K. Goldstein, pertains to the connection, still problematical, that exists between thinking and speech.

Specifically for this reason, aphasia is neither a pure disruption of the speech function nor a pure disturbance of thinking; the connection of the one and the other and their complex interrelations are disrupted. We could say that the stable, independent synthesis that develops in the thinking of the adolescent during the transition to forming concepts is damaged. Specifically for this reason, the study of aphasia has a great significance for the general problem of the relation between thinking and speech. Gelb and Goldstein studied the phenomena of amnesia connected with naming colors. The patient, forgetting names of colors as a result of a brain disease, but fully retaining the ability to distinguish between them, exhibits extremely curious changes in all his behavior with respect to colors.

We have here an experiment as if prepared by nature that shows what is changed in the thinking and behavior of a patient when he loses the ability to name colors. The patient frequently exhibits a transition to concrete-objective designations of color which are typical for normal adults in the sphere of olfaction and are observed in primitive peoples at an earlier stage of the development of their thinking. For example, the patient calls the color red of a certain shade, cherry; green, grassy; blue, violet; orange, the fruit; light blue, forget-me-not, etc. Here we see, as the authors note, a primitive method of verbal naming of colors characteristic for early stages of development of speech and thinking.

The following circumstance is especially interesting. The patient was able to select from a bundle of colored threads shades that corresponded to a given object. For each object, he unfailingly selected the color corresponding to it. But because he lacked the concept of color, he could not select a color that was somewhat similar to that of the object but only belonged to the same category. In our experiments, we observed how an aphasic in selecting extremely fine shades and tones of color refused to select a corresponding color when he saw no shade of that color before him. He was able to select precisely the same shade of red, but could not select red of a different shade and behaved much more concretely than a normal person.

For this reason, classification of colors and selection of different colors with respect to an identical basic range of shades presents an insoluble problem for this patient. Experiments show that the patient seems to lack the principle of grouping and that he always selects according to some present, concrete experience of similarity or connection. Gelb and Goldstein believe that perhaps this method of behavior could be designated as irrational, concrete-visual, biologically primitive, and more elemental. The authors characterize the difference between the behavior of the normal person and the aphasic in this situation as follows. In sorting colors, the normal person establishes a certain direction for his attention with the help of the instruction; according to the instruction, he considers only the sample (in terms of its basic color regardless of the intensity and purity in which the shade appears). He perceives each concrete color as a representative of a concept—red, yellow, blue. The colors relate to each other on the basis of their belonging to the same category, to one concept of the color red, but not on the basis of their concrete identity in experience. The authors call this behavior categorical behavior. It is curious that patients cannot voluntarily isolate any specific property of color just as they cannot direct their attention to any one thing for any time.

What is the essence of these diseases? The authors believe that in itself, the absence of the word cannot be considered as causing the difficulty in categorical relation to an object or making it impossible. But evidently, words themselves must lose something that they have in the normal state which makes it possible to use them in connection with a categorical relation.

From the following, the authors infer that in patients, words lost specifically that property. Patients know that colors have names familiar to them. But these names were converted for them into an empty sound and stopped being a sign of a concept for the patients. Categorical relations and the use of words in their significative meaning are expressions of one and the same basic type of behavior and cannot be considered as cause or effect of each other. Disrupting the basic type of behavior and, corresponding to it, dropping to a more primitive vital behavior are specifically the disruption that explains all separate symptoms observed in the patient.

Thus, we see that a consideration of aphasia compels the conclusion that thinking in concepts connected with speech is a single function in which no separate, independent action of concept and action of word can be distinguished. Specifically this unity is disrupted and disintegrates in aphasia. Comparative studies show that the word affects the threshold of perception of color and thus changes and alters the process of perception itself. The object is changed each time the patient previously says different names of colors and accidentally hits on a correct name.

These phenomena can be applied also to amnesic aphasia with respect to naming objects as a whole. All of these disruptions are internally connected to each other and can be reduced, as we have said, to difficulty in the area of categorical thinking. In amnesic aphasia, most striking is the fact that the aphasic forgets words relating specifically to concrete objects. In the opinion of A. Kussmaul, the more concrete the concept, the easier it is to lose the word that signifies it. Thus, disturbances evident in aphasia were usually considered as a transition from more concrete to more abstract designations.

This is undoubtedly a contradiction of the picture that we have just presented of the process that is just exactly the transition of the aphasic to a purely concrete method of perceiving and thinking.

A number of studies have shown that when the aphasic replaces concrete names with more general names, he has in mind not at all the relation of the given object to a certain group of objects, that is, not the concept, but a certain completely definite relation to the object that is expressed for the most part either in an indefinite expression, "thing," "little thing," "this," or in signifying an action done in connection with the object. The more or less general words that the aphasic uses for naming a concrete object do not serve to designate species or genus concepts. The experiment shows that words that have nothing abstract in intention can be used with an abstract meaning.

The authors quite justifiably compare this phenomenon to the fact well known in child psychology when a child assimilates a general word, "flower," for example, before the name of different kinds of flowers. It would be a mistake, however, to assume that by the word "flower," the child understands something common to all flowers. On the contrary, he has in mind something completely concrete. Stern emphasizes especially that at this stage, the child does not determine the application of separate words logically. Thus, it seems that common names can be applied without actually having anything general in mind.

In the life of the adult, we also frequently observe general expressions that pertain to completely specific and concrete objects. If we take this into account, we see that what occurs in the amnesic aphasic is also a general drop in thinking to a level more primitive, concrete, and close to reality. In excellent agreement with this is the fact that not all the speech activity of the aphasic is disrupted, that he can correctly select objects matching words he names, and, on the contrary, if a number of names are given for a familiar object, the aphasic will select the correct word so that in the opinion of the authors, this operation does not require in essence either understanding the word that is a sign of the concept or the categorical relation to the object itself.

We know from the history of the development of children's speech that words, long before they begin to represent concepts, can serve another function, specifically, they can be associatively connected with situations according to the principle of a syncretic image or a simple complex.

The basic disruption in aphasia consists not in that the patient forgets some words, but in that all words, including those that are retained, stop serving him as signs of concepts. The complex unity, which is the basis of the concept, and the complex of judgments, which is applied in it as a certain synthesis, disintegrate, and a complex system of connections that have never been established around the word that are its base, in its associative substratum, come to the foreground. In order to understand the role of complex thinking when the concept begins to disintegrate, we must recall the law of preservation of lower functions as a subordinate factor in higher functions and the emancipation of lower functions when the higher functions disintegrate or are damaged.

In the complex thinking of aphasics the same thing happens as with hypobulic mechanisms in hysterics. Both make up an early stage in the structure of higher complex functions and both are preserved as a substratum in a cryptic form, as an auxiliary subordinate factor in the composition of a single higher function. We all carry within us the mechanisms that appear in aphasia and in hysteria, but in us, they are a certain part of more complex mechanisms; in disease, they are isolated and begin to act according to their primitive laws.

Without an associative substratum, no theory of thinking is possible. A stage passed in development, such as complex thinking, does not disappear. Actually, where could connections established during the course of a child's life go? They lie at the base of other, higher units constructed over them. But the more elementary, lower connections are preserved even when the higher units of which they are a part disintegrate. Thus, the complex is maintained within the concept as its removed substratum. Thinking in concepts has its substratum in complex thinking. For this reason complex thinking is not a rudiment, not an accessory mechanism, but an internal component part of thinking in concepts. Isolation of this factor also occurs in aphasia. As Gelb and Goldstein believe, this phenomenon causes difficulty with categorical thinking or makes it impossible; it is not in itself simply not being able to find a word, but all words are lacking in something that they have in a normal state that makes them a means of categorical thinking.

On the basis of our observations, we are inclined to think that the base of this is the disintegration of complex unified structures that we call concepts and the dropping of the word to a genetically earlier function in which it was a sign of a complex or a family name. Specifically from this point of view, aphasia is an instructive example of development opposite to that which we observe during the transitional age. At that time, concepts are being constructed; in this case, they are disintegrating. There a transition is made from complex thinking to thinking in concepts; here—the opposite transition from thinking in concepts to complex thinking. In this sense, Gelb and Goldstein are entirely correct when they maintain unity of the function that suffers in aphasia and determine that this function is not purely intellectual, not purely a speech function, but a function generated by the connection of thinking and speech.

Thus, the genetic key to understanding the behavior of the aphasic is the assertion that his categorical thinking is disrupted and yields to a more primitive, genetically earlier stage of concrete-visual relation to reality. The word as a sign of a concept is converted into the word as a sign of a complex. From this all reality begins to be thought of in completely different systems of connections, in another relation that differs sharply from the ordered thinking in concepts.

Above we considered in detail what the transition from complex thinking to thinking in concepts means, and we could easily imagine what the reverse way of thinking, from concepts to complexes, would mean. For this reason, we need not consider in detail a description of the features of the aphasic's thinking. We shall only say that the features exhibit the basic patterns of complex thinking described and established above. We are interested in the following question: what is the nature of the process of the emancipation of more primitive layers of thinking, since that may give us the solution to understanding the nature of the development and structure of its higher layers.

Gelb and Goldstein believe with respect to the physiology corresponding to this form of behavior, that there is a basic function of the brain, about whose essence we can say scarcely anything definite. In general, we might discuss it only within the framework of the general theory of brain functions. Together with activation of the function, categorical thinking develops simultaneously with the word in its significative meaning. With damage to this function, naming, in the sense of a subordinate designation, and categorical behavior are disturbed in aphasia patients.

In this sense, the authors return again to the general formulation, saying that all disruptions observed in aphasia are internally connected with each other and are an expression of one and the same basic damage, which from the psychological aspect is characterized as difficulty in categorical behavior, and from the physiological aspect, as disruption of a certain basic brain function.

Here we were confronted for the first time by a serious contradiction of the representations of the nature of thinking in concepts at which we had arrived in the process of studying its development. On the basis of data on the development of this form of thinking, could we really think that the development of some kind of definite basic and single brain function that appears only during the transitional age lies at the base of the development of the concept? Neither the physiology of the brain nor the history of the development of children's thinking provides any kind of basis for such assumption.

At the time when striving to find the anatomical localization of all mental functions was dominant, C. Wernicke[88] assumed the existence of a special center for concepts, not strictly delineated, it is true, which the scientist divided into two parts: one, for the receptive images connected with the sensory field of speech, and the other, for purposeful representations connected with the field of motor projection. We have moved far from the time in psychoneurology when special centers were postulated, special organs for each mental function, when a parallelism was assumed between the structure of separate parts of the brain and the development of different functions, when W. Wundt placed the center of apperception in the frontal lobes, and when a primitive representation not corresponding to reality, seemingly separate functions of behavior, were developed by separate brain centers similarly to the way separate glands produce different secretions. A complex interweaving of functions, their complex structure, the appearance of new syntheses in the process of development, the development based on complex cooperation of centers and various physiological processes in the brain were not taken into account in this case. Now in science, there is a completely opposite position when the idea of such a crude localization has been abandoned, when, in the expression of K. Monakow,[89] the very fact of wishing to localize spatially a process that occurs in time seems to us to be self-contradictory.

Using this author's comparison, we might say that where a complex function is disrupted in the course of time, it is impossible to ask where this function is localized, just as one must not ask where a melody in a music box is localized. Ever greater significance is being attributed to the idea of chronogenic localization, which consists of a complex function being understood as an operation carried out by a number of mechanisms and segments of the brain acting in a certain sequence in an act and forming in their sequential flow a certain melody, a certain process that has its own configuration, structure, and patterns. In the expression of Monakow, a chronogenic synthesis develops that forms the base of every complex function.

From the point of view of the history of development and structure of higher functions, this representation seems to us singularly correct. In the process of development there occurs an integration of functions in the nervous system. Monakow says that the matter concerns the sequential appearance during phylogenesis and ontogenesis of different functions that find their chronogenic localization. For this reason it seems to us to be a mistake and a contradiction of the history of the development of function to assume a direct parallelism between the appearance of a new brain function and the formation of thinking in concepts, as Gelb does. In essence, this takes us back to parallelism, but not to anatomical, but to physiological parallelism. Must we assume that the basis of historical development of forms of behavior is the acquisition by the brain of new physiological functions? Of course, the human brain, having a ready inventory, did not produce thinking in concepts itself at primitive stages of development of humanity and the child; of course, there was a time when thinking in concepts was a form unknown to humanity. Even now, there are tribes that do not have this form of thinking. We ask, should we assume that they, like the aphasics, are suffering from a disturbance of the basic brain function?

We have tried to show that the development of higher historically developed forms of behavior occurs according to a type completely different from the development of elementary functions. For some authors, the main thing is that the significative function of the word is a basic physiological function. Thus, concept formation is excluded from cultural development. The concept is considered as a function of the brain, that is, a natural, eternal law. For us, a concept is a historical, not a biological category in the sense of the function that produces it. We know that primitive man had no concepts. In the aphasic, in the area of thinking the same thing occurs as in the primitive, that is, a drop to a lower level of cultural-historical development of behavior and not to what happens in an animal, that is, not a drop to a lower biological level. A return to archaic, old functions occurs here not according to a biological, but according to a historical ladder. It is understood that thinking in concepts has its correlate in brain functions, but this correlate consists in chronogenic synthesis, in a complex temporal combination and uniting of a number of functions that are basically characterized by two factors.

First, it is distinguished by its secondary and derivative quality. This means that development of brain functions does not in itself result in the appearance of chronogenic synthesis. The brain left to itself outside cultural development of the personality would never come to the development of this kind of combination of functions. Let us recall what was said above on the formation of logical forms of behavior. We saw that the logical figure in thinking is nothing other than forms of a person's practical inferences reflected and fixed in thinking. Thus, the historical development of human experience and historical development of human thinking

connected with it are the true source of the development of logical forms of thinking, the function of concept formation, and other higher mental functions. The brain
did not of itself generate logical thinking, but the brain assimilated the form of
logical thinking in the process of the historical development of man. For this, there
is no need to assume the existence of a special basic function in the brain. It is
enough to assume that in the structure of the brain and in the system of its basic
functions there are the possibilities, the conditions for the development and formation of higher syntheses.

It seems to us that we should think of the development of historically evolved
human functions specifically in such form—in phylogenesis and ontogenesis—since
we are considering the relation of these functions to the brain.

Second, what distinguishes chronogenic synthesis is what distinguishes the
parts, the sum of the elements from the whole, from the structure. From the point
of view of physiology, specifically not one basic brain function in the form of inhibition, stimulation, etc., but a multitude of various functions in a complex combination and union, in a complex temporal sequence, is the basis of concept
formation. But the patterns and properties that appear in the process of concept
formation may and must be derived not from the properties of these separate partial
processes, but from the properties of their synthesis as a single, independent whole.

We found profound confirmation of this in the fact that disruptions of behavior
in aphasics involve far from just the sphere of their thinking, but the youngest and
highest functions, the whole upper story of behavior. In this sense, we believe that
H. Head provides a functionally more correct definition of the disruptions that are
observed in aphasia. It is his opinion that the basis for these disruptions is damage
to the function that he calls the formulation and expression of symbols, understanding by these words a method of behavior in which the symbol—verbal or
other—is brought forward between the beginning of any act and its definite exe-
cution. This formula includes a multitude of methods of behavior that usually are
not considered as a form of speech behavior and must be established purely empirically.

J. Jackson has shown that in essence in aphasia, the potential for forming intentions and voluntary decisions is disrupted since these presume a preparatory
formulation of action in a symbolic form. The structure of a voluntary act is closely
connected to symbolic formulation. Jackson says that a preconception is present in
all voluntary operations—the act is generated before it is done. Before realization,
an act is as if preliminarily undertaken in a dream. In these acts there is a duality.
This is why voluntary acts also are disturbed in aphasia; the function of forming
intentions suffers just as does the function of forming concepts.

Head and other authors have shown that in aphasia, there is a complex disturbance not only of the intellect, but also of all of behavior as a whole, which
changes because of the disturbance of the function of forming concepts. Perception
drops to a more primitive level. The aphasic is much more a slave to his visual
field than a speaking person. Voluntary attention undergoes a complex change. According to Gelb, wherever we experience a disjunction in the definite direction of
attention elicited by the word, in the aphasic patient, there is a deviation from
normal conditions. He is dominated by concrete impressions and does not control
his attention. This is especially clearly evident in motor aphasia, in which isolating
parts of a certain intricate complex of impressions or executing some operation
that requires a sequential change of separate parts becomes extremely difficult.

Monakow says that the aphasic is not capable of so-called voluntary attention.
This is actually a substantial disruption. Memory in concepts is disrupted and drops
again to concrete memory that depends on direct impressions. Complex practical

action is also disrupted if it requires preliminary formulation of a plan and intention in concepts to be implemented.. So simple acts of imitation are possible for the patient when he copies the movements of the experimenter that he sees in a mirror. But when he has to copy these movements sitting opposite the experimenter, and thinks all the time of the necessity of transferring movements of right and left arms, he cannot carry out this operation since it requires preliminary formulation of intention and plan.

However, we believe that even this interpretation requires a substantial correction. The fact is that the aphasic does not at all exhibit a complete inability with respect to symbolic formulation. No, using signs, using the words that remain, he creates appropriate formulations, but only when these formulations do not require thinking in concepts. In this sense, we must remember the substantial difference pointed out by Gelb of which we spoke above. When the aphasic names an object presented, to him, this does not at all require categorical thinking on his part. This means that the word can be used with various meanings and by no means only as a sign of a concept. In the aphasic, those forms of behavior suffer that are connected with verbal formulation and depend on concepts. Words as signs of complexes are preserved, and thinking within limits and forms corresponding to this primitive stage is done more or less well.

Thus, the study of aphasia shows that our hypothesis regarding unity of all changes that occur in the psychology of the adolescent is fully confirmed in the history of the disintegration of these functions. We proposed that the development of such functions as perception, memory, attention, and action in their higher forms is derived from the development of the basic function—the formation of concepts.

Aphasia confirms that the disintegration of the function of forming concepts entails a drop of all functions to a more primitive stage. Not only thinking, but behavior as a whole, perception and memory, attention and actions of the aphasic, regress to the time that the adolescent left behind when he entered the period of sexual maturation. As Gelb says, the word makes man a man. It emancipates him from subordination to the situation and endows his perception and his action with freedom.

The aphasic pronounces any word when this is required by a comprehended situation, but he cannot do this when he must pronounce the named action voluntarily. Here are some simple examples. Gelb's patient, who could not remember the word "box" when he was shown this object, when asked what he did not know replied: "I don't know what the box is called." This case alone shows that the essence of the disease is not that representations of words are lost, but that the word loses some one of its functions, and that it is one of its higher functions.

Head's patient could use the words, "yes" and "no" as responses to a question, but he could not pronounce these words when he was asked to do so. During the experiment, he was asked to repeat the word, "no"; he shook his head negatively and said: "No, I can't do that." As Gelb says, instead of objects, for the aphasic there are operative states. His memory goes from memory in concepts and returns to memory of operative situations. This is most clearly expressed in experiments with classification of various objects.

The processes of classification suffer in aphasia. The patient has no principle of classification or relation of objects. For him, as for the primitive, an object in a different operative situation seems to be a different object. In classification, the patient simply reconstructs previous situations and supplements them, but does not classify objects according to a certain characteristic. He distributes various objects as being related to each other purely according to a concrete characteristic. Experiments with classification disclose more homogeneous complexes constructed for the most part on the basis of a collection or similarity of impression. Thus, the aphasic places the most varied metallic objects in one group and wooden objects, in another. He puts objects with each other in such a way that in each case there is some kind of concrete, factual association or similarity between the one and the other so that a group might include objects with various characteristics. For him, unity of connection is not required.

The second conclusion we might reach from the study of aphasics is that we again find a confirmation of our hypothesis on the genetic continuity of the concept and the complex. Just as in development we find a transition from the complex to the concept, in reverse development and disintegration, the path is from concept to complex. Genetic continuity of these two stages finds full confirmation in the study of aphasia.

Finally, the following: the essence of complex thinking and the nature of other intellectual functions that dropped to a more primitive level exhibit a similarity to the state of those same functions prior to the period of sexual maturation.

We might formulate our conclusion thus: in amnesic aphasia, the essence of the disruption consists not of the dropping out of individual words, but in a change in the method of using words as signs of a concept. This change is called disturbance of categorical thinking or symbolic formulation. The patient may lose very few words, but the disruption may reach very far, and vice versa. How does this happen? Complex combinations, unique in content and form, which are the base of the concept (systems of judgment, structure of traits), are disrupted, and since for every person, complex connections in ontogenesis precede concepts and are preserved within the concepts as a removed category, as a subordinate factor, complex thinking is emancipated and acts in the foreground. This is why hysteria and aphasia have a common mechanism. We see one pattern in various types of damage, one mechanism in a different form. This should not surprise us. We know, for example, that a symptom such as increased temperature is observed in various illnesses. The move to the foreground of complex thinking may be observed in the same way in various forms of neural diseases.

Traditional studies of aphasics and even newer attempts to study them suffer from a substantial inadequacy: because of formalism that is still dominant in this area, only disturbance of forms of manifestation of some functions or others is studied and, consequently, general changes in the content of experience, consciousness of reality, and consciousness of self of the personality are studied very little. Moreover, we have seen that consciousness of reality and consciousness of self of the personality also are based on external and internal experience systematized in concepts. For this reason, complex disintegration of experience of reality in itself, complex change of object and personal consciousness that accompany aphasia remain outside the field of study of the investigators. Here we find a predominance of functional over morphological analysis, oblivion with respect to unity of form and content, ignoring of the fact that thinking in concepts means not only a new step in the forms of thinking, but also a conquest of new areas in the content of thinking.

9

A similar, but reverse mistake is made by psychiatry, which finds itself under the exclusive dominance of morphological analysis of experience, forgets about the change in form, and is interested only in changes in consciousness of reality and in the consciousness of self of the personality. This one-sidedness is expressed in the classical teaching on schizophrenia, in the light of which the transitional age was frequently considered. As is known, on the basis of the fact that the pathology is an exaggerated norm, many pedologists compared the temperament of the adolescent as it appears in the transitional age with the schizophrenic temperament and thinking of a patient. There is no boundary between the normal and the abnormal.

Kretschmer says that people who for decades carried out their official responsibilities as eccentric and exceptional personalities may accidentally disclose that they hid within themselves fantastic and nonsensical ideas.

What is eccentricity and what is a nonsensical system?

Man changes especially openly during sexual maturation, and schizophrenia occurs predominantly during this period. Must we consider people who change greatly during this period as psychopathic personalities or never consider them as afflicted schizoids? During the period of sexual development, schizoid traits are found in full bloom. We do not know, however, whether, in mild cases, we are confronted by the development of schizophrenic psychosis, whether psychosis has already occurred, or, finally, whether this is all only a stormy and odd development of a schizoid personality. Kretschmer concludes that, of course, normal affects of the period of sexual development—timidity, awkwardness, sentimentality, emotional eccentricity—are closely related to certain traits of temperament in schizoids.

The situation arises when, in the expression of Kretschmer, we cannot identify the schizoid, when the boundaries between the normal and the afflicted are erased, when closely related traits of the schizoid temperament and the adolescent temperament appear. In the expression of one of the psychologists, it is not for nothing that schizophrenia was formerly called early or juvenile feeble-mindedness.

We also think that we can recognize certain essential traits in the psychology of the adolescent if we make a comparative study of them and similar traits of schizophrenia. But, as we have said, understanding the relation between the one and the other is substantially different from that which is presented in the traditional formulation of this problem.[90]

We are interested not in the relationship based on external similarity of the disease process and the process of development, but in what pertains to the essence of the matter, the very nature of the phenomena studied, the reversibility of the processes of development, which is observed in both cases. Just as aphasia was studied primarily from the aspect of disturbances of the function of forming concepts and not from the aspect of changes in consciousness of reality and consciousness of self of the personality, so was the study of schizophrenia limited to a description only of the content of thinking and consciousness. Morphological analysis was not accompanied by genetic and functional analysis.

Recently, attempts have been made to move to studying the connection that undoubtedly exists between the disruption in content of consciousness and disruption in activity of certain functions in schizophrenia. A comparison of functional and morphological analysis makes it possible for the first time to change the traditional presentation of the comparative study of the transitional age and schizophrenia to its direct opposite. The bridge for comparing morphological and functional analysis of thinking of schizophrenics, the transition from studying the content of their thinking to a study of its form is, in this case as in all other cases, the historical point of view, the method of genetic analysis that reveals the unity and mutual dependence in the development of form and content of thinking. It reveals in schizophrenia what we already found in hysteria and aphasia, specifically, the drop to a genetically more primitive level of development, regression, movement backward, reverse movement of the processes of development. Only in the light of this kind of understanding will we be able to approach one period or another of development and construction of the functions and their disintegration in general if we want to depend not on external, phenotypic similarity but on similarity that is internal, essential, rooted in the nature of the compared phenomena, in their relationship.

As an epigraph to the work on genetic analysis of schizophrenia, A. Storch (1922) takes the words of Carus, who says that to the extent that disintegrations of mental activity in disease are a reflection of diseases of the organism and develop more and more distinctly, it is possible to that extent to understand and identify the essence of the disease itself in its deepest significance, and, specifically, as a repetition of the special organic life in a form that is considered normal at lower levels of organic nature.

Storch tries to compare phenomenological and genetic analysis of the experience of schizophrenics. He is interested in the question of interrelations between schizophrenic and primitive-archaic thinking. The path to this research has been suggested repeatedly in the conclusion we presented: pathology is the key to understanding development, and development is the key to understanding pathology.

F. Nietzsche and S. Freud believed that in sleep and in dreams we again do the mental work of preceding humanity that is the basis on which the mind in each person developed and still continues to develop. Dreams transfer us to remote states of human culture and give us the means to understand those states better. These authors believe that dreams preserved for us an image of primitive and rejected work of the mental apparatus, rejected because of its inappropriateness. That which at one time dominated the wakeful state, when mental life was still young and inexperienced, has been as if exiled into the life of the night. This reminds us that in childhood we find long discarded, primitive tools of the adult person—the bow and arrow. K. Jung compared these views of dreams with the views of schizophrenic thinking. Jung assumes that if the dreamer spoke and acted like a wakeful person, we would have a picture of early feeble-mindedness. Storch also proceeds from the basic position that states that abnormal processes are primitive processes.

Traditional psychiatry usually studies schizophrenia from the aspect of changes in consciousness and personality. The investigator was interested in the first place in a number of changes in thinking, consciousness, and experiences of reality in patients, but these changes were taken primarily from the aspect of content. Experiences of the patient were subjected to morphological analysis; in the studies, functional and genetic analysis usually was not applied at all.

The special feature of the disease, as we know, is that a splitting of consciousness, a personality change, comes to the forefront, but the basic psychological functions (memory, perception, orientation) are preserved. Specifically this was the basis for ignoring the disintegration and change in forms of thinking, of intellectual functions, and turning directly toward analysis of delusion, split consciousness, and broken associations of the patient.

As we have indicated, in this respect, pedology followed the path opposite that of psychiatry and was satisfied with a simple comparison of the features of the schizothymic temperament with the temperament of the adolescent. Through Kretschmer, it announced that there are no boundaries between the turbulently occurring sexual maturation of the schizoid personality and the schizophrenic process, that the phenomena of sexual maturation and schizophrenic changes in the personality are related.

Just as in aphasia, the internal world of the patient—consciousness of reality and consciousness of self of the personality—was not studied, but only functions, only forms of thinking were studied, in this case, the opposite error was committed, but the one-sided approach to the phenomenon either from the aspect of form or from the aspect of content remained unchanged in principle. Only recently have we seen attempts to approach schizophrenia with the help of genetic and functional analysis. In the work of Storch, we see an attempt to compare the changes in the mind in schizophrenia to archaic-primitive thinking that was dominant at early stages of mental development. The basic conclusion that the author reaches in his study is that in schizophrenia, certain mental constants of developed consciousness disintegrate, for example, a precisely delineated consciousness of "I" and objective consciousness, and these are replaced by more primitive forms of experience, undifferentiated, aggregate complexes. More penetrating analysis showed that in schizophrenia, from the formal aspect, not all functions remain unchanged. Only elementary or lower functions remain relatively unchanged in the form of perception, orientation, and memory; the function of forming concepts suffers substantially in schizophrenia, specifically the function of maturation that constitutes the main content of intellectual development during the transitional age.

E. Bleuler (1927)[91] emphasized that the essential trait of schizophrenic thinking is the abundance of images and symbols. The tendency to represent experiences in a visual form is actually the distinguishing trait of this thinking. Because of its visual quality, primitive thinking appears close to pathological thinking. True, even in the thinking of the normal person there are some auxiliary devices in the form of visual diagrams that serve as support points for the thinking process, but they always have a significance only as a means of symbolic, visual representation.

Storch maintains that in schizophrenic thinking, on the other hand, the images fulfill not just the function of representation; rather we must assume that in the schizophrenic, consciousness may be wholly absent, that one image or another replaces or represents a certain idea. The schizophrenic is not conscious that a correlation exists here. In general, the formation of concepts in the schizophrenic is fed to a much greater extent by visual elements than the formation of concepts in ordinary thinking. This is one of the most essential differences between the formation of concepts in developed thinking and the formation of concepts at a primitive mental stage. Our developed concepts were liberated to a greater extent from the visual elements that were the basis for their development.

Storch continues: in our concepts, together with a visual foundation, there are more or less abstract elements of knowing and judgment. For the primitive formation of concepts, however, especially impressive visual traits were the key factors. Since consciousness of relations such as similarity and difference is still not completely developed, the child can unite in one concept things that have a direct visual interconnection if only in one common impressive trait. In precisely this way, concepts formed in schizophrenia are connected mainly from the visual and affective-active impression. Consciousness of connections and relations takes the background. One, single, general impressive trait is enough to unite the most varied representations.

A. Storch is fully justified in comparing this method of concept formation with the method that is dominant at the early stage of development in the child and in primitive man. Actually, we see that this author describes the formation of concepts in the schizophrenic in almost the same expressions in which we described the features of complex thinking in the child. The possibility of the historic point of view of schizophrenia, its genetic analysis, opens before us. We begin to understand the changed world experienced by the schizophrenic not simply as an unformed, chaotic mass of deluded ideas, without order, without any sense, without any structure, where segments, pieces of broken-up, disjointed thinking, are collected. We have before us not chaos, not a pile of broken glass, in the expression of one of the psychologists; we have before us a patterned move backward, a drop to a lower, more primitive stage in the development of thinking. This is regression, well known to us and consisting in that functions and forms of thinking, earlier in the history of development and actually preserved in the form of subordinate factors, are emancipated and begin to act according to their primitive laws when the higher unity in which they are included disintegrates.

The higher unities, or concepts, disintegrate in schizophrenia and complex thinking is emancipated which, as a substrate, always is preserved within concepts, and complex connections begin to control thinking. But since all consciousness of reality and all consciousness of one's own personality in a developed, normal person are represented in a system of concepts, it is natural that together with the disintegration and break-up of concepts, the whole system of consciousness of reality and the whole system of personal consciousness disintegrates. The changes in content of thinking are the direct result of the disruption and disintegration of the function of thinking.

We have said many times that not all content can be adequately accommodated in any form. Content is not indifferent to the form of thinking; it does not fill it purely in an external mechanical way as a liquid fills a vessel. Studying the development of the function of concept formation, we saw that the transition to a higher stage in mastering the new form of thinking opens to the adolescent new areas in the content of thinking also. These new areas are closed to the schizophrenic, and the content of his consciousness returns to the primitive complex system of connections that correspond to that form of thinking, and these connections cannot but seem to be confusion to a consciousness for which thinking in concepts is very proper. Confusion arises because such regression—transition to complex thinking—is never complete.

In the words of Storch, these patients live in a dual world: on the one hand, in a primeval world of visual images, magical connections and participations, and on the other hand, in a world of past, partly preserved thinking corresponding to experience. This is the source of the break-up in the consciousness of the schizophrenic, who accepts his primitive experiences as direct reality, then recognizes and considers them as fantastic reality. For this patient, the whole world and his own experiences disintegrate into two spheres. This is the source of the complex interweaving of old and new connections, and the source of the confusion, disjointedness, and disruption of associated thinking that is always noted as the most characteristic trait of schizophrenic thinking.

Capers, who spent much time on the anatomical study of schizophrenia, developed a hypothesis according to which the second, third, and fourth cortical layers of the brain, which carry out intracortical functions, are the most affected. He believes that this is the basis for the explanation of the origin of associative disjunction while perceptions, orientation, and memory are retained, that is, a central disruption is primary in the mind of the schizophrenic. In the light of his hypothesis, the author considers this disease as anatomical regression. He believes that an anatomically reverse course of the history of the brain leads also to psychological regression and a return to archaic, primitive thinking and behavior. From his point of view, the predominance in mental schizophrenia of elements of this kind of thinking can be explained by damage to those segments of the cortex that develop later in onto- and phylogenesis and are carriers of higher, later intellectual functions. This is why in schizophrenia, the attitude to the surrounding world changes wholly, and more primitive forms of thinking are brought forth.

The historical view of schizophrenia, as we see, is confirmed in both anatomical and psychological analysis. It is understood that the essence of schizophrenia is not exhausted by this, but the essence of the mechanisms of thinking that come forward in schizophrenia is disclosed quite clearly. We tried to define the essence of the disease as an emancipation and coming to the foreground of the complex forms of thinking that were preserved as a substrate when the synthetic unities that we call concepts disintegrate. The transition from thinking in concepts to complex thinking is the central cause of all the changes in the content of consciousness and thinking of the schizophrenic. We explained above how damage to the function of concept formation disrupts all the systems of experience of reality and self-consciousness of the personality and how confusion and break-up of consciousness arises.

The self-recognition of schizophrenics confirms the indeterminate character of this thinking. A 24-year-old schizophrenic teacher complains: "My thoughts are so diffuse, everything is so unstable, for me nothing is definite, everything is so unclear, so impregnated with emotion. Everything merges for me, one object turns into another, as in a dream, I cannot concentrate on anything." Such undifferentiated, aggregate complexes are found also in the animal world and in the normal person in his peripheral perceptions. Here moments of perceptions of various elements and emotional moments are tightly fused with one another in one mental amalgam.

As an analogy to this confused, indeterminate thinking of the schizophrenic, A. Storch cites the diffuse, merged physical and emotional factors in the feeling of cold and refers to the work of Volkelt, who in a study of ideas of animals, showed that the ideas of some groups of animals, for example, spiders, have no objective character. The basic traits of objectivity, dependence, closure, articulation, and shape are absent in their perception. Their perceptions are not shaped, are without structure, and are diffuse: they are similar to emotions.

As we know from the experiments of Volkelt, the spider watching for a fly, reacts to its appearance only when the whole complex of stimuli connected with catching the prey develop. When the fly begins to buzz and shake the spider web, the reaction of the spider to this situation is quite adequate, but when the investigator, using tweezers, takes the fly caught in the spider web and places it directly in front of the spider, the hungry spider seems to fail to recognize his prey, moves away from it, and never carries out in a more direct way what he otherwise usually does. The fly outside the situation, taken out of the spider web, separated from the diffuse complex of impressions in which it is usually included, stops being a stimulus—food for the spider. For the spider, the fly is not an object, but is an entire operative situation as a whole of which the fly is only a part. Taken out of the situation, it loses its sense, its meaning.

Volkelt's experiments brilliantly confirmed the point made above that consciousness of a stable and shaped object develops relatively late and mainly in connection with the word, and that perception at primitive stages pertains not so much to the object in the sense in which we understand the word with respect to the thinking of man, as with consciousness of operative situations.

Only the word leads us to objective thinking and consciousness. This idea does not seem at all new for those who study schizophrenia. Comparing schizophrenic thinking with archaic-primitive forms of thinking and creating a conception of the archaic mind of the schizophrenic belongs to the psychoanalytical school. We have already cited the opinion of Jung that if a dreamer walked along the street, talking and acting, we would have before us a clinical picture of schizophrenia. In his last paper on this question, on the basis of analysis of motor manifestations in schizophrenia, I. P. Pavlov (1930) also compares these phenomena with hypnosis from the physiological aspect and with the diffusion of internal inhibition, which plays a decisive role in dreams also.

We believe that a serious mistake was made here. It is not that ancient forms of thinking are comparable to forms of thinking in schizophrenia, but that the authors leap over a number of historical stages in the development of thinking. They forget that between the thinking of the spider and thinking in concepts, between thinking in dreams and the abstract-logical thinking of modern man, between thinking in hypnosis and purposeful thinking in a normal state, there are a number of historical stages that fill the process of the development of this function. The polar points come together here. From the last link of the historical chain of development of thinking, a transition is made instantly to its initial link, and all the intermediate links are omitted. Moreover, if we consider primitive man, we will note that his thinking least of all resembles thinking in dreams. In the process of thinking, the primitive man adapts to external nature and to the social environment. Thinking occurs according to laws other than dreaming, and besides, it is not really thinking in concepts. Precisely so does the thinking of the child at various stages of development differ sharply from the thinking of the spider or thinking in dreams. It still is not thinking in concepts. Thus, there is no basis for assuming that with the disintegration of concepts, there is a sliding at once to the very bottom, to the very depths of historical development, to its initial forms.

It is sufficient to assume (and facts support the assumption) that the schizophrenic makes a transition to the closest genetic stage in thinking, specifically to complex thinking. But here again we fall under the spell of a word with a double meaning. The word "complex" has so many meanings and is used with such varied meanings in modern psychology that the danger develops of leaping over a number of important stages in the history of the development of thinking. Actually, if we call the thinking of the spider described above complex thinking and if we describe the thinking of the child before the beginning of sexual maturation with the same words, we consider two very different things as being identical and ourselves follow the path of complex thinking. A number of investigators make this same error.

For them, archaic means initial, all stages of historical development of thinking merge into one for them. They forget the substantial difference between thinking done with the help of the word and the nonverbal thinking of animals. The logic of the one thinking and the other is completely different. For this reason, we can understand that schizophrenia must be compared not with the nonverbal thinking of the spider or the nonverbal thinking in dreams, but with complex thinking based on a unique use of words as characteristic names for similar groups of objects. Only by introducing this correction will we be able to find the historically correct place and the correct point of support for comparing the diseased with the primitive forms of thinking.

Storch's second error is that in genetic analysis also, he mainly follows the path of analysis of the content of concepts. He successfully supplements morphological analysis with genetic analysis, but he lacks functional analysis. For this reason, the changes of which he speaks seem to us to be unfounded, incomprehensible, internally unconnected and problematical, as they have always seemed. Actually, how can we explain the fact that in the sphere of undisturbed mental functions, perception, orientation, and memory are preserved, the method of action, state, and structure of basic forms of thinking remain unchanged, but the content represented in concepts changes so sharply and profoundly? The psychological picture is completely confused and problematical.

Only an assumption of primary damage to the function itself of concept formation (isolation and emancipation of older mechanisms included in it) followed by disintegration of the complex synthesis that developed relatively late in developmental history introduces comprehension and clarity into the whole picture. We have seen that concept formation develops when all elementary mental functions are mature and that the function of concept formation does not occupy a position beside them, but above them and represents their complex and unique combination.

For this reason, it is quite understandable that with the disintegration of this higher unity, all the elementary mental functions may be preserved and an impression may develop of an undamaged, not disintegrated functional system of thinking as in aphasia. Of course, the legend persisted for a long time in psychology that thinking in aphasia remains untouched. Upon examination, it develops that such functions as perception and memory in schizophrenics do not remain untouched. Their higher development, which we elucidated earlier and which is carried out under the controlling effect of the function of concept formation, also exhibits a reverse movement, a reverse course in schizophrenia. Perception in concepts, like memory in concepts, disintegrates and yields to earlier, more primitive forms of perception and memory.

We see evidence of this in that in the schizophrenic, not only the content of separate concepts changes, not only separate connections are disrupted, but all perceptions of reality, all experiences of the external world are disturbed. We said above that for the adolescent, only with the transition to thinking in concepts does a systematized picture of the world that surrounds him develop. In the schizophrenic, his experience of the world, his world perception, is disturbed.

Storch briefly formulates his conclusions regarding the modified structure of the schizophrenic objective consciousness. For the schizophrenic, the objective world in many cases is not objectively shaped as it is for us. The world of internal experiences is ordered for him corresponding to a relatively isolated groups of ideas. Certain concepts are replaced by visual, diffuse, complex qualities analogous to concepts. The schizophrenic lacks mental constants that make possible the development of strictly defined complexes of people and things, conclusive groups of experiences, and formation of precise concepts. Objective consciousness loses shape and stability. According to the thinking of Storch, from the point of view of developmental psychology, it drops to an earlier stage of complex qualities.

This is a fact of paramount importance. It speaks with indisputable clarity of the fact that the very consciousness of reality is changed, and this means that the function of perception is also changed. Exactly as in the schizophrenic the experience of the world is changed, his consciousness of self is also changed. In schizophrenia, the experience of the break-up of the "I" into separate partial components is observed extremely frequently, and a similarity to more primitive stages in the development of the personality is exhibited.

As studies show, in primitive man, his "I," the personality, is not yet as definitive as it is in the developed man. The personality consists of separate heterogeneous components that have not yet merged into a single whole. For the primitive man, the "I" coincides more or less with the idea of the body made up of separate parts and organs and of the forces and spirits assumed to be in it. Karutz believes that primitive man is more conscious of the function of the organs, of the eyes, the sexual apparatus, etc., than he is of the unity of his personality. The mind of the body is not disjointed into the minds of the organs, but the emanations of the organs are merged into an emanation of the organism. The idea of multiple minds in one individual is quite widespread among primitive peoples.

In the schizophrenic, the "I" frequently exhibits the primitive structure of a complex of partial components not united into a single whole. The return to a more primitive-structure "I" is exhibited not only in the break-up of the personality into separate parts, but also in the loss of boundaries between the "I" and the external world. The break-up of consciousness of reality goes in parallel with the break-up of consciousness of the personality. Both are experienced together and have an internal connection.

Storch believes that the patterns that he established for objective consciousness and for consciousness of the "I" are parallel to each other. The potential for the merging between the "I" and the external world is based on an inadequate development and an inadequate stability and closure, which distinguish the primitive consciousness of the "I" as opposed to the consciousness of the "I" in developed man.

The schizophrenic teacher, whose statements we mentioned, complains that he is in a sexual union with a girl who is at a great distance from him. He says that this girl was Eve to his Adam, but at the same time, he was also the serpent and exhibited this by always walking in sinuous lines and circles. At the same time, he knew that he was himself. Of course, everyone knows something more about himself. But he, obviously, was Eve also. This is evident from the fact that he felt a jab in his heart that meant a pain in the uterus. He added that all of this seemed unclear to him, as if instinctive, in the form of a feeling.

The loss of unity of the personality corresponds completely to the loss of unity of the external world. The one and the other is rooted in the disintegration of the function of concept formation and in the transition to complex thinking. That this complex thinking differs substantially from the thinking of the spider can be seen in the examples of Tuczek, who published an analysis of the phenomena of speech confusion in catatonia. The patient called a bird "the song," summer, "the heat," the cellar, "the spider," or "the breaking-up" (a cobweb is easily broken). In all these cases, the replacement words are signs for complex thinking for which parts of a whole are not yet differentiated traits, for which the actual connection between the spider and the cellar, between the bird and the song make it possible to classify them in one and the same complex. This pattern in language reaches such a degree that the investigator learns to understand the patient as a whole, and each separate word, when he unravels the complex connections that form its base.

Speech, seeming a delusion from the point of view of thinking in concepts, becomes clear and comprehensible when we understand the complex significance of the word. Understanding is especially difficult because the actual connection that is the base of the complex is sometimes hidden and can be disclosed only when we establish the concrete experience that actually forms the basis of the given designation and placing of a given object in a complex. An especially odd obviousness is exhibited in Tuczek's patient when he replaces the word "doctor" with the word "the dance," because during his visit, the doctor "dances" around the professor.

In Werner's words, what we observe here is only an extreme expression of verbal replacements and symptomatic metaphors, which we observe in children's thinking and in the thinking of primitive man. For example, a crocodile is called "rare teeth" in some primitive tribes, and the word "debt" is replaced by the word "yellow" with which it is connected by the auxiliary concept "gold." Tuczek himself called attention to the similarity between the speech of the child and speech in dreams and the coded speech of the patient.

Summarizing our consideration of schizophrenia, we can refer to Storch. He believes that as in the area of objective consciousness, in the schizophrenic the abnormality is based on the loss of the stable elements that provide differentiation, shaping, and a definite structure to the picture of the world for the developed man, so in the area of personal experiences the schizophrenic experiences a similar loss of stability in the sense of the "I." In the first case, nondifferentiated visual complex qualities replace the world of shaped things and other concepts, and in the second, the definitive sense of the "I" takes up a complex coexistence of its partial components and the elimination of the boundaries of the "I" which makes possible the various, diffuse merges and participations with other individuals.

To the words of Storch, from our point of view, we must add one very important point: the disruption of the function of concept formation is the basis for the break-up of the consciousness of reality, of the experience of the picture of the world and the sense of self. This assertion contains the basic and central idea of all the comparative study of schizophrenia in connection with the psychology of the transitional age.

We see that schizophrenic thinking presents a picture of reverse development of the process whose direct development we studied in the psychology of the adolescent. What develops there is disrupted here. Comparing the structure and disruption of one and the same function, we confirm the real genetic connection between the two stages of the construction of thinking—complex thinking and thinking in concepts. Schizophrenic thinking when concepts disintegrate drops to the stage of complex thinking, which serves as a direct confirmation of the genetic connections of these two stages, which we established in our analysis in the study of the development of concepts.

Further, we find a confirmation of the position that the new form of thinking is also connected with new content, and the disintegration of this form leads to the disintegration of ordered consciousness of reality and of personality.

But most important is the following conclusion that we can make on the basis of a comparative study of direct and reverse processes of development: the function of concept formation is connected not only with the development of other functions—memory, attention, perception of reality—as we have shown above, but also with the development of personality and world view. An integrated picture of the world and an integrated picture of a consciousness of personality disintegrate together with the loss of the function of concept formation.

It would be a mistake to assume that such patients return completely to prelogical thinking, just as it would be a mistake to think that a normal, educated person would make all of his thoughts completely logical. Storch says that patients of this kind live in a *dual world*; on the one hand, in a primitive world of visual images, magical connections and participations, and on the other hand, in a world of their former, still partially preserved thinking corresponding to experience.

But the former thinking—thinking in concepts—ceases to be the dominant form, together with the disintegration of the function of concept formation and consciousness of reality reflected in the system of concepts, in the system of logical connections and consciousness of personality, which also is developed on the basis of thinking in concepts. As in development, so also in disintegration, thinking is the central, leading function.

Storch assumes that in schizophrenics, as a result of the disease process, there is a *weakening of the intellectual superstructure*, "the higher cerebral function" (Groos), the higher intentional sphere (Berze, A. Kronfeld); as a result of this weakness, the synthesis of *mental functions into a single, definitive personality* is disrupted. Wernicke has spoken of the destruction of the merging of all higher connections into a certain unity, into an "I," of the disintegration of individuality. According to Stern, the loss of stability and definiteness in the structure of things, the disintegration of the consciousness of the "I," and the elimination of boundaries of the "I"—such is the phenomenological expression of the basic dynamic disruption.

Reiss expresses the same idea of the central significance of the disintegration of the function of concept formation in schizophrenia and of the connection between this disintegration and the disintegration of the activity of the will and the consciousness of the personality, and the changes in affective life caused by the disease; he places this dependence at the base of the *theory* of schizophrenic disruption of thinking. He maintains that the disintegration in schizophrenic thinking is based on disruption of the logical superstructure, which includes—together with abstract thinking—the function of combining affects and creating unity of personality, the functioning of which is connected with activity of the will. If tendencies that emerge from the unconscious are not subjected to this action, but also penetrate into consciousness, we have before us schizophrenic break-up. Berze, who made a special study of the psychology of schizophrenia, also points to the development of inadequacy of the intentional function and to the absence of uniting tendencies into a relatively stable system.

Thus, schizophrenia opens before us a picture of disintegration of those higher syntheses, the higher unities, the structure and formation of which make up the main content of the whole process of mental development during the transitional age. All higher mental functions—logical memory, voluntary attention, processes of the will—take essentially *one and the same* historical path in the process of maturation of the adolescent and in the process of schizophrenic disintegration, but in opposite directions. In schizophrenia, all higher functions, all higher psychological syntheses, including consciousness of reality and consciousness of self of the personality, follow a reverse path, and this path *repeats* in reverse order the whole path of direct development and construction of the syntheses during sexual maturation.

Coincidence in composition, structure, sequence, and interdependence of functions in the processes of development and disintegration belongs to the number of the most astonishing, most remarkable facts established by modern psychoneurology on the basis of comparative-genetic study of the normal and the pathological personality. In both the one and the other, at the center of the disintegration and construction of the personality stands the function of concept formation. In this sense, schizophrenia helps us understand *the whole* psychology of the transitional age, just as the transitional age provides a key to the understanding of the psychology of schizophrenia, but not in the old sense of comparing processes of construction and disintegration of the personality on the basis of external resemblance and similarity in a number of secondary symptoms, but in the sense of relatedness of the mental nature, the connections and interdependencies of the higher functions of the personality in diametrically opposed processes of development and dissociation. The disintegration of a complex whole uncovers and discloses the laws of its construction, just as the history of the construction of the whole predetermines the laws of its disintegration. In this lies the *greatest* theoretical significance of the study of schizophrenia for pedology of the transitional age.

10

We have tried above to disclose the internal dependence of these two series of phenomena and perhaps, what is most important, what the study of schizophrenia provides for us—the discovery of the internal connection that exists between thinking in concepts and the personality and world view—the higher syntheses that develop during the transitional age. In this sense, the significance of schizophrenia for the understanding of common patterns of the construction of the personality goes far beyond the limits of the study of this form of disease and takes on a great significance for general psychology. We can join K. Schneider (1930), who in the study of speech and thinking of schizophrenics was convinced that schizophrenia is a psychopathological concept and not a medical-diagnostic concept. It is more likely that it encompasses a certain type of pathological changes in the personality and world view than a definite form of mental illness, a certain nosological unity, a definite clinical picture. Together with this, we obtain the key to the pre-eminent and most difficult problem of the transitional age—to understanding the development of personality and world view and their internal connection with the function of concept formation.

That which disintegrates in schizophrenia arises and develops during the transitional age. This is how we might summarize the basic relations between the series of phenomena that we discovered. The function of concept formation, maturing during the transitional age, leads not only to a change in all the functional apparatus of thinking, as has been shown above, not only to a change in the whole content of thinking, but also to the construction of the personality and world view—the higher syntheses that first appear during the period of sexual maturation.

"The formation of (abstract) concepts and operating with them *already* includes in itself the idea, the conviction, the *consciousness* of the regularity of the objective connection of the world," states V. I. Lenin in notes to Hegel's *The Science of Logic.* "It is preposterous to take causality out of this bond. It is impossible to deny the objective quality of concepts, the objective quality of the general in the separate and in the particular. Hegel is more profound and consistent than Kant and others in tracing the reflection of the movement of the objective world in the movement of concepts. As a simple form of cost, the separate act of exchange of one given piece of merchandise for another already includes in itself in an unexpanded form *all* the main contradictions of capitalism—in the same way the simple *generalization*, the first and simplest formation of a *concept* (judgment, conclusion, etc.) signifies the man's recognition of an ever more profound *objective* connection of the world. Here we must seek the true sense, the significance and role of Hegelian Logic. . ." (*Complete Collected Works*, Vol. 29, pp 160-161).

Thus, the concept brings with it for the first time a recognition of reality in the true sense of that word because it suggests a pattern of the phenomenon being recognized. The concept in reality takes the child from the stage of experiencing to the stage of cognition. For this reason, only with the transition to thinking in concepts does the definitive separation and development of the personality and world view of the child occur.

One of the basic and most important general conclusions of the work of Piaget is the idea that the difference between thinking and the external world is not innate in the child, but develops and is constituted slowly. In the very beginning of development, as Piaget's experiments show, the child still does not distinguish his own movements from the movements that occur in the outside world and reacts to both in exactly the same way. At the last stages of separating himself from the surrounding world, the child develops true relations to the environment gradually through a number of stages qualitatively different from each other in the development of consciousness of his personality and its unity on the one hand, and in the development of consciousness of [outward] reality and its unity on the other hand.

We call these two syntheses that arise in the thinking of the child personality and world view.

The child only gradually arrives at the formation of these syntheses and specifically only in connection with the formation of concepts does this become possible. "Instinctive man, the savage, does not separate himself from nature," says Lenin. "Conscious man does separate . . ." (*Complete Collected Works*, Vol. 29, p. 85). Some modern investigators conclude that consciousness is impossible without thinking in concepts. In any case, there is no doubt about one thing—without thinking in concepts, consciousness is impossible in man.

If we try to trace the steps of development during the transitional age, how the personality and world view are put together and constructed, we will see that on the basis of the changes in forms and content of thinking that we described above, on the basis of the transition to thinking in concepts, the bases of personality are established in the child.

We recall that internal speech is shaped definitively and socialized during the transitional age, that introspection is still only slightly accessible to the child of early school age, that logical thinking only develops in the child when he begins to be conscious of external processes and to control them, that the basis of logical thinking is the mastery of his own internal operations, completely analogous to the mastery of external movements that develops in the child quite early. Because of this, a systematized, ordered world of external consciousness of the personality also develops, as does the special form of need that we call free will.

Engels says: "Hegel was the first to present correctly the correlation of will and necessity. For him, freedom is recognition of necessity. *'Necessity is blind only to the extent that it is not understood.'* Freedom does not consist of an imagined independence of laws of nature, but in recognizing those laws and in the possibility based on this knowledge of systematically setting into motion the laws of nature to act toward a certain purpose. This refers both to laws of external nature and to laws that govern the bodily and spiritual life of man himself—two classes of laws which we can separate one from the other is the greatest thing in our ideas, but not at all in reality" (K. Marx and F. Engels, *Works*, Vol. 20, p. 116).

Even in this definition, we see to what extent the development of freedom of will is connected with thinking in concepts because only the concept raises cognition of reality from the stage of experience to the stage of understanding patterns. And only this understanding of necessity, that is, pattern, is the basis of freedom of the will. Necessity becomes freedom through understanding.

Hegel expressed this beautifully when he said that it is wrong to consider freedom and necessity as mutually exclusive. It is true that necessity as such is not yet freedom, but freedom has necessity as its precursor and contains it within itself as a release. Without the function of concept formation, there is no recognition of necessity and consequently, no freedom. Only in the concept and through the concept does man acquire a free relation to things and to himself.

Engels says: "Freedom, therefore, consists in the management of ourselves and of external nature based on recognizing the necessities of nature (*Naturnotwendigkeiten*); for this reason it is a necessary product of historical development. The people who first emerged from the animal kingdom were on the whole no more free than the animals themselves; but each step forward along the path of culture was a step toward freedom" (ibid.).

Categorical thinking develops precisely at that time. In the words of Gelb, for the adolescent, the world develops in place of the environment that existed for the child. The adolescent enters into the inheritance of the spiritual experience of all of mankind, the bases of world view are established in him, in the expression of J.-J. Rousseau who said that man is born twice: first to exist, and then to continue the genus, which pertains to the time of sexual maturation; and he justifies himself in application to both psychological and cultural development of the adolescent. Only here, at this juncture, does the adolescent actually begin to continue the life of mankind, the life of the genus.

In this sense, the distinction between the child and the adolescent may be expressed best of all in the statement of Hegel, who drew a distinction between things in themselves and things for themselves. He said that all things are at first in themselves, but the matter does not stop there, and in the process of development, the thing turns into a thing for itself. Thus, he said, man in himself is a child whose task is not to remain in that abstract and undeveloped "in himself," but in becoming also for himself what he is thus far only in himself, specifically, to become a free and rational being.

This is the conversion of the child from a man in himself into an adolescent—a man for himself—and this makes up the principal content of the whole crisis of the transitional age. This is the time of maturation of the personality and world view, the time of higher syntheses on the basis of the crisis of becoming, and maturation of those higher formations that are the foundation of the whole conscious existence of man. But we will speak of this at the conclusion of the whole course, in the chapter in which we will consider the dynamics and structure of the adolescent's personality.

Chapter 4
IMAGINATION AND CREATIVITY IN THE ADOLESCENT[92]

1

E. Cassirer (1928) tells of a patient with complex disturbances of higher intellectual functions whom he observed in a Frankfurt neurological institute. This patient could previously repeat a phrase he heard with no difficulty, but could now relate only real situations that matched his own concrete, sensory experience. One time during a visit in clear and bright weather, he was asked to repeat the sentence, "The weather today is bad and rainy." He could not do this. The first words were pronounced easily and confidently, then the patient became confused, stopped and could not finish the sentence as it was said to him. He always made a transition to another form that agreed with reality.

In the same institute, another patient, suffering from serious paralysis of the entire right side of his body, could not move his right hand; he was unable to repeat the sentence, "I can write very well with my right hand." Every time, in place of the word "right," which was false for him, he invariably used the correct word, "left."

Patients who suffer from a complex disturbance of other higher mental functions that are constructed on the basis of speech and thinking in concepts display very clearly complete dependence on direct concrete perceptions. One such patient was able to use objects of daily life properly when he came upon them in usual circumstances and under usual conditions, but he could not do so when the circumstances changed. During dinner, he used a spoon and a glass like a normal person, but at other times, he did things with these implements that were completely senseless. Another patient who could not pour himself a glass of water when told to do so, did this very well when he was motivated by thirst.

In all these cases, the complete dependence of behavior, thinking, perception and action on the concrete situation is obvious. This dependence is exhibited with precise regularity every time the higher mental functions are disrupted, when the mechanism of thinking in concepts is disturbed and a genetically older mechanism of concrete thinking replaces it.

What we have in these cases in a clear and sharp form, seemingly ultimate in expression, can be considered as the complete antithesis of fantasy and creativity. Should we want to find a form of behavior that would contain in itself absolutely no elements of imagination and creativity, we would have to point to the examples we have just given. A person who is able to pour himself a glass of water from a bottle when he is moved by thirst but cannot carry out the same operation at other times, a person who cannot say that the weather is bad when it is good—all of this shows us much that is important and essential in understanding what lies at the base of fantasy and creativity and what connects these with the higher mental functions that are disturbed and disrupted in this case.

We could say that the behavior of the patients strikes us mainly as not being free. A person cannot do anything that he is not moved to do by a concrete situation. To create a situation, change its appearance, to be free of the direct influence of external and internal stimuli is beyond his capability.

As we have already said, pathological cases are interesting for us because they illuminate the same patterns that occur in the normal development of behavior. Pathology is the key to understanding development and development is the key to understanding pathological changes. In precisely the same way, we can find the same zero point of imagination and creativity in the process of the development of behavior in the young child and in primitive man. Both are at the stage of development at which the mechanism of lack of freedom and complete dependence of behavior on the concrete situation, complete determination of behavior by the external environment, complete connection with stimuli present is normal, a mechanism that serves as a manifestation of disease in the cases cited above.

K. Lewin, who recently performed a number of studies of the process of forming intention, calls attention to the very interesting problem of the possibility of forming any intention. Lewin thinks it curious that a person has unusual freedom to carry out any, even senseless, intended actions. This freedom is characteristic for the cultured person. For children and probably for primitives also, it is accessible to an immeasurably lesser degree and probably distinguishes man from animals close to him to a much greater degree than does his higher intellect. This difference probably coincides with the problem of mastering one's own behavior. The behavior of the patients we spoke of is striking specifically because of their inability to form any intentions. Not without reason is this phenomenon found most often in disruption of the higher mental functions that are based on thinking in concepts. This is especially clearly manifested in aphasia, that is, in the disease consisting of disruptions of speech activity and thinking in concepts.

In our studies, we observed how patients like these meet with difficulties they cannot solve: when they are asked to do something, say something, draw something, they ask each time to be told what to do, what to say; otherwise they cannot cope with the task. It is precisely so when an aphasic is asked to do something that he can begin from either end; the problem is insoluble for him, as H. Head noted, because the aphasic cannot find the departure point and he does not know where to start. The point must be selected voluntarily and this is his main difficulty. In our experiments we repeatedly observed how difficult it was for some aphasics to repeat a sentence that contained something that was not true from the point of view of a concrete impression, a confirmation.

Thus, the patient would repeat without error dozens of sentences, but could not repeat the sentence, "Snow is black." He could not succeed in this task regardless of multiple promptings on the part of the experimenter.

The patient experiences these kinds of difficulties when, in response to a given word, he must contradict what the given thing is or what it does. The aphasic deals easily with the opposite task if he is allowed to formulate his response in the following way: "Snow is not black." But simply to name a color that is not right, a property or action that is not true, is a task that exceeds his ability. Even harder for the aphasic is naming incorrect colors or action when looking at a concrete object of a different color or an object that is meant for another action. To transpose properties of things, to replace some with others, to combine properties and actions, is an impossible task for the patient. He is firmly and stably connected to the concretely perceived situation and cannot escape it.

We have spoken of the fact that thinking in concepts is connected with freedom and intention of actions. A. Gelb formulates this same idea paradoxically, but completely correctly when he recalls the statement of J. Herder that the language of thinking is a free language. Gelb carries this idea further, saying that only man is capable of doing something senseless. This is absolutely true. An animal cannot do anything senseless from the point of view of the concrete situation or operation. An animal does only what he is moved to do by internal prompting or external stimuli. Doing what is voluntary, intentional, free, senseless from the point of view of the situation is impossible for the animal.

We note in passing that in philosophical arguments on freedom of the will and in ordinary thinking our ability to do something senseless, absolutely unnecessary, not elicited by either the external or internal situation, has long been considered as the clearest manifestation of voluntariness of intention and freedom of an action carried out. For this reason, the incapacity of the aphasic for senseless action also indicates manifestation of his incapacity for free action.

We believe that the examples presented are quite enough for elucidating the simple idea that imagination and creativity connected with free processing of elements of experience and with their free combination absolutely require as a precursor the internal freedom of thinking, action, and cognition that can be attained only by one who has already mastered the formation of concepts. Not without reason do imagination and creativity drop to zero with the disturbance of this function.

2

We intentionally used this small psychopathological digression as a preface to the consideration of fantasy and creativity in the transitional age. We were guided by the desire to stress clearly and sharply from the very outset that in the light of our personal understanding of the psychology of the adolescent, this problem takes on an entirely new formulation opposite to that which might be considered traditional and generally accepted in the pedology of the transitional age.

The traditional point of view considers this function as the central, leading function of the mental development of the adolescent, it moves imagination to the forefront as characterizing all of the intellectual life of the adolescent. The traditional point of view attempts to subordinate all the other factors in the behavior of the adolescent to this basic function, assuming it to be the primary and independent manifestation of fundamental and dominant factors of the whole psychology of sexual maturation. This is not just an erroneous distortion of proportion and an erroneous representation of the structure of all intellectual functions of the adolescent, but the process itself of imagination and creativity in the transitional age is given a false interpretation.

The false interpretation of fantasy consists in the fact that it is considered from one aspect alone, as a function connected with emotional life, with life of drives and attitudes; its other aspect, related to intellectual life, remains in the shadow. Moreover, according to the valid observation of A. S. Pushkin, imagination is as necessary in geometry as it is in poetry. Everything that requires creative recreation of reality, everything that is connected with the interpretation and construction of something new, needs the indispensable participation of fantasy. In this sense, some authors correctly contrast fantasy as the creative imagination of memory with fantasy as reproducing imagination.

Also, what is substantially new in the development of fantasy during the transitional age is contained precisely in the fact that the imagination of the adolescent enters into a close connection with thinking in concepts; it is intellectualized and included in the system of intellectual activity and begins to fulfill a completely new function in the new structure of the adolescent's personality. T. Ribot (1901), noting the curve of development of the adolescent's imagination, pointed out that the transitional age is characterized by the fact that the curve of development of imagination, which up to that time moved separately from the curve of development of intelligence, now approaches the latter and moves parallel to it.

If we correctly defined the higher development of the thinking of the adolescent as a transition from rational to judicious thinking and if we determined correctly the intellectualization of such functions as memory, attention, visual perception, and willful action, then in the same logical sequence we must reach the same conclusion with respect to fantasy. Thus, fantasy is not a primary, independent and leading function in the mental development of the adolescent; its development is the result of the function of forming concepts, the result which completes and crowns all the complex processes of changes that all of the intellectual life of the adolescent undergoes.

The character of the imagination during the transitional age still serves as a subject of debate among psychologists of different specializations. Many authors, like C. Bühler, indicate that in the adolescent, with the transition to abstract thinking, all the elements of concrete thinking begin to be accumulated, as if at the opposite pole, in his fantasy. Here fantasy is considered not only as a function independent of thinking in concepts, but even as opposed to it. Thinking in concepts is characterized by the fact that it moves in an abstract and general plane and imagination moves in the plane of the concrete. And since fantasy during the transitional age, yielding to the productivity of the mature fantasy of the adult, surpasses the latter with respect to intensity and primacy, then, this author maintains, we are right to consider fantasy as a function that is the polar opposite of the intellect.

In this respect, most interesting is the fate of the so-called eidetic images studied recently by E. Jaensch and his school. Those visual representations that are produced by the child with hallucinatory clarity after he perceives some visual situation or picture are usually called eidetic images. Similar to the way the adult fixates on a red square, then subsequently sees its image in a complementary color on a gray or white background, the child looking at a picture for a short time continues to see this picture on a blank screen even later when it is removed. This is a seemingly permanent inertia of visual excitation that continues to act after the source of the stimulation has disappeared.

Just as a loud sound seems to ring in our ears after we have actually stopped perceiving it, the eye of the child retains for some time a strong visual stimulation, as if a trace of it, its lasting echo.

It is not our task at present to analyze in any detail the teaching on eidetism and all the facts that have been discovered through experimental research. For our purposes, it is enough to say that these graphic visual representations are, according to the teaching of Jaensch, as if a transitional stage from perception to representation. They usually disappear with the end of childhood, but do not disappear without a trace, but are converted, on the one hand, into a visual basis of ideas and on the other, enter into perception as component elements. Some authors indicate that eidetic images are found most frequently during the transitional age.

Since these phenomena are evidence of the visual, concrete, sensory character of remembering and thinking, since they lie at the base of graphic perception of the world and graphic thinking, doubts arose immediately as to whether they are actually distinctive symptoms of the transitional age. Recently this question was reconsidered by a number of investigators who were able to establish that eidetic visual images are typical for childhood; specifically, there is a basis for assuming that they are most proper to very early childhood. The very young child is an eidetic in the sense that his recollections, his imagination, and his thinking still directly produce genuine perception in all the fullness of experience and in all the richness of concrete details, with the vitality of hallucinations.

With the transition to thinking in concepts, eidetic images disappear, and we must assume a priori that they disappear before the period of sexual maturation since the latter marks the transition from the visual concrete method of thinking to abstract thinking in concepts.

Jaensch maintains that not only in the ontogenesis, but also in the phylogenesis of memory were eidetic images dominant at the primitive stage of human culture. Gradually, together with cultural development of thinking, these phenomena disappeared, yielding their place to abstract thinking, and were preserved only in primitive forms of the thinking of the child. In later development, according to Jaensch, the significance of the word became more and more universal and abstract. Probably, hand in hand with the interest in concrete images, eidetic tendency moved to the background, and the change in the character of language resulted in eidetic instincts being pushed back farther and farther. The pushing back of this aptitude in cultured man must be the result of the appearance of cultured language with its common meanings of words which, in opposition to individual verbal knowledge of primitive languages, limit more and more the attention directed to sensorially perceived fact.

Just as in the genetic plan, the development of language and the transition to thinking in concepts in its time marked the demise of eidetic features, so in the development of the adolescent, the period of sexual maturation is characterized by two internally mutually connected factors: increase in abstract thinking and disappearance of eidetic, visual images.

With respect to the peak attained by the development of eidetic images, there are thus far serious differences among various authors. While some refer the flowering of this phenomenon to early childhood, others are inclined to put the peak of the curve at the transitional age, and a third group puts it in the middle, approximately at the beginning of primary school age. In recent times, however, we can consider it to be definitively established that at the transitional age, there is not a steep rise, but a steep drop in the curve of development of visual images. The change in intellectual activity of the adolescent is connected very closely with the change in the life of his ideas also. We must stress quite urgently that subjective visual images are not symptoms of the period of maturation, but are essential traits of childhood. This is what the expert investigator of eidetism, O. Kroh, says (1922).

This note is necessary because again and again attempts are made to turn eidetic images into a symptom of the period of maturation. In opposition to this, we must note that even the first studies of the author pointed to the strong drop in the curve of development of eidetic images at the onset of sexual maturation. Other investigators demonstrated that the maximum frequency of the phenomenon occurs at age 11-12 and drops with the onset of the transitional age. It is Kroh's opinion that for this reason we must decisively reject all attempts to consider visual images as a symptom of the transitional age derived directly from the psychological lability of this age. Also, it is understood that visual images do not disappear in an instant, but are preserved, as a rule, for quite a long time during the period of sexual maturation. But the sphere of origin of these images is more and more compressed and specialized, being determined basically by dominant interests.

We spoke in the preceding chapter of the radical changes that memory undergoes during the transitional age. We tried to show that memory makes a transition from eidetic images to forms of logical memory, and that internal mnemotechnique becomes the main and basic form of memory in the adolescent. For this reason, it is characteristic for eidetic images that they do not disappear entirely from the sphere of intellectual activity of the adolescent, but are moved as if into a different sector of the same sphere. As they cease being the basic form of the processes of memory, they come to serve imagination and fantasy, thus changing their basic psychological function.

On a solid basis, Kroh indicates that during the years of adolescence, so-called waking dreams, daydreams, appear that occupy a middle ground between real dreaming and abstract thinking. In waking dreams, the adolescent usually weaves a long, imaginative poem connected in separate parts and more or less stable over the course of long periods, with distinct sudden changes, situations, and episodes. This is seemingly creative dreaming produced by the imagination of the adolescent and experienced by him in waking dreams. These daydreams, this dream-like thinking of the adolescent, are frequently connected with visual eidetic images spontaneously evoked.

Kroh says that for this reason, spontaneous visual images at the beginning of maturation frequently appear even when voluntarily evoked images do not appear at all. To the question as to the main reason why eidetic images disappear from the sphere of memory and make a transition to the sphere of imagination, which is the basic factor in the change of their psychological function, Kroh's answer, in complete agreement with Jaensch, is: in ontogenesis just as in phylogenesis, language, becoming the means of forming concepts, automatizes speech and thinking in concepts and this is the basic reason.

In the concepts of the adolescent, the essential and nonessential, which are mixed in eidetic images, are found in a separated form. This is why the general conclusion of Kroh that subjective visual images disappear beginning at age 15-16 corresponds completely with his position that during this period, concepts begin to occupy the place of former images.

Thus, we come to the conclusion which seems to confirm the traditional assertion that establishes the concrete character of imagination during the transitional age. We must recall that the presence of elements that bring these images close to fantasy was already established in the investigation of eidetic images in children. The eidetic image does not always arise as a strict and true continuation of the perception that evokes it. Very frequently this perception changes and is reworked in the process of eidetic reproduction. Thus, it is not the inertia alone of visual stimulation that is the basis of eidetic tendency and feeds it, but in eidetic images, there is also the complex function of processing of the visual perception, the selection of what is interesting, reconstruction and even a unique generalization.

The exceptional merit of Jaensch is the discovery of visual concepts, that is, generalizing visual eidetic images that are as if analogs of our concepts in the sphere of concrete thinking. The great significance of concrete thinking cannot but be underestimated, and Jaensch is absolutely right when he says that intellectualism, which has long been dominant in school, has developed the child from one aspect and approached the child from one aspect, seeing in him primarily a logician and making logic the underlying principle of the system of his psychological operations. Actually, the thinking of the adolescent is still to a significant degree concrete.

Concrete thinking is preserved also at a higher stage of development in mature age. Many authors identify it with imagination. And actually, it would seem that in this case, visual reprocessing of concrete sensory images occurs, and this was always regarded as a basic trait of imagination.

3

The traditional view considers the visual character of the images that make up the content of fantasy to be its integral and distinctive trait. With respect to the transitional age, it is usually pointed out that all the elements of concrete, graphic, visual representations of reality that are gradually being pushed out of the sphere of the adolescent's abstract thinking are concentrated in the area of fantasy. We have already seen that such a statement is not entirely correct, in spite of a number of factual corroborations that support it.

It would be incorrect to consider the activity of fantasy exclusively as a visual, graphic, concrete activity. It has been pointed out quite correctly that on the one hand, this kind of visual quality is proper also to images in the memory. On the other hand, activity of fantasy of a sketchy or only slightly visual character is possible. J. Lindworsky believes that if we limit fantasy exclusively to the area of visual representations and completely exclude from it moments of thinking, then it would be impossible to designate poetic work as a product of the activity of fantasy. In precisely this way, E. Meumann objects to the point of view of W. Lay, who saw the distinction between thinking and fantasy to be that fantasy operates with visual images and that elements of abstract thought are absent from it. Meumann believes that elements of abstract thought are never absent from our ideas and perceptions. They cannot be completely absent because in the adult, all the material of ideas exists in a form processed by abstract thinking. The same idea was expressed by W. Wundt in raising objections to the view of fantasy as the work of purely visual representations.

As we shall see later, one of the essential changes that fantasy undergoes during the transitional age is actually a liberation from purely concrete, graphic factors and, together with this, a penetration into it of elements of abstract thinking.

We have already said that the essential trait of the transitional age is the closeness of fantasy to thinking and the fact that the imagination of the adolescent begins to depend on concepts. But this closeness does not mean that fantasy is fully absorbed by thinking. The one function approaches the other, but they do not merge, and the expression of R. Müller-Freienfels, who says that productive fantasy and thinking is one and the same thing, is not borne out by the way things really are. As we shall see, there are some points that characterize the activity of fantasy and corresponding experiences that distinguish fantasy from thinking.

So we have before us the problem of finding the unique relations between abstract and concrete factors that are characteristic for imagination during the transitional age. In the imagination of the adolescent, we actually have a kind of collection of all the elements of concrete, visual thinking that move to the background of his thinking. In order to understand correctly the significance of concrete factors in the adolescent's fantasy, we must take into account the connection that exists between the imagination of the adolescent and the play of the child.

From the genetic point of view, imagination during the transitional age is the successor to child's play. In the correct expression of one of the psychologists, no matter how interesting it is, the child distinguishes very well between the world he has created in play and the real world, and willingly seeks support for the imagined objects and relations in tangible, real objects of real life. The child stops playing as he approaches adolescence. He replaces play with imagination. When the child stops playing, he really rejects nothing other than seeking support in real objects. In place of play, he now fantasizes. He builds castles in the air, creates what we call daydreams.

It is understood that fantasy, which is the successor of child's play, separated itself only a short while ago from the support it found in tangible and concrete objects of real life. For this reason, fantasy so willingly seeks support in concrete representations that replace these real objects. Images, eidetic pictures, visual representations begin to play the same role in imagination that a doll representing a child or a chair representing a steam engine play in the child's game. This is the source of the striving of the adolescent's fantasy for support from concrete, tactile material, the source of the tendency toward graphic quality, visual quality. It is remarkable that these visual and graphic qualities have completely changed their function. They stopped being a support for memory and thinking and moved to the sphere of fantasy.

A clear example of this tendency toward concretization can be found in the novel of J. Wassermann, *The Maurizius Case*. One of the heroes of the novel, Etzel, a 16-year-old adolescent, is thinking of the unfair verdict imposed on Maurizius, who, because of a legal error, languished in prison for 18 years. The idea of an innocent person being sentenced possesses the adolescent, and in an agitated state when he thinks of the fate of this person, his fired up brain draws pictures while Etzel demands exclusively logical thinking from it.

"But he cannot always compel the thinking apparatus to carry out its function. He computes that eighteen years and five months is two hundred twenty-one months or approximately six thousand six hundred thirty days and six thousand six hundred thirty nights. They must be divided: days are one thing, nights, another. But at this point he stops to consider that what remains is a number that says nothing; he literally stands before an ant hill trying to count the swarming insects. He tries to imagine what this means, he wants to fill this number with content—six thousand six hundred thirty days. He draws in his imagination a house with six thousand six hundred thirty steps—it's a little difficult; a matchbox with six thousand six hundred thirty matches —hopeless; a wallet with six thousand six hundred thirty pennies—impossible; a train with six thousand six hundred thirty cars—unnatural; a stack of six thousand six hundred thirty sheets (note: sheets, not pages—two pages to each sheet to correspond to day and night).

"Finally, he arrives at a visual representation; he gets a stack of books from the shelf; the first book has one hundred fifty sheets, the second one hundred twenty-five, the third, two hundred ten; not one has more than two hundred sixty; he overestimated the possibilities; having accumulated twenty-three volumes, he had a total of four thousand two hundred twenty sheets. In amazement, he gave up this work. Just think, every day lived has to be counted. His own life had scarcely amounted to five thousand nine hundred days, and how long it seemed to him, how slowly it had passed; a week seemed a hard passage along cart-track roads, a day stuck like an irremovable dab of tar to the body.

"Then too—while he slept, read, went to school, played, talked to people, made plans, winter came, spring came, the sun shone, rain fell, night came, morning came—and the whole time he [Maurizius] was there; time came, time went, and he was always there, always there, always there. Before Etzel was born (infinite, mysterious word, suddenly—he was born), the first, the second, the five hundredth, the two thousand two hundred thirty-seventh day—he already had been and still remained there." (J. Wassermann, 1929).

From this example, it is easy to see how closely the adolescent's fantasy is still connected to the concrete support that it finds in perceptible representations. In this sense, the genetic fate of visual or concrete thinking is extremely interesting. Visual thinking does not disappear altogether from the intellectual life of the adolescent as abstract thinking develops. It is only moved to another place, to the sphere of fantasy, changes partially under the influence of abstract thinking and rises, like all other functions, to a higher level.

Special studies on the relation between visual thinking done with the aid of eidetic images and the intellect at first led investigators to contradictory results. Some found that dominance of visual thinking and eidetic tendencies were characteristic of retarded and primitive children. Others, on the contrary, saw a connection between this trait and intellectual giftedness. Schmitz's most recent study showed that there is no clear connection between the intellect and eidetic tendency. A strongly expressed eidetic tendency may be combined with any degree of intellectual development. However, a more detailed study showed that timely development of concrete thinking is an unalterable condition for the transition of thinking to a higher level. Schmitz is fully justified in citing the studies of T. Ziehen, who established that gifted children remain at the stage of concrete representations longer than those that are not gifted, as if the intellect at first had to be saturated with visual content which created in this way a concrete base for subsequent development of abstract thinking.

4

The study of so-called visual concepts is of special interest. Recently special studies were conducted in the school of Jaensch on the formation of concepts in visual thinking. The author understands the formation of concepts in visual thinking to be the special uniting, combining, and merging of images into new structures analogous to our concepts. The studies were conducted with eidetic images, a very convenient material for this kind of study.

Let us recall that the eidetic image is a visual representation seen by the eye as if on a blank screen, the way we see a green square in the same place after fixating on a red square. The subject was presented with several pictures or images that had some similar and some different characteristics. Then a study was made of what the subject saw when the eidetic image appeared under the influence of one of a number of similar images. The study showed that in this case, the eidetic image was never constructed mechanically, like Galton's photographic film, picking up matching traits and erasing the nonmatching. In the eidetic image, traits that matched and were repeated several times were never isolated, and the nonmatching were never concealed. Experiments showed that from a number of concrete impressions, the eidetic image creates a new whole, a new combination, a new image.

The investigators described two basic types of similar visual concepts. The first type is the so-called fluxion, in which the eidetic image is a dynamic combination of separate concrete images. The eidetic sees one of a number of presented objects on the screen, and this begins to take on different shapes and to be replaced by another, similar object. One image is converted to another and the other, to a third image. Sometimes this goes full circle, and the whole series of objects is combined in a dynamic change in the image that reflects each of the separate objects. For example, the subject is presented with a red carnation and rose of the same size. The subject at first sees the last flower shown. Then its shapes and forms are erased and merged into an indefinite colored spot that is a kind of average of the two flowers presented. When the subject is presented with two other flowers, at first he sees the image of the rose which changes into a diffuse red spot. Gradually it acquires a yellow color. Thus one image is transposed into another. The authors of this study say that, as a rule, the intermediate image that appears before a certain stage is close to the picture that traditional logic considers as the base of the concept in that the images similar to the spot described above actually contain the traits common to both single objects.

In this respect, it is extremely instructive to turn our attention to what actually would happen in the formation of concepts if it were to occur according to the plan devised by formal logic. Some kind of spot, confused, indefinite in form, with no individuality and no similarity to the real object—this is what the visual image, generated by two similar flowers, is converted into. Such a spot is also the concept of formal logic which sees the function of the concept to be the loss of a number of traits, and its formation to result in the fortunate gift of oblivion.

In contrast to this meager picture, the combination of images of the fluxion type conveys all the riches of reality. While, in comparison with reality, the colored spot actually discloses only the loss of traits, fluxions present really new formations, new forms consisting of the fact that the traits of single objects unite in a new synthesis that was not provided earlier. An image of a leaf that is evoked after several leaves similar to each other are presented may serve as an example of fluxion. This image moves, is constantly transformed from one to the other and changes form.

Composition is another new combination of images in visual thinking. In this case, the subject forms a new comprehended whole constructed according to a certain constructive trait or the selected traits of concrete objects. For example, the subject is shown an image of a taxi and an image of a donkey. On the screen, he sees the image of a police dog. The composition differs from fluxion in that the combination of images in it is given not in a moving, fluctuating form, but in a resting and stable form. For example, if images of three houses are presented to the subject, he sees one house that combines in itself various traits of all the images presented. The studies of Jaensch and Schweicher graphically demonstrate to what extent the idea that concepts develop by a simple addition or combination of images is without a solid base. Jaensch's visual concept is a uniting of images. A concept in the true sense of the word, however, is not a uniting of images, but a uniting of judgments, their certain system. The most essential difference of the one from the other is that there we have a direct and here an indirect knowledge and judgment of the object.

Using Hegel's well-known distinction, we can say that in the area of visual thinking, we are dealing with the product of common sense, and in the area of abstract thinking, with the product of the intellect. The thinking of the child is common sense thinking. This view of the concept definitively solves one of the most difficult problems of experimental psychology, the problem of nonvisual thinking. The concept is a kind of cluster of judgments, a key to the whole complex, their structure. From this, it is understandable that the concept has a nonvisual character, and develops in way different from simply combining representations.

The studies of which we just spoke definitively eliminate the question of the possibility of the appearance of anything like a true concept in processes of visual thinking. The highest thing to which a combination of representations can be brought is fluxion and combination. Together with this, we must wholly agree with authors who maintain that visual thinking must be considered as a special form of thinking that has great significance in the development of the intellect. According to our observations, visual thinking, the development of which seemingly ends with the formation of concepts, finds its continuation in fantasy, where it begins to play a substantial role. But even there, as shall see, it does not continue to exist in its previous form, as exclusively visual thinking. It undergoes a great transformation under the influence of concepts, which cannot be excluded from the activity of the imagination. Here again, we have a confirmation of the words cited above that to think without words, humanly, means basically to be supported by the word.

5

Of what does the essential difference between the fantasy of the adolescent and the fantasy of the child consist, what is new here?

We have already indicated what is most essential when we noted that the child's play ends in the fantasy of the adolescent. Thus, regardless of the concrete and real quality, the imagination of the adolescent is different from the play of the child in that it breaks the connection with real objects. Its support remains concrete, but less visual than that in the child. Nevertheless, we must note the progressing abstractness of his fantasy.

There is a widespread opinion that the child has greater fantasy and that the time of early childhood is a time of the flowering of fantasy. Regardless of how extremely widespread this opinion is, it is erroneous. As Wundt correctly states, the fantasy of the child is not as extensive as has been thought. On the contrary, it is satisfied with very little. Whole days are filled with thoughts of a horse that pulls a cart. And the scenes imagined deviate very little from reality.

In the adult, similar activity would be called absolute absence of fantasy. The lively fantasy of the child does not use the riches of his ideas, but has its root in the great intensity and the easier excitability of his feelings. In this respect, Wundt is inclined to extreme conclusions maintaining that combining fantasy is completely absent in the child. We can dispute this statement, but the basic idea is true that the child's fantasy is significantly poorer than the adolescent's fantasy, that only owing to the easy excitability of feelings, the intensity of experience, and uncritical quality of judgments does it occupy a greater place in the behavior of the child and for this reason seems to us to be richer and well developed. Thus, we see that the fantasy of the adolescent does not become poorer, but becomes richer than the child's fantasy.

Wundt is right when he points to the exceptional paucity of creative moments in the child's fantasy. The fantasy of the adolescent is more creative than the fantasy of the child. True, C. Bühler is fully justified in maintaining that it is nonproductive in the sense in which we use this word with respect to adult imagination. One recently developed fact on artistic creativity attests to this.

In the opinion of these authors, of all the creative products of the adolescent, only the love ideal that the adolescent creates for himself is noteworthy. But the same author notes the exceptional range of creativity in the form of journals and writing of poetry during the transitional age. Bühler says that it is striking how even people without a grain of poetry begin to write it in the transitional age. Obviously, this is not accidental, and the internal gravitation toward creative fulfillment, the internal tendency toward productivity, is a distinctive trait of the transitional age.

In addition, we see inconsistencies in two assertions that have just been made. The adolescent's fantasy is more creative than the child's fantasy and it is less productive than the adult's fantasy. This happens because the creative character first becomes inherent in fantasy only during the transitional age. From this, it is understandable that creativity has a rudimentary form and that this is not yet a fully developed creativity. As C. Bühler correctly points out, the adolescent's fantasy is closely connected with the new needs that arise during the transitional age and because of this, images acquire definite traits and an emotional tone. This is how the fantasy of the adolescent works.

Later we shall have the occasion to consider the connection between fantasy and needs and emotions. Now we are interested in another problem: the relation of the adolescent's fantasy to intellect. Bühler maintains that experiment shows that abstract thinking and visual imagination are separate from each other in the adolescent. They still do not cooperate in any creative activity. Internal images colored by feeling and experienced intensely alternate, but creative thinking does not influence them through selection or by connecting them. Thinking is done abstractly without any visual quality.

Again, if we take this assertion in terms of genesis and introduce into it a correction from the point of view of development, it will not contradict the position given above which states that specifically the coming together of intellect and imagination is the distinctive trait of the transitional age. Two lines of development proceeding separately thus far, meet at one point, as T. Ribot has shown, during the transitional age and continue their course closely interwoven. But specifically because this meeting, this drawing together first occurs only during the transitional age, it does not result instantly in a complete merging, in a complete cooperation of both functions, and the estrangement between thinking and imagination proposed by Bühler arises.

Also, we have seen that many authors attempt not so much to establish separation of thinking and imagination during the transitional age as to find traits that separate thinking from imagination. E. Meumann sees the distinction in the fact that in the activity of the imagination, we direct our attention predominantly to the content itself of the ideas and thoughts, and in thinking, we direct it to the logical relations within the content. In Meumann's opinion, the activity of fantasy consists in the fact that we attend to the content itself of an idea, sometimes predominantly analyzing it and sometimes predominantly forming new combinations from it. In thinking, however, the purpose of the activity is to establish logical relations between the content of ideas.

From our point of view, this definition does not lead to a sufficiently precise distinction between imagination and thinking. We do not even believe it is possible to make such a precise distinction. Where the matter stands in itself makes it impossible: the most substantial change in the adolescent's imagination consists precisely of its external drawing together with thinking in concepts. Like all other functions of which we have spoken in the preceding chapter, the adolescent's imagination changes substantially and is reconstructed on a new basis under the influence of thinking in concepts.

We can illustrate the internal dependence of the imagination on thinking in concepts with examples of the behavior of aphasia patients given at the beginning of this chapter. Imagination disappears together with the loss of speech as a means of forming concepts. The following is extremely curious: in aphasics, we very frequently observe the inability to use and understand metaphors, words with a figurative meaning. We have seen that thinking with metaphors becomes accessible only during the transitional age. A schoolchild finds it very difficult to compare a proverb and a sentence that have identical meanings. It is extremely significant that in aphasia a precisely similar disruption occurs. One of our subjects afflicted by aphasia could not at all understand any symbolic expressions. When he was asked what is meant when it is said of a person that "he has golden hands," the aphasic responded: "It means that he knows how to melt gold." The patient usually interpreted a figurative expression with an absurdity. He was not able to understand a metaphor. Comparing a proverb or another allegorical expression with a sentence expressing the same idea in a direct form was impossible for him.

Together with the disappearance of thinking in concepts, imagination also drops to zero. This too is understandable. We have seen that the zero point for the imagination and absolute absence of fantasy develops as follows: the person is in no condition to divert himself from the concrete situation, to change it creatively, to regroup the characteristics and to free himself from its influence.

In precisely the same way we see in this example how the aphasic cannot free himself from the literal meaning of the word and how he is unable to combine creatively the various concrete situations into a new image. In order to do this, he would have to have a certain freedom from the concrete situation, but, as we have seen above, this freedom is possible only with thinking in concepts. Thus, thinking in concepts is the most important factor that makes creative fantasy during the transitional age possible. However, it would be a mistake to assume that fantasy in this case merges with abstract thinking and loses its visual character. Specifically in the unique relation of abstract and concrete factors, we see the most important feature of fantasy during the transitional age. This can be understood as follows: thinking that is purely concrete, completely devoid of concepts, is also without fantasy. The formation of concepts brings with it, first of all, liberation from the concrete situation and the possibility of creatively reprocessing and changing its elements.

6

It is characteristic for imagination that it does not stop at this point, that for it, the abstract is only an intermediate link, only a stage on the path of development, only a pass in the process of its movement to the concrete. From our point of view, imagination is a transforming, creative activity directed from the concrete toward a new concrete. The movement itself from a given concrete toward a created concrete, the feasibility of creative construction is possible only with the help of abstraction. Thus, the abstract enters as a requisite constituent into the activity of imagination, but is not the center of this activity. The movement from the concrete through the abstract to the construction of a new concrete image is the path that imagination describes during the transitional age. In this respect, J. Lindworsky points to a number of factors that distinguish fantasy from thinking. In his opinion, the relative novelty of the results obtained is the characteristic that distinguishes fantasy. We think that not novelty in itself, but novelty of the concrete image of the idea produced distinguishes this activity. We believe that in this sense, the definition of B. Erdmann is more correct when he says that fantasy creates images of imperceptible objects.

The creative character of embodying something in the concrete, constructing a new image, this is characteristic for fantasy. Its conclusive point is concreteness, but this concreteness is attained only with the help of abstraction. The fantasy of the adolescent moves from the concrete, visual image through a concept to the imagined picture. In this respect, we cannot agree with Lindworsky, who sees the absence of a definite task as the characteristic that distinguishes fantasy from thinking. True, he makes the reservation that absence of a definite task should not be confused with involuntariness of fantasy. He indicates that in the activity of fantasy, the influence of the will on the unfolding of the ideas participates to a significant degree. We think that specifically for the adolescent, typical is a transition from the passive and imitative character of the child's fantasy, which Meumann and other investigators note, to the active and voluntary fantasy that marks the transitional age.

It seems to us that the most essential trait of fantasy during the transitional age is its division into subjective and objective imagination. Strictly speaking, fantasy is first formed only during the transitional age. We agree with the assertion of Wundt, who assumed that the child has no combining fantasy. This is true in the sense that only the adolescent begins to isolate and be conscious of this form as a special function. The child has no strictly separate function of imagination. The adolescent, however, is conscious of his subjective fantasy as subjective and objective fantasy, cooperating with thinking and he also is conscious of its real limits.

As we have already said, separating subjective and objective points and forming the poles of personality and world view characterize the transitional age. The same separation of subjective and objective points characterizes the adolescent's fantasy as well.

Fantasy is divided as if into two streams. On the one hand, it begins to serve emotional life, needs, attitudes, and feelings that crowd the adolescent. It is a subjective activity that gives personal satisfaction resembling the child's play. As a psychologist that we have cited states correctly, it is by no means the happy person who fantasizes, but only one who is dissatisfied. Unsatisfied desire is the stimulus that arouses fantasy. Our fantasy is a fulfillment of desire, a corrective for activity that is not satisfying.

This is why almost all authors agree in noting this feature of the adolescent's fantasy: it first turns to the intimate sphere of experiences that is usually hidden from others and becomes an exclusively subjective form of thinking, thinking exclusively for oneself. The child does not hide his play, the adolescent hides his fantasies and conceals them from others. Our author correctly says that the adolescent hides them as an innermost secret and would sooner admit his faults than disclose his fantasies. Specifically the secrecy of the fantasy indicates that it is closely connected with internal desires, incentives, drives, and emotions of the personality and begins to serve this whole aspect of the adolescent's life. In this respect, the connection between fantasy and emotion is extremely significant.

We know that some emotions always evoke a certain flow of ideas in us. Our feeling strives to be poured into certain images in which it finds its expression and its discharge. And it is understood that certain images are a powerful means of evoking and arousing a certain feeling and its discharge. This is what constitutes the close connection that exists between the lyric and the feeling of the person that perceives it. The subjective value of fantasy consists in this. The circumstance that, in Goethe's expression, feeling does not deceive, judgment deceives, has long been noted. When we use fantasy to construct any nonreal images, these are not real, but the feeling that they evoke is experienced as real. When the poet says: "I will shed tears over a fantasy," he recognizes the fantasy as something that is not real, but the tears he sheds belong to reality. Thus, in fantasy the adolescent lives out his rich internal emotional life, his impetuosity.

In fantasy, he finds a vital means for directing and mastering his emotional life. Just as the adult, when he perceives an artistic work, let us say a lyrical poem, gets in touch with his own feelings, so precisely the adolescent, with the help of fantasy, illuminates and clarifies himself and turns his emotions, his tendencies into a creative image. Life that is not lived out finds expression in creative images.

Thus, we can say that creative images produced by the adolescent's fantasy fulfill the same function for him that an artistic work fulfills for the adult. It is art for oneself. It is for oneself, in the mind, that poems and novels are produced, dramas and tragedies are acted out, and elegies and sonnets are composed. In this sense, Spranger is very right in contrasting the fantasies of the adolescent with the fantasies of the child. This author says that although the adolescent is still half child, his fantasy is of a completely different type than that of the child. It gradually approaches the conscious illusion of adults. About the difference between the child's fantasy and the imagination of the adolescent, Spranger graphically says that the child's fantasy is a dialogue with things and the fantasy of the adolescent is a monologue with things. The adolescent is conscious of his fantasy as a subjective activity. The child does not yet distinguish between his fantasy and the things with which he plays.

Together with the stream of fantasy which serves mainly the emotional sphere of the adolescent, his fantasy develops another stream of purely objective creativity. We have already said: wherever in the process of understanding or in the process of practical activity, the creation of some kind of new concrete structure, new image of activity is necessary, a creative embodiment of some idea, there fantasy comes forward as a basic function. Not only artistic works are produced with the help of fantasy, but also all scientific inventions and all technical constructions. Fantasy is one of the manifestations of man's creative activity, and specifically in the transitional age, approaching thinking in concepts, it undergoes broad development in this objective aspect.

It would be incorrect to think that the two streams in the development of fantasy during the transitional age are widely separated from each other. On the contrary, both concrete and abstract points and subjective and objective functions of fantasy occur during the transitional age frequently in a complex interweaving each with the other. Objective expression is colored with bright emotional tones, but even subjective fantasies are frequently observed in the area of objective creativity. As an example of the drawing close of one stream to the other in the development of the imagination, we could point to the fact that specifically in fantasy, the adolescent gropes for the first time for his life plan. His strivings and confused motives pour out in the form of certain images. In fantasy he anticipates his future and, consequently, also creatively approaches its construction and implementation.

7

With this, we can close the circle of our discussion of the psychology of the adolescent. We began with a consideration of this most serious change which occurs at the transitional age. We established that on the basis of sexual maturation, a new and complex world arises with new tendencies, strivings, motives, and interests, new movers of behavior and its new directions; new motive forces push the thinking of the adolescent forward, and new tasks open before him. We saw further that these new tasks lead to the development of the central and leading function of all mental development—to the formation of concepts—and we saw how on the basis of the formation of concepts, some completely new mental functions develop, how on the new base, perception, memory, attention, and practical activity of the ado-

lescent are restructured, and what is the main thing, how they unite in a new structure, how gradually a foundation is laid for higher syntheses of personality and
world view. Now, with an analysis of imagination, we see again how these new
forms of behavior, bound in their origin to sexual maturation and connected with
it by drives, serve the emotional strivings of the adolescent, how in creative imagination, the emotional and intellectual aspects of the adolescent's behavior find a
complex synthesis, how in it are synthesized abstract and concrete points, how sexual
drive and thinking are complexly combined in a new unit—in the activity of this
creative imagination.

Chapter 5
DYNAMICS AND STRUCTURE OF THE ADOLESCENT'S PERSONALITY

1

We are approaching the end of our study. We began with a review of the changes that occur in the structure of the organism and its most important functions during the period of sexual maturation. We were able to trace the complete restructuring of the whole internal and external system of activity of the organism, the radical change in its structure and the new structure of organic activity that is connected with sexual maturation. Tracing many stages, passing from drives to interests, from interests to mental functions, and from these to the content of thinking and to creative imagination, we have seen how the new structure of the adolescent's personality, which differs from the structure of the child's personality, is formed.

Then we considered briefly certain special problems of pedology of the transitional age and were able to trace how the new structure of the personality is manifested in complex, synthetic, vital actions, how the social behavior of the adolescent changes and rises to a higher level, how it arrives internally and externally at one of life's decisive moments—the selection of a vocation or profession, and, finally, how the unique, vital forms, the unique structure of the personality and world view of the adolescent are developed in the three main classes of contemporary society. Many times during our study, we came upon separate elements for constructing a general teaching on the personality of the adolescent. Now it remains for us to correlate what has been said and to try to give a graphic picture of the structure and dynamics of the adolescent's personality.

We deliberately unite these two sections of the study of personality since we believe that traditional pedology of the transitional age has given much attention to purely descriptive representation and study of the adolescent's personality. To do this, it used self-observation, journals, and poetry of adolescents and tried to recreate the structure of the personality on the basis of separate documented experiences. We think that the most plausible path would be the simultaneous study of the adolescent's personality from the aspect of its structure and dynamics. More simply put, in order to answer the question of the unique structure of the personality during the transitional age, it is necessary to determine how this structure develops, how it is constituted, and what the principal laws of its construction and change are. We shall now proceed to do this.

The history of the development of personality can be encompassed by a few basic patterns which have been suggested by all of our foregoing study.

The first law of the development and structure of higher mental functions which are the basic nucleus of the personality being formed can be called the law

167

of *the transition from direct, innate, natural forms and methods of behavior to mediated, artificial mental functions that develop in the process of cultural development.* This transition during ontogenesis corresponds to the process of the historical development of human behavior, a process, which, as we know, did not consist of acquiring new natural psychophysiological functions, but in a complex combination of elementary functions, in a perfecting of forms and methods of thinking, in the development of new methods of thinking based mainly on speech or on some other system of signs.

The simplest example of the transition from direct to mediated functions may be the transition from involuntary remembering and remembering that is guided by the sign. Primitive man, having first made some kind of external sign in order to remember some event, passed in this way into a new form of memory. He introduced external, artificial means with which he began to manage the process of his own remembering. Study shows that the whole path of historical development of man's behavior consists of a continuous perfecting of such means and of the development of new devices and forms of mastering his own mental operations, and here the internal system of one operation or another also changed and sustained profound changes. We shall not consider the history of behavior in detail. We shall only say that the cultural development of the behavior of the child and the adolescent is basically of the same type.

Thus we see that cultural development of behavior is closely linked to the historical or social development of humanity. This brings us to the second law, which also expresses certain traits common to phylo- and ontogenesis. The second law can be formulated thus: considering the history of the development of higher mental functions that comprise the basic nucleus in the structure of the personality, we find *that the relation between higher mental functions was at one time a concrete relation between people; collective social forms of behavior in the process of development become a method of individual adaptations and forms of behavior and thinking of the personality.* Every complex higher form of behavior discloses specifically this path of development. That which is now united in one person and appears to be a single whole structure of complex higher internal mental functions was at one time made up of separate processes divided among separate persons. Put more simply, higher mental functions arise from collective social forms of behavior.

We might elucidate this basic law with three simple examples. Many authors (J. Baldwin, E. Rignano, and J. Piaget) demonstrated that the logical thinking of children develops in proportion to the way in which argument appears and develops in the children's group.[93] Only in the process of working with other children does the function of the child's logical thinking develop. In a position familiar to us, Piaget says that only cooperation leads to the development of logic in the child. In his work, Piaget was able to trace step by step how in the process of developing cooperation and particularly in connection with the appearance of a real argument, a real discussion, the child is first confronted by the need to form a basis, to prove, confirm, and verify his own idea and the idea of his partner in the discussion. Further, Piaget traced that the argument, the confrontation that arises in a children's group is not only a stimulus for logical thought, but is also the initial form in which thought appears. The dying out of those traits of thinking that were dominant at the early stage of development and are characterized by absence of systematization and connections coincides with the appearance of argument in the children's group. This coincidence is not accidental. It is specifically the development of an argument that leads the child to systematizing his own opinions. P. Janet showed that all deliberation is the result of an internal argument because it is as if a person were repeating to himself the forms and methods of behavior that he applied earlier to others. Piaget concludes that his study fully confirms this point of view.

Thus, we see that the child's logical deliberation is as if an argument transferred to within the personality and, in the process of the child's cultural development, the group form of behavior becomes an internal form of behavior of the personality, the basic method of his thinking. The same might be said of the development of self-control and voluntary direction of one's own actions which develop in the process of children's group games with rules. The child who learns to conform and coordinate his actions with the actions of others, who learns to modify direct impulse and to subordinate his activity to one rule or another of the game, does this initially as a member of a small group within the whole group of playing children. Subordination to the rule, modification of direct impulses, coordination of personal and group actions initially, just like the argument, is a form of behavior that appears among children and only later becomes an individual form of behavior of the child himself.

Finally, in order to avoid multiplying examples, we might point to the central and leading function of cultural development. The fate of this function confirms as clearly as is possible the law of transition from social to individual forms of behavior, which might also be called the law of sociogenesis of higher forms of behavior: speech, being initially the means of communication, the means of association, the means of organization of group behavior, later becomes the basic means of thinking and of all higher mental functions, the basic means of personality formation. The unity of speech as a means of social behavior and as a means of individual thinking cannot be accidental. As we have said above, it indicates the basic fundamental law of the construction of higher mental functions.

As indicated by P. Janet (1930),[94] the word was at first a command for others, and then a change in function resulted in separating the word from action and this led to the independent development of the word as a means of command and independent development of action subordinated to the word. At the very beginning the word is connected with action and cannot be separated from it. It is itself only one of the forms of action. This ancient function of the word, which could be called a volitional function, persists to these times. The word is a command. In all its forms, it represents a command and in verbalized behavior, it is always necessary to distinguish the function of command which belongs to the word from the function of subordination. This is a fundamental fact. Specifically because the word fulfilled the function of a command with respect to others, it begins to fulfill the same function with respect to oneself and becomes the basic means for mastering one's own behavior.

This is the source of the volitional function of the word, this is why the word subordinates motor reaction to itself; this is the source of the power of the word over behavior. Behind all of this stands the real function of command. Behind the psychological power of the word over other mental functions stands the former power of the commander and the subordinate. This is the basic idea of Janet's theory. This same general theory may be expressed in the following form: every function in the cultural development of the child appears on the stage twice, in two forms—at first as social, then as psychological; at first as a form of cooperation between people, as a group, an intermental category, then as a means of individual behavior, as an intramental category. This is the general law for the construction of all higher mental functions.

Thus, the structures of higher mental functions represent a cast of collective social relations between people. These structures are nothing other than a transfer into the personality of an inward relation of a social order that constitutes the basis of the social structure of the human personality. The personality is by nature social. This is why we were able to detect the decisive role that socialization of external and internal speech plays in the process of development of children's thinking. As we have seen, the same process also leads to the development of children's ethics; the laws of construction here are identical to the laws of development of children's logic.

From this point of view, adapting the well-known expression, we might say that the mental nature of man is an aggregate of social relations transferred within and becoming functions of the personality, the dynamic parts of its structure. The transfer inward of external social relations between people is the basis for the structure of the personality, as has long been noted by investigators. K. Marx wrote: "In certain respects man resembles merchandise. Just as he is born without a mirror in his hands and is not a Fichtean philosopher: 'I am I,' man initially sees himself in another person as in a mirror. Only by relating to the man, Paul, as being similar to himself, does the man, Peter, begin to relate to himself as to a man. Also, Paul as such, in all his Paulian corporeality, becomes for him a form of manifestation of the genus 'man'" (K. Marx and F. Engels, *Works*, Vol. 23, p. 62).

The third law, connected with the second, may be formulated as the law of *transition of a function from outside inward.*

We understand now why the initial stage of the transfer of social forms of behavior into a system of individual behavior of the personality is necessarily connected with the fact that every higher form of behavior initially has the character of an external operation. In the process of development, the functions of memory and attention are initially constructed as external operations connected with the use of an external sign. And we can understand why. Of course, as we have said, initially, they were a form of group behavior, a form of social connection, but this social connection could not be implemented without the sign, by direct intercourse, and so here the social means becomes the means of individual behavior. For this reason, the sign always appears first as a means of influencing others and only later as a means of affecting oneself. Through others, we become ourselves. From this, we can understand why all internal higher functions were of necessity external. However, in the process of development, every external function is internalized and becomes internal. Having become an individual form of behavior, in the process of a long period of development, it loses the traits of an external operation and is converted into an internal operation.

According to Janet, it is difficult to understand how speech became internal. He believes this to be so difficult a problem that it is the basic problem of thinking and is being solved extremely slowly by people. Eons of evolution were required to implement the transition from external to internal speech, and Janet assumes that if we were to look closely, we would find that even now there are very many people who have not mastered internal speech. Janet calls the idea that internal speech is well developed in all people a great illusion.

We noted the transition to internal speech during childhood in one of the preceding chapters (Vol. 2, pp. 314-331) [Translator's note: this is probably Vol. 1, pp. 71-76 in the current series.] We showed that the child's egocentric speech is a transitional form from external speech to internal, that the child's egocentric speech is speech for himself that fulfills a mental function completely different from that of external speech. In this way, we showed that speech becomes internal mentally sooner than it becomes internal physiologically. Without further attention to the process of transition of speech from external to internal, we can say that this is the common fate of all higher mental functions. We have seen that transition inward is specifically the main content of the development of functions during the transitional age. Through a long process of development, function moves from an external to an internal form, and this process is concluded at this age.

The following point is closely connected to the formation of the internal character of these functions. As we have said repeatedly, the higher mental functions are based on mastery of one's own behavior. We can speak of the formation of the personality only when there is mastery of the person's own behavior. But as a prerequisite, mastery assumes reflection in consciousness, reflection in words of the structure of one's own mental operations because, as we have indicated, freedom in this case also signifies nothing other than recognized necessity. In this respect, we can agree with Janet, who speaks of the metamorphosis of language into will. What is called will is verbal behavior. Without speech, there is no will. Speech enters into volitional action sometimes cryptically and sometimes openly.

Thus, the will, being the basis of the structure of personality, is, in the final analysis, initially a social form of behavior. Janet says that in all voluntary processes there is speech and the will is nothing other than a conversion of speech into implementation, regardless of whether it is for another or for oneself.

The behavior of the individual is identical to social behavior. The higher fundamental law of behavioral psychology is that we conduct ourselves with respect to ourselves just as we conduct ourselves with respect to others. There is social behavior with respect to oneself and if we acquired the function of command with respect to others, applying this function to ourselves is essentially the same process. But subordinating one's actions to one's own authority necessarily requires, as we have already said, a consciousness of these actions as a prerequisite.

We have seen that introspection, consciousness of one's own mental operations, appears relatively late in the child. If we trace the process of development of self-consciousness, we will see that it occurs in the history of development of higher forms of behavior in three basic stages. At first, every higher form of behavior is assimilated by the child exclusively from the external aspect. From the objective aspect, this form of behavior already includes in itself all the elements of the higher functions, but subjectively, for the child himself who has not yet become conscious of it, it is a purely natural, innate method of behavior. It is only due to the fact that other people fill the natural form of behavior with a certain social content, for others rather than for the child himself, that it acquires the significance of a higher function. Finally, in the process of a long development, the child becomes conscious of the structure of this function and begins to control his own internal operations and to direct them.

Using the simplest examples, we can trace the sequence in the development of the child's own functions. Let us take the first pointing gesture of the child. The gesture is nothing other than an unsuccessful grasping movement. The child stretches out his hand toward a distant object and cannot reach it, but his hand remains stretched out toward the object. Here we have a pointing gesture with the objective meaning of a word. The movement of the child is not a grasping movement but a pointing movement. It cannot affect the object. It can affect only the people nearby. From the objective aspect, it is not an action directed toward the external world, but is really a means of social effect on people nearby. But the situation is such only from the objective aspect. The child himself strives for the object. His hand, stretched out in the air, maintains its position only because of the hypnotizing force of the object. This stage in the development of the pointing gesture can be called the stage of the gesture in itself.

Then the following occurs. The mother hands the child the object; for her rather than for the child, the unsuccessful grasping movement is converted into a pointing gesture. Because of the fact that she understands it in this way, this movement objectively turns ever more into a pointing gesture in the true sense of the word. This stage can be called the pointing gesture for others. Only significantly later does the action become a pointing gesture for the self, that is, a conscious and deliberate action of the child himself.

In exactly the same way, the child's first words are nothing other than an affective cry. Objectively, they express one need or another of the child long before the child consciously uses them as a means of expression. Again, as before, others, not the child, fill these affective words with a certain content. Thus, the people nearby create the objective sense of the first words apart from the will of the child. Only later are his words converted into speech for himself used deliberately and consciously.

In the course of our study, we have seen a number of examples of this kind of origin of functions through three basic stages. We have seen how speech and thinking intersect objectively in the child at first, apart from his intention in the practical situation, how at first a connection arises objectively between these two forms of activity, and how only later does it become a deliberate connection for the child himself. In development, every mental function passes through these three stages. Only when it rises to a higher level does it become a function of the personality in the true sense of the word.

We see how complex patterns appear in the dynamic structure of the adolescent's personality. What we have usually called personality is nothing other than man's consciousness of himself that appears specifically at this time: new behavior of man becomes behavior for himself; man himself is conscious of himself as a certain entity. This is the end result and central point of the whole transitional age. In a graphic form, we can express the difference between the personality of the child and the personality of the adolescent using different verbal designations of mental acts. Many investigators have asked: why do we attribute a personal character to mental processes? What should we say: I think or *It seems to me*? Why not consider the processes of behavior as natural processes that occur of themselves due to connections with all the other processes and why not speak of thinking impersonally, just as we say *it's getting dark* or *it's getting light*? To many investigators, such a manner of expression seemed to be solely scientific, and for a certain stage of development, this is actually so. Just as we say *mne snitsya* [the impersonal, idiomatic Russian expression, *it dreams to me*], the child says *it seems to me*. The course of his thought is as involuntary as our dreaming. But, in the well-known expression of L. Feuerbach, it is not thinking that thinks—man thinks.

This can be said for the first time only in application to the adolescent. Mental acts acquire a personal character only on the basis of a personality's self-consciousness and on the basis of their being mastered. It is interesting that this kind of terminological problem could never arise with respect to action.

No one would ever think to say *it acts to me* or doubt the correctness of the expression *I act*. Where we feel ourselves to be the source of a movement, we ascribe a personal character to our actions, but it is to specifically this level of mastery of his internal operations that the adolescent rises.

2

Recently in the pedology of the transitional age, much attention has been given to the problem of development of the personality. As Spranger has indicated, one of the basic features of the age as a whole is the discovery of one's own "I." This expression seems to us to be inaccurate since Spranger has in view the discovery of personality. It seems to us that it would be more correct to speak of the development of personality and of the conclusion of this development during the transitional age. Spranger justifies his formulation by the fact that the child too has his "ego." However, he is not conscious of it: Spranger has in mind the unique transfer of attention and internal reflection, that is, thinking directed toward oneself. Reflection appears in the adolescent; it is impossible in the child.

Recently, A. Busemann[95] did two special studies (1925, 1926) on the development of reflection and the self-consciousness connected with it during the transitional age. We shall briefly consider the results of his studies since they present rich *factual* material for understanding the dynamics and structure of personality during the transitional age. Busemann proceeds from an entirely correct position that self-consciousness is not something original. Lower forms of organisms live in interrelation with the environment, but not with themselves. The development of self-consciousness is accomplished extremely slowly, and we must seek its rudiments even in early animal forms. Engels noted that even in the organization of the nervous system, around which all the rest of the body is constructed, the first rudiment is given for the development of self-consciousness.[96]

We believe that Busemann is fully justified in considering the most primitive forms of interrelations with one's own organism as the biological roots of self-consciousness. When an insect, a beetle for example, smooths his wings with his feet, his extremities touch, stimulate each other, and are perceived as an external stimulation. Further, through a series of biological forms of development, this process rises to reflection directed toward one's own body, if under this word, we follow Busemann in understanding all transfer of experience from the external world to oneself.

The psychology of reflection, as the author correctly indicates, requires a radical review of a number of theoretical positions. The psychology which considers man as a natural being does not consider the problem of the development of self-consciousness. Only in taking into account the historical development of man and child do we approach a correct formulation of this problem.

Busemann set a goal of studying the development of reflection and the self-consciousness connected with it on the basis of free compositions of the child and the adolescent. The compositions disclosed to what extent the writer had mastered reflection or self-consciousness. The basic result of the study revealed a close connection between the environment and the adolescent's self-consciousness. In complete agreement with what we have said above, Busemann found that the vital form of the adolescent's personality depicted by Spranger refers only to an adolescent from a certain type of environment.[97] Its transfer to other social strata is not borne out by facts. Transferring this structure to proletarian and peasant youth is completely inadmissible. Busemann's first study showed a tremendous difference in the development and structure of self-consciousness and personality of the adolescent depending on the social environment to which he belongs. Children and adolescents wrote compositions on themes such as: "My good and bad qualities," "What kind of person I am and what kind I should be," and "Can I be pleased with myself (am I satisfied with myself)." The author was interested not in the plausibility of the responses, but in their character, which made it possible to judge the extent of the development or lack of development of the adolescent's self-consciousness.

One of the basic facts as expressed in the words of Busemann is the connection between social position and reflection. Another basic fact is that the process of self-consciousness is not some kind of fixed and constant ability that arises instantly in full measure, but one that undergoes a long development through various stages;

TABLE 5. Frequency of Mentioning Ethical Judgments Depending on Age, Sex, and Social Environment, % (according to A. Busemann)

Age, years	Boys			Girls		
	A	B	C	A	B	C
11	0	0	0	10	25	100
12	5	4	17	40	39	45
13	13	11	22	51	44	73
14	6	7	9	53	83	31

Note: A—uneducated workers; B—educated workers and lower-level employees; C—mid-level employees and officials, independent craftsmen, small farmers, and tradesmen.

this makes it possible to separate the stages of development and compare people in this respect. According to Busemann, the function of self-consciousness develops in six different directions which basically constitute the principal factors that characterize the structure of the adolescent's self-consciousness.

The first direction is simply growth and the appearance of a self-image. The adolescent begins to recognize himself more and more. This recognition becomes more firmly grounded and connected. There are many intermediate steps between the completely naive lack of knowledge of oneself and the rich, profound knowledge that is evident at another time toward the end of the period of sexual maturation.

The second direction in the development of self-consciousness takes this process inward from outside. Busemann says that at first children know only their own body. Only at age 12-15 is there a consciousness of the existence of an interior world in other people also. The adolescent's own self-image is transferred inward. At first, it encompasses dreams and feelings. It is important that the development in the second direction does not move in parallel with the increase in self-consciousness in the first direction. Table 5 presents the increase in transition inward at the beginning of the adolescent years and the dependence of this process on the environment. We see to what extent the village child remains at the stage of external self-consciousness for a significantly longer time (see Table 5).

The third direction in the development of self-consciousness is its internalization. The adolescent begins to recognize himself more and more as a single whole. In his consciousness, separate traits increasingly become traits of character. He begins to perceive himself as something whole and every separate development as a part of the whole. Here we can observe a number of stages qualitatively different from each other which the child passes through gradually depending on age and social environment.

The fourth direction in the development of the adolescent's self-consciousness is setting a boundary between his personality and the surrounding world, recognizing the differences and uniqueness of his own personality. Inordinate development of self-consciousness in this direction leads to reticence and to acutely painful alienation, which frequently marks the transitional age.

The fifth line in development consists of the transition to judging oneself on ethical scales,* which a child or adolescent begins to apply to evaluating his own personality; these scales are acquired from objective culture and not simply assimilated biologically. Busemann says that up to the age of 11, the child judges himself on a scale of strong—weak, well—sick, beautiful—ugly. Country adolescents, age 14-15, frequently still remain at this stage of biological self-evaluation. But in com-

*Editor's note: internal, moral criteria.

plex social relations, development moves forward very rapidly. The center of gravity is transferred to one capability or another. Following the stage of "Siegfried ethics" according to which corporal virtues and beauty are everything, the ethic of skills becomes part of the child's development. Busemann believes that the child takes pride in knowing how to do something which attracts the respect of adults.

Under the influence of adults who continuously repeat the formula, "You must obey us," the child enters the stage of evaluation, which is determined by what the adults require of him. Every so-called well-brought-up child goes through this stage. Many children, especially girls, remain at the stage of ethical obedience.

The next stage in development leads to group ethics and is attained by the adolescents only at the age of approximately seventeen, and not by all of them.

The sixth and last line of development of the adolescent's self-consciousness and personality consists of an increase in differences between individuals and increase in interindividual variation. In this respect, reflection orders the fate of the remaining functions. As instincts become more mature and the influence of the environment continues, people become less and less alike. Up to the age of 10, we find insignificant difference in the self-consciousness of the city and the rural child; at age 11-12, this difference becomes clearer, but only in the transitional age does the difference in environment bring the various types in the structure of the personality to a full expression.

3

The most substantial result of Busemann's study is that he established three factors that characterize reflection during the transitional age.

The first: reflection and the adolescent's self-consciousness based on it are represented in development. The appearance of self-consciousness is taken not only as a phenomenon in the life of consciousness, but as a much broader factor biologically and socially based on the whole preceding history. Rather than approaching this complex problem only phenomenologically, from the aspect of experience, from the aspect of analysis of consciousness, as Spranger had done, we obtain an objective reflection of the real development of the adolescent's self-consciousness.

On a solid base, Busemann says that the roots of reflection must be sought very deeply in the living world and that its biological bases are wherever there is a reflection not only of the external world, but also a self-reflection of the organism and a relation of the organism with itself that results from this. Spranger describes this change in the transitional age as a discovery of one's own "I," as a turning of the gaze inward, as an event of a purely spiritual order. In this way he takes the formation of the adolescent's personality as something primary, independent, and primordial and from this as from a root, he derives all further changes that characterize the age. Actually, what we have before us is not primary, but one of the very last, perhaps even the last link in the chain of the changes which constitute the characteristics of the transitional age.

We pointed out above that the potentials for self-consciousness are established even in the organization of the nervous system. Further, we tried to trace the long path of psychological and social changes that leads to the appearance of self-consciousness. We have seen that there is no instantaneous and unexpected discovery of a purely spiritual order. We have seen how of natural necessity all mental life of the adolescent is reconstructed so that the appearance of consciousness is only the product of the preceding process of development. This is the main thing, this is the essence.

Self-consciousness is only the last and highest of all the restructuring that the adolescent's psychology undergoes. For us, the formation of self-consciousness is nothing other, I repeat, than a certain historical stage in the development of personality that arises inevitably from preceding stages. Thus, self-consciousness is not a primary, but a derivative fact in the adolescent's psychology and appears not through discovery, but through a long development. In this sense, the appearance of self-consciousness is nothing other than a certain moment in the process of development of a consciousness being. This moment is part of all of the processes of development in which consciousness begins to play any perceptible role.

This concept corresponds to the pattern of development that we find in Hegel's philosophy. In contrast to Kant, for whom a thing in itself is a metaphysical entity not subject to development, for Hegel, the concept itself "in oneself" means nothing other than the initial moment or stage of development of the thing. Specifically from this point of view, Hegel considered a seedling as a plant in itself and a child as a man in himself. All things are in themselves from the beginning, Hegel said. A. Deborin (1923)[98] considers it interesting that in formulating the question in this way, Hegel inseparably connects the knowability of a thing with its development or, using a more general expression, with its movement and change. From this point of view, Hegel justifiably pointed to the fact that the "I" serves as the closest example of "life for oneself." "It can be said that the man differs from the animal and, consequently, from nature in general mainly by the fact that he knows himself as 'I'."

The concept of self-consciousness as developing definitively liberates us from the metaphysical approach to this central fact of the transitional age.

The second factor which facilitates our real approach to this process is Busemann's finding the connection between the development of self-consciousness and the social development of the adolescent. Busemann moves the discovery of the "I," which Spranger places at the beginning of the creation of adolescent psychology, from the heavens to earth and from the beginning of the mental development of the adolescent to the end when he indicates that the picture drawn by Spranger corresponds only to a certain social type of adolescent. Busemann maintains that transferring this image to proletarian and peasant youth would be a big mistake.

Most recently, Busemann conducted a study in which he again tried to elucidate the connection between the environment and the adolescent's self-consciousness. If, as the author himself believes, it was possible on the basis of his former work to elucidate the differences in self-consciousness between the city and the rural child, between pupils of higher, middle, and folk schools, not by the influence of social position, but simply by the educational effect of type of school, then the results of the new study contradict this. The great amount of material collected was processed. The statements of the adolescents were divided into four groups:

1. Representation of the conditions in which the child lives instead of his representation of his own personality. This was accepted as evidence of his own naive relation to the theme "Am I satisfied with myself."

2. Description of his own body, which also was evidence of a primitive understanding of this question.

3. Self-evaluation at the level of ethical knowledge.

4. Self-evaluation of actual ethical character (regardless of whether it referred to ethical compliance or to group ethics).

TABLE 6. Distribution of Naive Statements (First and Second Category in the Total) according to Sex and Social Groups, % (according to A. Busemann)

Sex	Social Groups		
	A	B	C
M	66	53	43
F	21	15	13

Note: Designations A, B, C as in Table 5.

The author presents the differences in self-consciousness of various social groups in Table 6. These differences cannot be explained exclusively by type of schooling since all the children studied were in the same school.

In itself, the *fact of the close connection* established by Busemann between the adolescent's social position and development of his self-consciousness seems to us to be completely indisputable. The interpretation of the factual data, however, seems to be so *erroneous* that even the simplest analysis would detect this.

If we compare the differences in stage of development of the self-consciousness of adolescents depending on their social position with the same difference depending on sex, we see to what extent sex differentiation exceeds social differentiation (Table 7). For example, while the number of naive responses indicating an undeveloped self-consciousness in boys in group A is only 1.5 times greater than the number of the same responses in group C, compared with responses of girls in the same social group, it is more than 3 times greater. The same thing holds for the rest of the social groups. Can we call this fact accidental? We think not. The difference in development of self-consciousness between the sexes is much more significant than between children of different social strata.

To explain this, Busemann constructs what is in our view an unsustainable theory: he assumes that even in unfavorable socioeconomic circumstances, girls develop a mature ethical self-consciousness while boys require especially favorable conditions in their domestic environment or a strong influence of school to do so. Busemann sees confirmation of this fact in that we have known for a long time that the feminine sector of proletarian youth is psychologically remarkably close to the type of youth found in the best social conditions.

Girls are ahead in the same way in everything that pertains to transfer inward and animation of the personality, and all influences of a particularly favorable environment, for example, attending higher school, only bring boys closer to the feminine type in this respect. Busemann says that a man of the cultured type, especially a man who is highly cultured intellectually, falls on the line of transition from the masculine to the feminine type of self-consciousness. Busemann believes that our culture is masculine according to origin, but strives toward feminization according to psychological direction of development.

It is difficult to imagine a less sustainable explanation dictated by trying to place the facts obtained into some kind of preconceived pattern. Busemann's error lies in the fact that he cannot bring to an end the point of view of development and the point of view of social dependence in questions of the origin of the adolescent's self-consciousness. For this reason he does not take note of two major facts.

First, the girl precedes the boy in sexual maturation and consequently also in mental development. Due to this, it is natural that a greater percentage of girls

TABLE 7. Distribution of All Types of Judgments according to Sex and Social Groups, % (according to A. Busemann)

Type of Judgment	Boys			Girls		
	A	B	C	A	B	C
Mentioning circumstances	40	34	25	18	11	13
Body	26	19	18	3	4	0
Skill	27	40	42	33	41	33
Ethical character	7	7	15	46	43	53

TABLE 8. Mention of One's Own Body in Statements of Rural and City Children of Different Ages, % (according to A. Busemann)

Age, years	Rural	City
9-11	63.2	15.5
12-14	40.8	4.7

will attain a higher stage of development earlier than boys. Thus, here we have not superiority of the feminine type over the masculine, but the fact of earlier onset of sexual maturation, a different rate and rhythm of development. In fine agreement with this is the fact that such a quantitative difference in rate and rhythm exists between children of different social strata. Since development of self-consciousness is the result mainly of social-cultural development of the personality, it is understandable that the differences in the cultural environment must also directly affect the rate of development of this higher function of personality in children living in unfavorable social-cultural conditions. It is completely understandable that this difference between children of different social groups is one-half the difference between boys and girls.

However, this does not at all mean that Busemann's position on the internal connection between environment and self-consciousness must be discarded. This is far from the case. But the connection must be sought not where Busemann seeks it. Not in quantitative delay in growth, not in lag in rate of development, not in arrest at an earlier stage, but *this difference lies in a different type, in a different structure of self-consciousness.* The quantitative differences that Busemann found are not the most essential for the required connection between the environment and self-consciousness.

With respect to self-consciousness, the working-class adolescent is not simply arrested at an earlier stage of development in comparison with the bourgeois adolescent, *but is an adolescent with a different type of personality development, with a different structure and dynamics of self-consciousness.* The differences here are not in the same plane as the differences between boys and girls. For this reason, the roots of these differences must be sought in the class to which the adolescent belongs and not in one degree or another of his material well-being. For this reason, putting adolescents who belong to different classes into one group, as Busemann does, seems to us to be wrong.

He makes the same mistake when he considers the effect of social environment in age brackets.

TABLE 9. Mention of One's Own Feelings in Statements of City and Rural Children of Different Age and Sex, % (according to A. Busemann)

Age, years	City		Rural	
	M	F	M	F
9-11	20	16	28	20
12-14	18	29	38	52

As Tables 9 and 10 show, a corresponding influence of environment begins to show extremely early, but it is insignificant in comparison with the differences that exist between boys and girls. This again convinces us that the differences Busemann found are primarily differences in rate of development in which, as we know, girls precede boys. This is a major fact in the light of which we must understand all of Busemann's results.

However, his basic conclusion seems to us to be correct. He maintains that the development of self-consciousness depends on the cultural content of the environment to an extent greater perhaps than any other aspect of internal life. In Busemann's attempt to deduce the features of self-consciousness of the adolescent from the vital needs of the social group to which this adolescent belongs, there is an enormous omission, but his methodology marks out a completely correct path of research. He believes that the adolescent who has passed all of his life in an atmosphere of physical work and material want, who is not trained to any skill, naturally considers himself from this point of view: body plus external conditions.

Children of educated workers have a different point of view. We should pay attention here to how much the percentage of self-evaluation based on skills increases. In this respect, the children of skilled workers surpass even the children of the next group: for a skilled worker, Busemann believes that skill is the most important. For this reason children assimilate this factor in self-evaluation, transferred from the external inward, from a social criterion it becomes individual, from a group factor it is converted to a factor of self-consciousness. Finally, children of the third group also reflect the ethical level of their own families in their self-evaluations.

In general, Busemann says that the character and method by which the child recognizes his own existence and activity depend to a high degree on how his parents consider and value themselves. Value scales of adults become the value scales of the child himself. Busemann urges that prejudgment be avoided as if everything had to be done consciously and with reflection so that it might be good. He says that it is not just in the area of ethics that the very best happens when the left hand does not know what the right hand is doing. There is the perfection of the unconscious person.

This hymn to limitedness definitely shows the falsity of the basic premise of the author. Instead of giving a qualitative analysis and disclosing qualitative differences between the adolescent's consciousness in different social environments, the author is satisfied with a simple establishment of a delay in the transition from one stage to another. But the matter obviously is *not in stages* but in *types* of self-consciousness and in the course of the process itself of development. In certain respects, for example, in the sense of being conscious of one's own personality from the social-class aspect, the working-class adolescent will, of course, reach a higher stage of self-consciousness than the bourgeois adolescent. In other respects, he is slower. But we cannot say anything in general on the lag and movement forward where the paths of development form completely immeasurable qualitatively different curves.

TABLE 10. Degree of Internalization of Representations of Oneself (% of Compositions on the Internal World of the Personality, Taking into Account the Total Number of Compositions, according to Busemann)

	Schools							
	City						Rural	
	Total		Higher		Folk		Folk	
Age, years	M	F	M	F	M	F	M	F
9	30	—	36	43	25	80	20	16
10	41	45	23	50	36	67	30	27
11	50	52	19	79	37	53	24	22
12	95	88	26	72	50	69	16	26
13	89	96	30	100	49	52	19	50
14	80	92	58	96	42	60	37	69
15	79	90	50	90	—	—	—	—
16	77	92	60	100	—	—	—	—
17	74	—	61	—	—	—	—	—

4

The third point in the work of Busemann that frees us from the metaphysical approach to self-consciousness is that self-consciousness is not taken as some kind of metaphysical essence that is not subject to analysis. Together with the aspect of development and social dependence, an aspect of empirical analysis of self-consciousness is introduced. The six points listed above that characterize the structure of self-consciousness in the plane of development are the first attempt at such empirical analysis of personality. Figure 5 presents the course of development of self-consciousness (assimilating internal criteria of evaluation). We can easily see the rise in the curve and the sharp rise during the period of sexual maturation.

Busemann's great achievement is that he realized the new point, the new stage in the development of the adolescent as being a qualitatively unique time in his maturation. The investigator was fully justified in calling attention to the fact that reflection on its part can affect the subject in a reconstructive way (self-shaping). This is the great significance of reflection for the psychology of individual differences. Together with the primary conditions of the individual cast of the personality (instincts, heredity) and secondary conditions of its formation (environment, acquired traits), there is a set of *third conditions* (reflection, self-shaping).

Busemann is on firm ground in posing the question: does the principle of convergence established by Stern also apply to relations between the given individuality and its self-shaping by consciousness? In other words, the question concerns the independence of this third group of traits that arise on the basis of the self-consciousness of the personality. Can we imagine development of this group of traits on the basis of the principle of convergence? In other words, does the process of development in this area follow the same principle as does the formation of secondary traits on the basis of interaction of innate instincts and the effect of the environment? We believe that posing this question is enough to give it a negative answer. Here a new acting persona enters the drama of development, a new, qualitatively unique factor—the personality of the adolescent himself. We have before us the very complex structure of this personality.

Busemann notes six different facets in its development. Each of them can develop at a different rate, and for this reason the personality may present very different forms at each stage of development, depending on the different interrelation

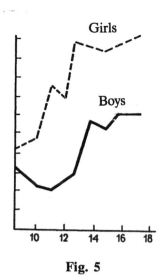

Fig. 5

and different structure of the basic six facets. For this reason, Busemann says that the most various forms are possible. On the one hand, there are people who know themselves very well, but at the same time, their self-evaluation does not include ethical scales to any significant degree. On the other hand, self-consciousness that is still vague may operate with such scales. For this reason Busemann believes that this matter is much more intricate than it may seem at first glance.

Specifically, it is an understanding of the qualitative self-image to the degree attained by the adolescent approaching self-consciousness that makes it possible for Busemann to evaluate the significance of reflection in the whole cycle of mental development at this age.

If we look at the significance of reflection for mental life as a whole, we will clearly see the profound difference between the structure of the personality that is nonreflecting, naive, on the one hand, and the structure that is reflecting on the other. True, the process of self-consciousness is a continuous process so there is no sharp boundary between naiveté and reflection.

Since the word, "naive," is used in still another sense, Busemann introduces a new term, "sympsychia," to designate a mental life complete, closed within itself and not divided by any kind of reflection. By this term, he understands the single attitude and activity of the primitive mind, an example of which may be the child wholly absorbed in play. An opposite example: the adolescent who reproaches himself in light of his own feelings. The state of this kind of division Busemann terms diapsychia. It is characteristic of reflection of a developed consciousness. The adolescent, according to the ideas of Busemann, is differentiated internally into the acting "I" and into another "I"—the reflecting "I."

The effect of reflection is not exhausted by just the internal change in the personality itself. In connection with the development of self-consciousness, it becomes possible for the adolescent to understand other people immeasurably more profoundly and broadly. The social development that leads to the formation of the personality acquires a support in self-consciousness for its further development.

Here we come in earnest to the last and most difficult and complex of all the questions connected with the structure and dynamics of personality. We have seen that the development of self-consciousness marks the transition to a new principle of development and to the formation of tertiary traits. We recall that the changes we noted above as changes characteristic of the mental development of the adolescent indicate this new type of development. We designated it as the cultural development of behavior and thinking. We saw that development of memory, attention, and thinking in concepts at this age consists not in a simple branching out of inherited instincts in the process of their realization under certain environmental conditions. We saw that the transition to self-consciousness and to mastery of internal control of these processes is the real content of the development of functions during the transitional age. If we were to try to determine more precisely what the new type of development consists of, we would see that it consists primarily of the formation of new connections, new relations, and new structural links between various functions. If the child did not see how others manage memory, he would not be able to master this process.

In the process of sociogenesis of higher mental functions, tertiary functions are formed based on the new type of connections and relations between separate processes. For example, we have seen that the development of memory is made up mainly of the new relation that is created between memory and thinking. We said that if for the child thinking means remembering, then for the adolescent, remembering means thinking. The same task of adaptation is resolved by different methods. The functions enter into new, complex relations with each other. This pertains also to perception, attention, and action.

All of these new types of connections and interrelations of functions presuppose reflection, reflection of his own processes as a substrate in the consciousness of the adolescent. We recall that logical thinking develops only on the basis of such reflection. Characteristic for mental functions in the transitional age is participation of the personality in each separate act. The child [using the idiomatic Russian expressions] would say impersonally, "it seems to me," and "it comes to my mind," but the adolescent would say, "I think" and "I remember." In the true expression of J. Politzer,[99] it is not the muscle, but the man that works. Precisely so we can say that it is not memory that remembers, but man. This means that the functions entered a new connection with each other through the personality. In these new connections, in these tertiary, higher functions, there is nothing mysterious or secret because, as we have seen, the law of their construction consists of the fact that what were at one time relations between people became psychological relations transferred to the personality. This is why this diapsychia, this distinguishing of the acting, reflecting "I," of which Busemann speaks, is nothing other than a projection of social relations to within the personality. Self-consciousness is social consciousness transferred within.

Using a very simple example, we can elucidate how the new tertiary connections of separate functions specific to the personality arise and how specifically in connections of this type, the personality finds its full embodiment, its adequate description, and how in connections of this type, instincts that characterize the personality (primary traits) and acquired experience (secondary traits) become a removed category, a subordinate instance. Connections that characterize the personality at the most primitive stage of development differ qualitatively from connections that are habitual for us to such a degree that their comparative study shows better than anything what the very nature of these connections and the type of their formation is. The study shows that connections of personality habitual to us are characterized by a certain relation between separate functions and, because they are new psychological systems, it is understandable that they are not something constant, everlasting, but are a historical formation characteristic for a certain stage and form of development.

Here is an example borrowed from the book on the primitive mind by L. Lévy-Bruhl (1930).[100] Dreams play a completely different role in the life of primitive man than they do for us. The connection of dreams with other mental processes and, derived from this, their functional significance in the general structure of the personality are completely different. Almost everywhere, dreams were at first a guide which was followed, an infallible companion, and frequently even a master whose commands were not disputed. What could be more natural than an attempt to compel this adviser to speak, to go for help to this master, to learn his commands in difficult situations. Here is a typical example of such a case. Missionaries insist that the leader of a tribe send his son to school, and he responds: "I will dream about it." He explains that the leaders of the Magololo** are very often guided by dreams in their actions. On a solid basis, Lévy-Bruhl maintains that the response of the leader of the primitive tribe expresses completely the state of his psychology. A European would have said, "I'll think about it"; the leader of the Magololo answers, "I'll dream about it."

Thus we see that in this kind of primitive man, dreams fulfill the function that thinking fulfills in our behavior. The laws of dreams are, of course, the same, but the *role* of dreams for the man who believes in them and is guided by them and for the man who does not believe in them is different. This is the source also of the different structures of the personality that are realized in the connections of separate functions with each other. For this reason, where we say, "*I dream*," a Kafir would say, "*I see a dream*."

The mechanism of behavior that is evident in this example is typical for tertiary traits, and what pertains to dreaming in this example, actually pertains to all functions. Let us take the thinking of modern man. As for Spinoza, for one, thinking is the master of passions, and for others (those described by Freud, people autistically oriented and closed within themselves), thinking is the servant of passions. And autistic thinking differs from philosophical thinking not in its laws, but in its *role*, in its functional significance in the total structure of the personality.

Mental functions change this hierarchy in various spheres of social life. For this reason, diseases of the personality are most often apparent in the change in the role of separate functions and the hierarchy of the whole system of functions. It is not the raving that distinguishes the mentally ill from us, but the fact that the person believes the raving and obeys it while we do not. On the basis of reflection, on the basis of self-consciousness and understanding our own processes, new groups and new connections of these functions with each other develop, and these connections which arise on the basis of self-consciousness and characterize the structure of the personality we call tertiary traits. The prototype of connections of this kind is the connection of the type that we illustrated with the dream of the Kafir. One set of internal convictions or another, one set of ethical standards or another, one set of principles of behavior or another—all of this in the last analysis is embodied in the personality through connections of this type specifically. The man who follows his convictions and does not decide on some complex and doubtful action before he considers it in the light of these convictions essentially sets in motion a mechanism of the same type and structure as the Kafir set in motion before deciding on what was for him the doubtful and complex proposal of the missionary. We call this mechanism a *psychological system*.

The transitional age is also a time of formation of tertiary connections, mechanisms of the type of the Kafir's dream. What is acting here is the law of transition from external to internal processes, which we have noted earlier. According to the

**Editor's note: Magololo and Kafir are names of African tribes.

determination of Kretschmer, one of the basic laws disclosed by the history of development is the law of transition from external to internal reaction. Kretschmer attaches great importance to the fact that in the higher living beings, reactions that involve selection move more and more inward. They depend less and less on peripheral organs of movement and, on the contrary, more and more on the nervous central organ. A new stimulation over a large area no longer evokes an apparent storm of arousal movements, but evokes an invisible sequence of mental states within the organism, the end result of which is an already prepared purposeful movement. Thus, attempts are now no longer made on the scale of the movements themselves, but only as if on the scale of an embryo of movement. The process of consciousness is connected with these physiological acts of selection in the nervous central organ. We call these volitional processes.

This law is also valid with respect to mechanisms of the new type of which we spoke above. They also develop initially as certain external operations, external forms of behavior, which then become internal forms of thinking and action of the personality.

5

E. Spranger was the first to turn his attention to an interesting fact that has substantial significance for understanding the structure and dynamics of the personality during the transitional age. He points out that no period in our life is remembered as are the years of sexual maturation. In recollections, significantly less is retained of the real rhythm of internal life during these years than of internal life at other age levels. This fact is really remarkable. We know that memory is the basis of what psychologists usually call unity and identity of the personality. Memory is the basis of self-consciousness. Disruption of memory usually indicates a transition from one state to another, from one structure of the personality to another. For this reason, it is typical that we do not remember our sickly conditions and our dreams very well.

There may be two explanations for disruption of memory. For example, let us take amnesia that involves early childhood. It can be explained on the one hand by the fact that memory at that stage is not connected with the word, with speech, and for this reason acts in a manner different from our memory. On the other hand, we see that the completely different structure of the infant's personality results in a development which makes nonseparability and heredity impossible in the development of the personality.

We have the same thing, but in a different form, in the transitional age. Here amnesia occurs again. Having lived through the transitional age, we forget it, and this is evidence of our transition to a different structure of personality, to a different system of connections between separate functions—here development is achieved not along a direct, but along a very complex and meandering curve. In the structure of the personality of the adolescent there is nothing stable, final, and immovable. Everything in it is *transition, everything is in flux*. This is the alpha and omega of the structure and dynamics of the adolescent's personality. This is, therefore, the alpha and omega of the pedology of the transitional age.

PART 2

PROBLEMS OF CHILD
(DEVELOPMENTAL) PSYCHOLOGY

Chapter 6
THE PROBLEM OF AGE[1]

1. The Problem of Dividing the Child's Development into Periods

According to theoretical bases, the schemes for dividing the child's development into periods proposed in science can be placed into three groups.

The first group includes attempts to divide childhood into periods not by separating the course itself of the child's development, but on the basis of a stepwise construction of other processes that are connected in some way with the child's development. As an example, we might cite the division of child development into periods that is based on the biogenetic principle. The biogenetic theory assumes that there is a strict parallelism between the development of humanity and the development of the child, that ontogenesis repeats phylogenesis in a brief and compressed form. From the point of view of this theory, it is most natural to divide childhood into separate periods conforming basically to the periods of the history of mankind. Thus, dividing childhood into periods is based on the division into periods of phylogenetic development. This group includes the proposals of Hutchinson and other authors on dividing childhood into periods.

Not all the attempts of this group are equally unfounded. For example, this group includes the attempt to divide childhood into periods corresponding to levels of training and education of the child, breaking up the system of national education accepted in a given country (preschool age, primary school age, etc.). In this case, breaking childhood up into periods is done not on the basis of internal breaking up of development itself, but, as we see, on the basis of training and education. This is where the error of this scheme lies. But since the processes of child development are closely connected with the teaching of the child, and the separation of teaching into levels depends on enormous practical experience, then naturally breaking childhood up according to a pedagogical principle brings us extremely close to a real division of childhood into separate periods.

Most of the attempts must be placed into a second group; these are directed toward isolating some single trait of child development as an arbitrary criterion for dividing it into periods. A typical example is the attempt of P. P. Blonsky (1930, pp. 110-111) to divide childhood into periods on the basis of dentition, that is, the appearance of teeth and their replacement. The trait serving as a basis for separating one period of childhood from another must be (1) an indicator for judgment on the general development of the child, (2) easily accessible visually, and (3) objective. Dentition meets precisely these requirements.

Dentition processes are closely connected with essential features of the constitution of the growing organism, specifically with its calcification and the activity of the glands of internal secretions. At the same time, these processes are easily accessible for observation and indisputably established. Dentition is a clear age trait. On the basis of dentition, postnatal childhood is divided into three periods: toothless childhood, the childhood of milk teeth, and the childhood of permanent teeth. Toothless childhood lasts until all of the milk teeth come through (from eight months to two or two and a half years). The childhood of milk teeth lasts to the beginning of tooth replacement (approximately age six and a half years). Finally, the childhood of permanent teeth concludes with the appearance of the third set of back molars (wisdom teeth). The period of breaking through of the milk teeth can in turn be divided into three stages: absolutely toothless childhood (the first half year), the stage of breaking through of the teeth (second half year) and the stage of breaking through of the canines and molars (the third year of postnatal life).

A similar attempt to divide childhood into periods on the basis of some single aspect of development is the scheme of C. H. Stratz, who proposed sexual development as the main criterion. Psychological criteria have been suggested in other schemes constructed along the same principle. This is the kind of division into periods proposed by W. Stern, who differentiates early childhood as the time during which the child displays only play activity (up to six years of age) followed by a period of conscious learning in which play and work are separated and a period of youthful maturation (age fourteen to eighteen) with the development of independence of personality and plans for subsequent life.

The schemes of this group are, first of all, subjective. Although as a criterion for dividing age levels, they do isolate an objective trait, the trait itself is taken according to subjective bases depending on which processes get the most attention. Age is an objective category and not an arbitrary, freely chosen, fictive value. For this reason, guideposts that mark age may be placed not at any points of the life of the child, but exclusively and only at those points at which objectively one age level ends and another begins.

Another inadequacy of schemes in this group is that they use a single criterion, some single trait, for separating all the age levels. What is forgotten here is that in the course of development the value, the significance, the indicative and symptomatic quality and importance of the selected trait changes. The trait that is indicative and substantive for making a judgment on the development of the child at one period loses its meaning in the following period since in the course of development, aspects that were primary earlier become secondary. Thus, the criterion of sexual maturation is significant and indicative for the age of puberty, but has no such meaning for the preceding age levels. The breaking through of teeth at the boundary between infancy and early childhood can be used as an indicative trait for the general development of the child, but the replacement of teeth at approximately seven years of age and the appearance of wisdom teeth cannot be compared in its significance for general development to the first appearance of teeth. These schemes do not take into account the reorganization of the process itself of development. Because of this reorganization, the importance and significance of any trait change continuously with the transition from age level to age level. This excludes the possibility of dividing childhood into separate periods according to a single criterion for all age levels. Child development is such a complex process that it cannot be determined at all completely according to one trait alone at any stage.

The third inadequacy of the schemes is their principal tendency to study external traits of child development and not the internal essence of the process. In theory, the internal essence of things and the external form of their manifestation do not coincide. ". . .If the form of manifestation and the essence of things coincided directly, then all science would be superfluous . . ." (K. Marx and F. Engels,

Works, Vol. 25, Part II, p. 384). For this reason, scientific research is an indispensable means for recognizing the reality that the form of manifestation and the essence of things do not coincide directly. At present, psychology is moving from a purely descriptive, empirical, and phenomenological study of phenomena to disclosing their internal essence. Until recently, the main problem was the study of symptom complexes, that is, the aggregate of external traits that differentiate the various periods, stages, and phases of child development. Symptom denotes trait. To say that psychology studies symptom complexes of different periods, phases, and stages of child development is to say that it studies its external traits. But the real problem consists of studying what lies behind these traits and determines them, that is, studying the process itself of child development in its internal patterns. With respect to the problem of dividing childhood into periods, this means that we must reject attempts of symptomatic classification of age levels and move on, as other sciences have done in their time, to classification based on the internal essence of the process being studied.

A third group of attempts to divide child development into periods is connected with the attempt to move from a purely symptomatic and descriptive principle to isolating substantial features of child development itself. However, in these attempts, the problem is formulated correctly but not solved. Attempts to solve problems always seem to be half-hearted, never proceed to the end, and are unsustainable with respect to the problem of periodicity. Methodological difficulties that result from an antidialectical and dualistic concept of child development are a fateful obstacle that prevents it from being considered as a single process of self-development.

Such, for example, is the attempt of A. Gesell to construct periodicity of child development on the basis of the change in the child's internal rhythm and tempo, on the basis of determining "the flowing stream of development." Based on essentially correct observations of the change in the rhythm of development related to age, Gesell arrives at separating all of childhood into separate rhythmic periods or waves of development united within themselves by a constancy of tempo over the whole duration of a given period and separated from other periods by a clear change in this tempo. Gesell presents the dynamics of child development as a process of gradual slowing of growth. Gesell's theory borders on the group of contemporary theories that, in his own expression, make early childhood the high point for the interpretation of the personality and its history. What is main and most important in child development, according to Gesell, is accomplished in the first years or even in the first months of life. Subsequent development taken as a whole does not equal one act of this drama that is maximally saturated with content.

What is the source of such delusion? It flows inevitably from the evolutionistic conception of development on which Gesell bases his theory and according to which nothing new arises in development, no qualitative changes occur, and only what is given from the very beginning grows and develops. Actually, development is not confined to the scheme, "more—less," but is characterized primarily and specifically by the presence of qualitative neoformations that are subject to their own rhythm and require a special measure each time. It is true that at early age levels, we observe maximum rates of development of those prerequisites on which subsequent development of the child depends. The basic, elementary organs and functions mature sooner than the higher. But it is not correct to assume that all development is exhausted by the growth of these basic, elementary functions which are the prerequisites for higher aspects of the personality. If we consider higher aspects, then the result will be the reverse; the tempo and rhythm of their establishment will be minimal during the first acts of the whole drama of development and will reach a maximum in its finale.

We cited Gesell's theory as an example of half-hearted attempts at periodicity which stop halfway in the transition from symptomatic to essential division of age levels.

What must the principles be for constructing a genuine periodicity? We already know where to look for its real basis: only internal changes of development itself, only breaks and turning points in its flow can provide a reliable basis for determining the main periods of formation of the personality of the child which we call age levels. All theories of child development can be reduced to two basic conceptions. According to one, development is nothing other than realization, modification, and combination of deposits. Nothing new develops here—only a growth, branching, and regrouping of those factors that were already present at the very beginning. According to the second conception, development is a continuous process of self-propulsion characterized primarily by a continuous appearance and formation of the new which did not exist at previous stages. This point of view captures in development something essential to a dialectical understanding of the process.

In its turn, it allows both idealistic and materialistic theories of personality construction. In the first case, it finds its embodiment in theories of creative evolution directed by an autonomous, internal vital surge of the purposefully self-developing personality, by the will toward self-affirmation and self-perfection. In the second case, it leads to an understanding of development as a process that is characterized by a unity of material and mental aspects, a unity of the social and the personal during the child's ascent up the stages of development.

From the latter point of view, no other criterion exists or can exist for determining the concrete periods of child development or age levels except for those neoformations that characterize the essence of each age level. We must understand that new type of structure of the personality and its activity, those mental and social changes which first appear at a given age level and which mainly and basically determine the consciousness of the child, his relation to the environment, his internal and external life, the whole course of his development during the given period as age-related neoformations.

But this alone is not enough for dividing child development into periods scientifically. We must also consider its dynamics and the dynamics of transitions from one age level to another. By purely empirical studies, psychology established that age-level changes may, in the words of Blonsky (1930, p. 7), occur abruptly and critically, or may occur gradually and lytically. Blonsky terms as *periods and stages* the times of the child's life that are separated from one another by more (periods) or less (stages) abrupt *crises*; *phases* are times of the child's life separated from each other lytically.

Actually, at certain age levels, development is marked by slow, evolutionary, or lytic flow. These are age levels of predominantly smooth and frequently unremarkable internal change in the child's personality, change that is accomplished by insignificant "molecular" attainments. Here, over a more or less long time that usually takes several years, no fundamental, abrupt shifts and alterations occur that reconstruct the child's whole personality. More or less remarkable changes in the child's personality occur here only as a result of a long-term cryptic "molecular" process. They appear outside and are accessible to direct observation only as a conclusion of long-term processes of latent development.[2]

During relatively firm or stable ages, development occurs mainly through microscopic changes in the child's personality that accumulate to a certain limit and then appear spasmodically in the form of some kind of neoformation of the age level.

Such stable periods make up the greater part of childhood, if judged purely chronologically. Since within them, development proceeds as if underground, great alterations in his personality are evident if a child is compared at the beginning and at the end of a stable period.

Stable age periods have been studied significantly more fully than those that are characterized by another type of development—crises. The latter are disclosed purely empirically and thus far have not been brought into the system, have not been included in the general division of child development into periods. Many authors even doubt that there is any internal need for their existence. They are more inclined to take them as "diseases" of development because of its deviation from the normal path. Almost none of the bourgeois investigators could theoretically realize their actual significance. For this reason, our attempt to systematize them and interpret them theoretically and include them in the general pattern of child development must be considered as almost the first such attempt.

None of the investigators can deny the fact itself of the existence of these unique periods in child development, and even authors with the most nondialectical frame of mind admit the need to allow, if only as a hypothesis, the presence of crises in the child's development even in earliest childhood.

From a purely external aspect, these periods are characterized by traits which are the opposite of the firm or stable age levels. During these periods, abrupt and major shifts and displacements, changes, and discontinuities in the child's personality are concentrated in a relatively short time (several months, a year or at most, two). In a very short time, the child changes completely in the basic traits of his personality. Development takes on a stormy, impetuous, and sometimes catastrophic character that resembles a revolutionary course of events in both rate of the changes that are occurring and in the sense of the alterations that are made. These are turning points in the child's development that sometimes take the form of a severe crisis.

The first feature of such periods consists, on the one hand, in the fact that the boundaries that separate the beginning and end of the crisis from adjacent age levels are not at all definite. The crisis arises imperceptibly—it is difficult to determine its onset and termination. On the other hand, an abrupt aggravation of the crisis, which usually occurs in the middle of this age period, is characteristic. The presence of a culmination point in which the crisis reaches apogee characterizes all critical ages and differentiates them clearly from the stable periods of child development.

The second feature of critical age levels served as a departure point for empirical study. The fact is that a significant proportion of children who experience critical periods of development are difficult children. These children seem to drop out of the system of pedagogical influence that until very recently provided a normal course for their training and education. In children of school age during critical periods, there is a drop in rate of success, a slacking of interest in school work, and a general decline in capacity for work. At critical age levels, the child's development frequently is accompanied by more or less sharp conflicts with those around him. The child's internal life is sometimes connected with painful and excruciating experiences and with internal conflicts.

True, it is far from always that all of this occurs. In different children, critical periods occur differently. During the passage of a crisis even in children most alike in type of development and in social situation, there is much greater variation than during the stable periods. Many children do not exhibit at all clearly any of the traits of difficult children or any decline in school success. The range of variation in the passage of these age levels in different children and in the influence of ex-

ternal and internal conditions on the course of the crisis itself is so great and significant that this caused many authors to question whether crises of child development in general are not a product of exclusively external unfavorable conditions
and whether they should therefore be considered the exception rather than the
rule in the history of child development (A. Busemann et al.).

It is understood that external conditions determine the concrete character of
manifestation and passage of critical periods. Dissimilar in different children, they
bring about a very mixed and diverse picture of variants of the critical age. But
neither the presence nor the absence of some specific external conditions, but internal logic of the process of development itself is responsible for the critical, disruptive periods in the life of the child. A study of comparative factors convinces
us of this.

Thus, if we move from an absolute evaluation of the difficult aspects of difficult
children to a relative evaluation based on a comparison of degrees of ease or difficulty of teaching the child during the stable period that either preceded or followed the crisis, we cannot help but see that *every* child at this stage becomes
relatively difficult in comparison with himself at a proximate age. In precisely the
same way, if we move from absolute evaluation of school success to a relative evaluation based on a comparison of the rate of movement of the child in the course
of teaching at different age periods, we will see that *every* child slows this rate
during the crisis period in comparison with the rate characteristic of the stable periods.

The third feature, perhaps most important but least clear from the theoretical
aspect and for this reason, one that impedes a correct understanding of the nature
of child development during these periods, is the negative character of development.
Everyone who wrote about these unique periods noted in the first place that development here is different from that in the stable ages and does destructive rather
than constructive work. Progressive development of the child's personality, the continuous construction of the new, which had been so prominent in all stable ages,
is seemingly attenuated or temporarily suspended. Processes of dying off and closure, the disintegration and breakdown of what had been formed at preceding stages
and distinguished the child of a given age move to the forefront. During the critical
periods, the child does not so much acquire as he loses some of what he had acquired earlier. The onset of these age levels is not marked by the appearance of
new interests of the child, of new aspirations, new types of activity, new forms of
internal life. The child entering a period of crisis is more apt to be characterized
by the opposite traits: he loses interests that only yesterday guided all his activity
and took the greater part of his time and attention but now seemingly die off;
forms of external relations and internal life developed earlier are neglected. L. N.
Tolstoy graphically and precisely called one such critical period of child development
the desert of adolescence.

This is what people have in mind primarily when they speak of the negative
character of the critical age levels. By this, they mean to express the idea that development seems to change its positive, creative significance, causing the observer
to characterize such periods predominantly from unfavorable, negative aspects.
Many authors are even convinced that the negative content exhausts the whole idea
of development during the critical periods. This conviction is fixed in the names
for the critical years (some call this age the negative phase, some, the phase of
obstinacy, etc.).

The concepts of separate critical ages were introduced into science by the empirical path and in a random order. The crisis of age seven was discovered and
described before the others (the seventh year in the life of the child is transitional

between the preschool and the adolescent periods). The seven- to eight-year-old child is no longer a preschooler, but not yet an adolescent. The seven-year-old differs from both the preschool child and from the school child and for this reason presents difficulties with respect to his teaching. The negative content of this age is apparent primarily in the disruption of mental equilibrium and in the instability of the will, mood, etc.

The crisis of the three-year-old, discovered and described later, was called by many authors the phase of obstinacy or stubbornness. During this period, limited to a short interval of time, the personality of the child undergoes abrupt and unexpected changes. The child becomes a difficult child. He exhibits obstinacy, stubbornness, negativism, capriciousness, and self-will. Internal and external conflicts frequently accompany the whole period.

The thirteen-year crisis was studied even later and described as the negative phase of the age of sexual maturation. As the very name indicates, the negative content of the period is most prominent and with superficial observation seems to be the whole idea of development in this period. The decrease in success, decline in capacity for work, lack of harmony in the internal structure of the personality, contraction and dying off of systems of previously established interests, and the negative, protesting character of behavior led Kroh to describe this period as the stage of such disorientation in internal and external relations in which the human "I" and the world are more divided than at any other periods.

Comparatively recently the idea has been recognized theoretically that the transition from infancy to early childhood, occurring at approximately age one, also presents an essentially critical period with its own differentiating traits known to us from the general description of this unique form of development; this transition has been thoroughly studied from the factual aspect.

To obtain a definitive chain of critical ages, we proposed including in it as an initial link, perhaps the most unique of all periods of child development, the newborn stage. This well-studied period stands alone in the system of other ages and is, by its nature, perhaps the clearest and least questionable crisis in the development of the child. The spasmodic change in conditions of development in the act of birth, when the newborn rapidly falls into a completely new environment, changes the whole tenor of his life and characterizes the initial period of extrauterine development.

The crisis of the newborn separates the embryonal period of development from infancy. The one-year crisis separates infancy from early childhood. The crisis at age three is a transition from early childhood to preschool age. The crisis at age seven is a link that joins preschool and school ages. Finally, the crisis at age thirteen coincides with the turning point in development at the transition from school age to puberty. Thus, an ordered picture opens before us. Critical periods alternate with stable periods and are turning points in development, once again confirming that the development of the child is a dialectical process in which a transition from one stage to another is accomplished not along an evolutionary, but along a revolutionary path.

If the critical ages had not been discovered through purely empirical means, the conception of them would have to be introduced into the pattern of development on the basis of theoretical analysis. Now it remains for theory only to become cognizant of and comprehend what has already been established by empirical studies.

At turning points of development, the child becomes relatively difficult due to the fact that the change in the pedagogical system applied to the child does not keep up with the rapid changes in his personality. Pedagogy during the critical ages is least developed in practical and theoretical respects.

As all life is at the same time also a dying (F. Engels),[3] so also child development—one of the complex forms of life—of necessity includes in itself processes of closure and dying off. The appearance of the new in development necessarily signifies the dying off of the old. The transition to a new age is always marked by the demise of the previous age. The processes of reverse development, the dying off of the old, are concentrated mainly during the critical ages. But it would be a great mistake to assume that this is the whole significance of the critical ages. Development never ends its creative work, and during critical periods too, we observe constructive processes of development. Moreover, processes of involution so clearly expressed during these periods, themselves are subordinate to processes of positive structuring of the personality, depend on them directly, and with them make up an indivisible whole. The disruptive work is done in these periods to the extent that is required by the need to develop properties and traits of the personality. Practical study shows that the negative content of development at turning points is only the reverse or shadow side of positive changes of the personality that make up the principal and basic sense of any critical age.

The positive significance of crisis at age three is evident in that here new character traits of the child's personality appear. It has been established that if the crisis for some reason passes sluggishly and is not clearly expressed, this leads to a serious delay in the development of affective and volitional aspects of the child's personality at a later age.

With respect to the crisis at age seven, all investigators noted that together with negative symptoms, during this period, there are a number of major achievements: the child becomes more independent and his relation to other children changes.

In the crisis at age thirteen, the decrease in productivity of mental work of the student is caused by a change from attention to what is obvious to understanding and deduction. The transition to a higher form of intellectual activity is accompanied by a temporary decrease in capacity for work. This is also confirmed for the rest of the negative symptoms of the crisis: behind every negative symptom is hidden a positive content consisting usually in the transition to a new and higher form.

Finally, there is no doubt that there is positive content in the crisis at age one. Here the negative symptoms are obviously and directly connected with positive acquisitions that the child makes by standing up and by learning to speak.

The same may pertain also to the crisis of the newborn. At this time, the child regresses at first even with respect to physical development: in the first days after birth, the newborn loses weight. Adaptation to the new form of life places such high demands on the vitality of the child that, in the words of Blonsky, man never stands as close to death as in the hours of his birth (1930, p. 85). Nevertheless, during this period more than at any of the subsequent crises, the fact is evident that development is a process of the formation and appearance of the new. Everything that we see in the child's development during the first days and weeks is a continuous neoformation. Negative symptoms that characterize the negative content of this period arise from the difficulties due specifically to the novelty of the form of life that arises for the first time and is much more complicated.

The most essential content of development at the critical ages consists of the appearance of neoformations which, as concrete research shows, are unique and specific to a high degree. Their main difference from neoformations of stable ages is that they have a transitional character. This means that in the future, they will not be preserved in the form in which they appear at the critical period and will not enter as a requisite component into the integral structure of the future personality. They die off, seemingly being absorbed by the neoformations of the subsequent, stable age and being included in their composition as subordinate factors that do hot have an independent existence, being dissolved and transformed in them to such an extent that without special and penetrating analysis, it is frequently impossible to detect the presence of this transformed formation of the critical period in the acquisitions of the succeeding stable age. As such, the neoformations of the crises die off together with the onset of the following age, but they continue to exist in a latent form within it, not living an independent life, but only participating in the underground development which leads to the spasmodic appearance of neoformations during the stable ages, as we have seen.

The concrete content of general laws on neoformations of stable and critical ages will be disclosed in subsequent sections of this work devoted to considering each age.

Neoformations must serve as the basic criterion for dividing child development into separate ages in our scheme. In this scheme, the sequence of age periods must be determined by the alternation of stable and critical periods. The times of stable ages that have more or less distinct beginning and end boundaries can most correctly be determined specifically according to these boundaries. Because of the different character of their passage, critical ages can be determined most correctly by noting the culmination points or peaks of the crisis and using as its beginning the preceding half year closest to this time, and for its conclusion, the closest half year of the subsequent age.

As was established by empirical study, stable ages have a clearly expressed two-member structure and can be divided into two stages, the first and the second. Critical ages have a clearly expressed three-member structure and consist of three interconnected lytic transitions of phases: precritical, critical, and postcritical.

It must be noted that our scheme of child development differs substantially from other similar schemes in the determination of basic periods of child development. In addition to using the principle of age-related neoformations as criteria, the following points are new in this scheme: (1) introducing critical ages into the scheme of division into periods; (2) excluding the period of embryonal development of the child; (3) excluding the period of development that is usually called youth, which includes the years after age seventeen to eighteen right up to the onset of final maturity; (4) including the age of sexual maturation among the stable, firm ages and not among the critical ages.[4]

We remove the embryonal development of the child from the scheme for the simple reason that it cannot be considered at the same level as extrauterine development of the child as a social being. The embryonal development is a completely special type of development subject to patterns other than development of the personality that begins at the moment of birth. Embryonal development is studied by an independent science, embryology, which cannot be considered a chapter of psychology. Psychology must take into account the laws of embryonal development of the child since the features of this period affect the course of subsequent development, but psychology does not include embryology in any way because of this. In precisely the same way, it is necessary to consider the laws and data of genetics, that is, the science of heredity, without turning genetics into one of the chapters of psychology. Psychology does not study either heredity or uterine development as such, but only the influence of heredity and uterine development of the child on the process of his social development.

We do not include youth in the scheme of age periods of childhood for the reason that theoretical and empirical studies equally compel opposition to stretching child development excessively and including in it the first twenty-five years of human life. In the general sense and according to basic patterns, the age eighteen to twenty-five years more likely makes up the initial link in the chain of mature age than the concluding link in the chain of periods of child development. It is difficult to imagine that human development at the beginning of maturity (age eighteen to twenty-five) could be subject to patterns of child development.

Including the age of puberty among the stable ages is a necessary logical conclusion from what we know about this age and what characterizes it as a period of enormous development in the life of the adolescent, as a period of higher syntheses effected in the personality. This arises as the necessary logical conclusion from the criticism that in Soviet science theories were imposed that reduced the period of sexual maturation to "normal pathology" and to a profound internal crisis.

Thus, we could present the division of age into periods in the following way[5]:

Crisis of the newborn.
Infancy (two months to one year).
Crisis at age one.
Early childhood (one to three years).
Crisis at age three.
Preschool age (three to seven years).
Crisis at age seven.
School age (eight to twelve years).
Crisis at age thirteen.
Age of puberty (fourteen to eighteen years).
Crisis at age seventeen.

2. Structure and Dynamics of Age

The task of this section is to establish the general states that characterize the internal structure of the process of development that we call the structure of age in each period of childhood.

The following is the most general state which we must indicate immediately: the process of development in each age period, regardless of all the complexity of its organization and composition, regardless of all the diversity of the partial processes that form it, that are disclosed by analysis, represents a single whole that has a certain structure; the structure and course of each partial process of development that is included in the constitution of the whole is determined by the laws of construction of this whole or by structural laws of the age level. An integral formation that is not made up entirely of separate parts, being a kind of aggregate, but itself determines the fate and significance of each of the parts that make it up is called a structure.

The age levels represent the integral, dynamic formation, the structure, which determines the role and relative significance of each partial line of development. At each given age period, development occurs in such a way that separate aspects of the child's personality change and as a result of this, there is a reconstruction of the personality as a whole—in development there is just exactly a reverse dependence: the child's personality changes as a whole in its internal structure and the movement of each of its parts is determined by the laws of change of this whole.

As a result of this, at each given age level, we always find a central neoformation seemingly leading the whole process of development and characterizing the reconstruction of the whole personality of the child on a new base. Around the basic or central neoformation of the given age are grouped all the other partial neoformations pertaining to separate aspects of the child's personality and the processes of development connected with the neoformations of preceding age levels. The processes of development that are more or less directly connected with the basic neoformation we shall call *central lines of development* at the given age and all other partial processes and changes occurring at the given age, we shall call *peripheral lines of development*. It is understood that processes that are central lines of development at one age become peripheral lines of development at the following age and conversely, peripheral lines of development of one age are brought to the forefront and become central lines at another age since their meaning and relative significance in the total structure of development changes and their relation to the central neoformation changes. Thus, in the transition from one stage to another, the whole structure of the age is reconstructed. Each age has a unique and singular structure specific to it.

We shall elucidate this with examples. If we stop to consider the consciousness of the child, understood as his "relation to his environment" (K. Marx),[6] and if we take consciousness generated by physical and social changes of the individual as an integral expression of higher and most essential features in the structure of the personality, then we shall see that in the transition from one age level to another, it is not so much separate partial aspects of consciousness, its separate functions or methods of activity that develop, as it is that primarily the general structure of consciousness changes which at each given age is characterized mainly by a certain system of relations and dependences between its separate aspects and separate forms of the individual's activity.

It is completely understandable that with the transition from one age level to another, together with a general reconstruction of the system of consciousness, the central and peripheral lines of development change places. Thus, when the development of speech appears in early childhood, it is so closely and directly connected with the central neoformations of the age that as soon as the child's social and objective consciousness appears in its most incipient configurations, speech development cannot but be attributed to the central lines of development of the period under consideration. But during school age, the continuing development of the child's speech is in a completely different relation to the central neoformation of this age and, consequently, must be considered as one of the peripheral lines of development. During infancy, when preparation for speech development in the form of babbling occurs, these processes are connected with the central neoformation of the period in such a way that they must also be placed in the peripheral lines of development.

Thus we see that one and the same process of speech development may act as a peripheral line in infancy, become the central line of development in early childhood, and again be converted to a peripheral line in subsequent age periods. It is completely natural and understandable that in direct and immediate dependence on this, speech development, considered as such, will in itself occur completely differently in each of these three variants.

The alternation of central and peripheral lines of development with the transition from age level to age level leads us directly to the second problem of this section—to the question of the dynamics of the appearance of neoformations. Once again, as in the problem of the structure of age, we must limit ourselves to the most general explanation of the concept, leaving the concrete disclosure of the dynamics of age changes for later chapters dealing with a survey of the separate periods.

The problem of the dynamics of age flows directly from the problem of the structure of age which we just noted. As we have seen, the structure of age is not a static, unchangeable, immobile picture. At each given age, the structure formed previously makes a transition to a new structure. The new structure appears and is formed in the course of the development of the age level. The relation between the wholes and the parts, so essential to the concept of structure, is a dynamic relation that determines the change and development of the whole and its parts. For this reason, the dynamics of development must be understood as an aggregate of all the laws that determine the period of the appearance, change, and connecting of structural neoformations of each age level.

The very initial and essential point in the general determination of the dynamics of age is to understand that the relations between the personality of the child and his social environment at each age level are mobile.

One of the major impediments to the theoretical and practical study of child development is the incorrect solution of the problem of the environment and its role in the dynamics of age when the environment is considered as something outside with respect to the child, as a circumstance of development, as an aggregate of objective conditions existing without reference to the child and affecting him by the very fact of their existence. The understanding of the environment that developed in biology as applied to evolution of animal species must not be transferred to the teaching on child development.

We must admit that at the beginning of each age period, there develops a completely original, exclusive, single, and unique relation, specific to the given age, between the child and reality, mainly the social reality, that surrounds him. We call this relation the *social situation of development* at the given age. The social situation of development represents the initial moment for all dynamic changes that occur in development during the given period. It determines wholly and completely the forms and the path along which the child will acquire ever newer personality characteristics, drawing them from the social reality as from the basic source of development, the path along which the social becomes the individual. Thus, the first question we must answer in studying the dynamics of any age is to explain the social situation of development.

The social situation of development specific to each age determines strictly regularly the whole picture of the child's life or his social existence. From this arises the second question which confronts us in the study of the dynamics of any age, specifically the question of the origin or genesis of central neoformations of the given age. Having elucidated the social situation of development that occurred before the beginning of any age, which was determined by relations between the child and his environment, we must immediately elucidate how, of necessity, neoformations proper to the given age arise and develop from the life of the child in this social situation. These neoformations that characterize the reconstruction of the conscious personality of the child in the first place are not a prerequisite but a result or product of development of the age level. The change in the child's consciousness arises on a certain base specific to the given age, the forms of his social existence. This is why maturation of neoformations never pertains to the beginning, but always to the end of the given age level.

Once the neoformations have appeared in the conscious personality of the child, they bring about a change in the personality itself, which cannot but have the most substantial influence on further development. If the preceding task in the study of the dynamics of age determined the path of the direct movement from the social existence of the child to a new structure of his consciousness, now the following task arises: finding a path of reverse movement from the changed structure of the child's consciousness to a reconstruction of his existence. The child, having changed the structure of his personality, is already a different child whose social existence cannot but differ in a substantial way from the existence of the child of an earlier age.

Thus, the next question that confronts us in the study of the dynamics of age is the question of the consequences that result from the fact of the development of age-related neoformations. With concrete analysis, we can see that these consequences are so comprehensive and great that they encompass the whole life of the child. The new structure of consciousness acquired at a given age inevitably signifies a new character of perceptions of external reality and activity in it, a new character of the child's perceiving his own internal life and the internal activity of his mental functions.

But to say this means at the same time to say something else also, which brings us directly to the last point that characterizes the dynamics of age. We see that as a result of the age-related development, the neoformations that arise toward the end of a given age lead to a reconstruction of the whole structure of the child's consciousness and in this way change the whole system of relations to external reality and to himself. Toward the end of the given age, the child becomes a completely different being than he was at the beginning of the age. But this necessarily also means that the social situation of development which was established in basic traits toward the beginning of any age must also change since the social situation of development is nothing other than a system of relations between the child of a given age and social reality. And if the child changed in a radical way, it is inevitable that these relations must be reconstructed. The former situation of development disintegrates as the child develops and to the same extent, with his development, a new situation of development unfolds in basic traits, and this must become the initial point for the subsequent age. Research shows that this reconstruction of the social situation of development makes up the content of the critical ages.

Thus we come to elucidating the basic law of the dynamics of age levels. According to the law, the forces moving the child's development at one age or another inevitably lead to rejection and disruption of the base of development of the whole age, with internal necessity determining the annulment of the social situation of development, the termination of the given period of development, and a transition to the following, or higher age level.

In a general outline, this is the scheme of age-related dynamic development.

3. The Problem of Age and the Dynamics of Development

The problem of age level is not only central to all of child psychology, but is also the key to all the problems of practice. This problem is directly and closely connected with the diagnostics of age-related development of the child. Systems of research devices that are intended to determine the actual level of development attained by the child are usually called diagnostics. The actual level of development is determined by that age, that stage or phase within a given age that the child is experiencing at the time. We already know that the child's chronological age cannot serve as a reliable criterion for establishing the actual level of his development. For this reason, the determination of the actual level of development always requires special study which serves to establish a diagnosis of development.

Determining the actual level of development is the most essential and indispensable task in resolving every practical problem of teaching and educating the child, checking the normal course of his physical and mental development, or establishing disturbances of one kind or another in development that upset the normal course and make the whole process atypical, anomalous, and in some cases pathological. Thus, the determination of the actual level of development is the first and basic task of the diagnostics of development.

The study of symptomatology of age levels in children is a basis for identifying a number of reliable traits which can be used to determine the phase and stage of each age of the process of the child's development just as a doctor diagnoses an illness on the basis of one set of symptoms or another, that is, identifies the internal pathological process that is manifested in the symptoms.

In itself the study of some age symptom or group of symptoms and even precise quantitative measuring of these still cannot be a diagnosis. Gesell said that there is a great difference between measuring and diagnosis. It consists in the fact that we can make a diagnosis only if we are able to disclose the sense and significance of the symptoms found.

The tasks confronting the diagnostics of development may be resolved only on the basis of a profound and broad study of the whole sequence of the course of child development, of all the features of each age, stage, and phase, of all the basic types of normal and anomalous development, of the whole structure and dynamics of child development in its many forms. Thus, in itself, determining the actual level of development and quantitative expression of the difference between chronological and standardized age of the child or the relation between them expressed in a coefficient of development is only the first step along the way toward diagnostics of development. In essence, determining the actual level of development not only does not cover the whole picture of development, but very frequently encompasses only an insignificant part of it. In establishing the presence of one set of symptoms or another in determining the actual level of development, we actually determine only that part of the total picture of development of the processes, functions, and properties that have matured by that time. For example, we determine growth, weight, and other indicators of physical development that are characteristic of an already completed cycle of development. This is the outcome, the result, the final attainment of development for the period passed. These symptoms indicate rather how development occurred in the past, how it was concluded in the present, and what direction it will take in the future.

It is understood that knowing the outcome of yesterday's development is a necessary point for making a judgment on development in the present and in the future. But this alone is certainly not enough. Figuratively speaking, in determining the actual level of development, we determine only the fruits of development, that is, that which has already matured and completed its cycle. But we know that the basic law of development is that different aspects of the personality and its different properties mature at different times. While some processes of development have already borne fruit and concluded their cycles, other processes are only at the stage of maturation. A genuine diagnosis of development must be able to catch not only concluded cycles of development, not only the fruits, but also those processes that are in the period of maturation. Like a gardener who in appraising species for yield would proceed incorrectly if he considered only the ripe fruit in the orchard and did not know how to evaluate the condition of the trees that had not yet produced mature fruit, the psychologist who is limited to ascertaining what has matured, leaving what is maturing aside, will never be able to obtain any kind of true and complete representation of the internal state of the whole development and, consequently, will not be able to make the transition from symptomatic to clinical diagnosis.

Ascertaining the processes that have not matured at the time, but are in the period of maturation is the second task of the diagnostics of development. This task is accomplished by finding the *zones of proximal development.* We will explain this concept, most important from both the theoretical and practical aspect, using a specific example.

In psychology, to determine the actual level of the child's intellectual development, most of the time a method is used in which the child is asked to solve a number of problems of increasing difficulty and standardized for the child's chronological age level. The study always determines the level of difficulty of the problems that the given child can solve and the standard age corresponding to it. The mental age of the child is determined in this way. It is assumed that independent solving of the problems only and exclusively is indicative of the mind. If in the course of solving a problem, the child is asked a leading question or given a direction as to how to solve the problem, such a solution is not accepted in determining mental age.

The basis for this idea is the conviction that nonindependent solving of the problem is devoid of significance for judging the mind of the child. Actually, this conviction distinctly contradicts all the data of contemporary psychology. It was based on the old, incorrect, and now completely discredited idea that imitating any kind of intellectual operation may be a purely mechanical, automatic act that says nothing about the mind of the imitator. The incorrectness of this view was initially exposed in animal psychology. In his famous experiments with humanlike apes, W. Köhler established the remarkable fact that animals can imitate only such intellectual actions as lie within the zone of their capabilities. Thus, the chimpanzee can reproduce sensible and purposeful action that it is shown only if this operation relates in type and degree of difficulty to the same category as do sensible and purposeful activities that the animal can do independently. The animal's imitation is strictly limited by the narrow boundaries of its capabilities. The animal can imitate only that which it is capable of doing.

With the child, the situation is much more complex. On the one hand, at different stages of development, the child may imitate far from everything. His capability for imitation in the intellectual sphere is strictly limited by the level of his mental development and his age-related potentials. However, the general law is that unlike the animal, the child can enter into imitation through intellectual actions more or less far beyond what he is capable of in independent mental and purposeful actions or intellectual operations. This difference between the child and the animal can be explained by the fact that the animal cannot be taught in the sense in which we apply this word to the child. The animal is adaptable only to dressage. It can only develop new habits. By exercise and combination, it can perfect its intellect, but is not capable of mental development, in the true sense of the word, through instruction. This is why all experimental attempts using instruction to develop in higher animals new intellectual functions not proper to them but specific to man inevitably meet with failure, as did the attempt of R. Yerkes to graft human speech into ape offspring or the attempts of E. Tolman to train and instruct chimpanzee offspring together with human children.

Thus we see that, aided by imitation, the child can always do more in the intellectual sphere than he is capable of doing independently. At the same time, we see that his capability for intellectual imitation is not limitless, but changes absolutely regularly corresponding to the course of his mental development so that at each age level, there is for the child a specific zone of intellectual imitation connected with the actual level of development.

Speaking of imitation, we do not have in mind mechanical, automatic, thoughtless imitation but sensible imitation based on understanding the imitative carrying out of some intellectual operation. In this respect, on the one hand, we restrict the meaning of the term, using it only in the sphere of operations that are more or less directly connected with mental activity of the child. On the other hand, we extend the meaning of the term, applying the word "imitation" to all kinds of activity of a certain type carried out by the child not independently, but in cooperation with adults or with another child. Everything that the child cannot do independently, but which he can be taught or which he can do with direction or cooperation or with the help of leading questions, we will include in the sphere of imitation.

With this kind of definition of this concept we can establish the symptomatic significance of intellectual imitation in the diagnosis of mental development. What the child can do himself, with no help on the side, reveals his already mature capabilities and functions. These are the ones that are established with tests usually used for determining the actual level of mental development since the tests are based exclusively on independent problem solving.

As we have said, it is always important to ascertain not only the mature processes but also those that are maturing. With respect to the child's mental development, we can solve this problem by determining what the child is capable of in intellectual imitation if we understand this term as defined above. Research shows a strict genetic pattern between what a child is able to imitate and his mental development. What the child can do today in cooperation and with guidance, tomorrow he will be able to do independently. This means that by ascertaining the child's potentials when he works in cooperation, we ascertain in this way the area of maturing intellectual functions that in the near stage of development must bear fruit and, consequently, be transferred to the level of actual mental development of the child. Thus, in studying what the child is capable of doing independently, we study yesterday's development. Studying what the child is capable of doing cooperatively, we ascertain tomorrow's development.

The area of immature, but maturing processes makes up the child's zone of proximal development.[7]

Using an example, we shall elucidate how the zone of proximal development is determined. Let us assume that as a result of a study, we established that two children are the same in age and mental development. Let us say that both are eight years old. This means that both independently solve problems of the level of difficulty that corresponds to the standard for age eight. In this way, we determine the actual level of their mental development. But we continue the study. Using special devices, we test to what extent both children are able to solve problems that are beyond the standard for age eight. We show the child how such a problem must be solved and watch to see if he can do the problem by imitating the demonstration. Or we begin to solve the problem and ask the child to finish it. Or we propose that the child solve the problem that is beyond his mental age by cooperating with another, more developed child or, finally, we explain to the child the principle of solving the problem, ask leading questions, analyze the problem for him, etc. In brief, we ask the child to solve problems that are beyond the limits of his mental age with some kind of cooperation and determine how far the potential for intellectual cooperation can be stretched for the given child and how far it goes beyond his mental age.

It develops that one child solves problems cooperatively that standards relate to, let us say, age twelve. The zone of proximal development moves his mental age forward by four years. The other child moves forward with cooperation only to the standard age level of a nine-year-old. His zone of proximal development is only one year.

Are these children identical in age according to the actual level of development attained? Obviously their similarity is limited to the area of already mature functions. But with respect to maturing processes, one went four times further than the other.

We explained the principle of immature processes and properties with the example of the mental development of the child.

It is completely understandable that in determining the physical development of the child, the method of study which we have just described with respect to intellectual development is completely inapplicable. But in principle, the problem pertains to this aspect of development as it does to all others in completely the same way. It is important for us to know not only the child's already attained limits of growth and of the other processes of which his physical development consists, but also the progress of the process of maturation itself which will be evident in later development.

We will not stop to consider determination of the zone of proximal development that applies to other aspects of the child's personality. We shall elucidate only the theoretical and practical significance of this determination.

The theoretical significance of this diagnostic principle consists in that it allows us to penetrate into the internal causal-dynamic and genetic connections that determine the process itself of mental development. As has been said, the social environment is the source for the appearance of all specific human properties of the personality gradually acquired by the child or the source of social development of the child which is concluded in the process of actual interaction of "ideal" and present forms.

A closer source of the development of internal individual properties of the child's personality is cooperation (this word understood in the broadest sense) with other people. Thus, by applying the principle of cooperation for establishing the zone of proximal development, we make it possible to study directly what determines most precisely the mental maturation that must be realized in the proximal and subsequent periods of his stage of development.

The practical significance of this diagnostic principle is connected with the problem of teaching. A detailed explanation of this problem will be given in one of the closing chapters.[8] Now we consider only the most important and initial moment. We know that there are optimum times in the child's development for each type of teaching. This means that teaching a given subject, given information, habits, and skills is easiest, efficient, and productive only at certain age periods. This circumstance has for a long time dropped out of sight. The lower boundary for optimum times for teaching was established earliest. We know that an infant of four months cannot be taught to speak, or a two-year-old be taught to read and write, because at those times, the child is not mature enough for such teaching; this means that the child has not yet developed those properties and functions that are prerequisites for this kind of teaching. But if only the lower limit existed for the potential for teaching at a certain age, we could expect that the later the respective teaching begins, the more easily it will be conveyed to the child and will thus be more productive because at a later age, there will be a greater degree of maturity of the prerequisites needed for the teaching.

Actually, this is not true. The child beginning to learn to speak at three years and to read and to write at twelve, that is, somewhat late, also seems to be in unfavorable conditions. Teaching that is a little late is also difficult and unproductive for the child, just like that which is a little too early. Obviously, there is also an upper threshold of optimum times for teaching from the point of view of the child's development.

How can we explain the fact that a three-year-old child in whom we find a great maturity of attention, alertness, motor ability, and other properties that are necessary prerequisites for learning speech, acquires speech with more difficulty and with less advantage than a child of a year and a half in whom these same prerequisites are undoubtedly less mature? Obviously the reason for this is that teaching is based not so much on already mature functions and properties of the child as on maturating functions. The period of maturation corresponding to the functions is the most favorable or optimum period for the corresponding type of teaching. It is also understandable, if we take this circumstance into account, that the child develops through the very process of learning and does not conclude the cycle of development. First the teacher teaches the pupil not what the child can already do independently, but what he still cannot do alone, but can do with the help of teaching and guidance. The process of teaching itself is always done in the form of the child's cooperation with adults and represents a partial case of the interaction of the ideal and the present form, of which we spoke above, as one of the most general laws of social development of the child.

In greater detail and more concretely, the problem of the relation between teaching and development will be presented in one of the last chapters dealing with school age and with teaching in school. But now it must be clear to us that since teaching depends on immature, but maturing processes and the whole area of these processes is encompassed by the zone of proximal development of the child, the optimum time for teaching both the group and each individual child is established at each age by the zone of their proximal development.

This is why determining the zone of proximal development has such great practical significance.

Determining the actual level of development and the zone of proximal development also comprises what is called *normative age-level diagnostics*. With the help of age norms or standards, this is meant to elucidate the given state of development characterized from the aspect of both the finished and the unfinished processes. In contrast to symptomatic diagnostics depending only on establishing external traits, diagnostics that attempts to determine the internal state of development that is disclosed by those traits is called *clinical diagnostics* in analogy to medical studies.

The general principle of all scientific diagnostics of development is the transition from symptomatic diagnostics based on the study of symptom complexes of child development, that is, its traits, to clinical diagnostics based on determining the internal course of the process of development itself. Gesell believes that normative data must not be applied mechanically or purely psychometrically, that we must not only measure the child, we must interpret him. Measurement, determination, and comparison to standards of symptoms of development must appear only as a means for formulating the diagnosis of development. Gesell writes that diagnosis of development must not consist only of obtaining a series of data by means of tests and measurements. Diagnostics of development is a form of comparative study using objective norms as points of departure. It is not only synthetic, but analytical as well.

The data from testing and measuring make up the objective basis for a comparative evaluation. The patterns of development yield standards of development.

But the diagnosis in the true sense of this word must be based on a critical and careful interpretation of the data obtained from various sources. It is based on all the manifestations and facts of maturation. The synthetic, dynamic picture of these manifestations, the aggregate of which we call personality, enters as a whole into the framework of the study. We cannot, of course, precisely measure the traits of personality. We can only with difficulty determine what we call personality, but from the point of view of diagnostics of development, as Gesell assumes, we must observe how personality is made up and matures.

If we limit ourselves only to determining and measuring symptoms of development, we will never be able to go beyond the limits of a purely empirical establishment of what is obvious to persons who just observe the child. In the best case, we will be able only to increase precision of the symptoms and confirm them with measurement. But we can never explain the phenomena we observe in the development of the child nor predict the further course of development, nor indicate what kind of measures of a practical nature must be applied with respect to the child. This kind of diagnosis of development, fruitless with respect to explanation, prognosis, and practical applications can be compared only to those medical diagnoses that doctors made at the time when symptomatic medicine prevailed. The patient complains of a cough, the doctor makes a diagnosis: the illness is a cough. The patient complains of a headache, the doctor makes a diagnosis: the illness is a headache. This kind of diagnosis is essentially empty since the investigator adds nothing new to what he knew from observations of the patient himself and plays back to the patient his own complaints, supplying them with scientific labels. The empty diagnosis cannot explain the observed phenomena, can predict nothing relative to their fate and cannot give practical advice. A true diagnosis must provide an explanation, prediction, and scientific basis for practical prescription.

The matter is precisely the same with respect to symptomatic diagnosis in psychology. If a child is brought in for consultation with complaints that he is developing poorly mentally, has a poor imagination and is forgetful, if after investigation, the psychologist makes the diagnosis: the child has a low intelligence quotient and mental retardation, the psychologist also explains nothing, predicts nothing, and cannot help in any practical way, like the doctor who makes the diagnosis: the illness is a cough.

It can be said with no exaggeration that definitely practical measures on safeguarding the development of the child, his teaching and education, since they are connected with the features of one age or another, necessarily require diagnostics of development. The application of diagnostics of development to solving endless and infinitely varied practical problems is determined in each concrete case by the degree of scientific development of the diagnostics of development and the demands that confront it in the resolution of each concrete practical problem.[9]

Chapter 7
INFANCY[1]

1. The Newborn Period

The development of the child begins with the critical act of birth and the critical period that follows it, the newborn period. At the moment of birth, the child separates physically from the mother, but because of a number of circumstances, biological separation from the mother does not quite occur at that moment. In basic vital functions, the child remains a biologically dependent being for a long time. During this whole period, the vital activity and existence itself of the child is of such a unique character that this alone is a basis for identifying the newborn period as a special age with all the distinctive traits of a critical age.

If we try to describe the principal feature of the age, we might say that it is rooted in that unique situation of development that is created by the fact that the child at the moment of birth separates from the mother physically but not biologically. As a result of this, the whole existence of the child during the newborn period occupies a kind of middle position between intrauterine development and the subsequent periods of postnatal childhood. The newborn period is as if a connecting link between intrauterine and extrauterine development and it contains traits of the one and the other. This link is in a true sense a transitional stage from one type of development to another that is radically different from the first.

The transitional or mixed character of the life of the child during this period may be traced by several basic features that set it apart.

We shall begin with feeding. Immediately after birth there is a drastic change in the child's feeding. S. Bernfeld says that with birth, in the course of several hours the mammal is converted from a water-breathing being with a variable temperature, fed only osmotically in the manner of a parasite, into an air breather with a constant temperature using liquid food. In the expression of S. Ferenczi, after birth, the child is converted from an endoparasite to an exoparasite. He thinks that just as the physical environment of the newborn is to a certain degree intermediate between the environment of the fetus (placenta) and the environment of later childhood (bed), the communication of the newborn represents at least in part a kind of continuation, weakened and of a different kind, of the bond between the fetus and the pregnant woman. The direct physical bond between the child and the mother is absent, but it continues to be fed by the mother.

Actually, we cannot but see that the feeding of a newborn is of a mixed type. On the one hand, the child feeds as animals do: he perceives external stimuli, responds to them with purposeful movements which help him to access and obtain food. His whole digestive apparatus and the complex of sensory-motor functions that serve it play a major role in feeding. However, the child is fed with the colostrum of the mother and later with her milk, that is, an intraorganic product of the maternal organism. Thus, feeding the newborn represents a kind of transitional form, as if an intermediate link between the intrauterine and the subsequent extrauterine feeding.

This duality and this intermediate character we find without difficulty in the basic form of existence of the newborn that differs primarily by its inadequate differentiation between sleep and wakefulness. As studies show, the newborn spends approximately 80% of his time in sleep. The main feature of the sleep of the newborn is its polyphasic character. Short periods of sleep alternate with islets of wakefulness inserted into them. Sleep itself is inadequately differentiated from the wakeful state and for this reason, in the newborn, a middle state between waking and sleep can be observed most closely resembling a state of somnolence. Regardless of the long duration of sleep, it seems, according to the observations of C. Bühler and H. Hetzer, that its periods are quite short: uninterrupted sleep lasting nine to ten hours occurs only at the seventh month. The average number of periods of sleep in the first quarter of the first year is twelve.

The most remarkable distinction of the sleep of the newborn is its restless, intermittent, and superficial character. The sleeping newborn makes many impulsive movements, sometimes he even eats without waking. This again indicates that his sleep is inadequately differentiated from waking. The newborn is capable of falling asleep with his eyes half open and conversely, waking, he often lies with his eyes closed and is in a somnolent state. According to the data of D. Canestrini, the curve of the brain pulse of the newborn does not form a noticeable boundary between sleep and waking. The criteria of sleep which we obtain in observing the sleep of an adult or a child older than six months is not valid for the first week of life.

Thus, the general vital state of the newborn may be described as an average somnolent state from which states of sleep and waking are gradually developed for short periods. For this reason, many authors, like J. Lermite and others, come to the conclusion that in the first days of extrauterine existence, the child seems to continue uterine life and retains its mental traits. If we combine this with the fact that the child retains the embryonal pose both while he sleeps and frequently during waking, the intermediate character of his vital activity becomes entirely clear. The favorite position of the child in sleep remains embryonal. The child takes the same position even in a resting waking state. Only when the child is four months old can we observe another position during sleep.

The sense of this unique life state leaves no doubt regarding its nature. In the mother's womb, the life activity of the child was almost totally made up of vegetative functions, and animal functions were reduced to a minimum. But even sleep is a state in which vegetative processes are in the forefront and animal functions are arrested more or less drastically. The sleep of the newborn is evidence of the comparative dominance of the vegetative system. The abundance and frequency of sleep of the newborn are to a certain degree evidently a continuation of the behavior of the fetus, the usual state of which, as far as we know, is more similar to sleep than anything else. From the genetic point of view, sleep is the most primitive vegetative behavior. Genetically, it precedes waking which develops from sleep. Thus, sleep of the newborn, like his feeding, occupies an intermediate place between the stage of embryonal and postnatal development.

Finally, animal functions of the newborn also leave no doubt that the child of this age stands as if at the border between intra- and extrauterine development. On the one hand, he already has a number of motor reactions that appear in response to internal and external stimuli. On the other hand, he still has no basic animal features—specifically the ability to move independently through space. He has the ability to move independently, but cannot move through space except with an adult's help. His mother carries him, which also indicates a seemingly intermediate position between movement of the fetus and the child rising to his feet.

Motor features of the newborn recall a number of instructive biological parallels. F. Doflein divides mammalian offspring according to the decreasing degree of their extrauterine dependence on the mother into four groups. He places marsupials in the first group; their offspring are placed by the mother in an external womb and pass the beginning of their childhood in the pouch. Here we have a kind of grossly anatomic expression of the transitional stage from intrauterine development to independent existence. Next are the offspring of hibernating animals, which are born helpless, frequently blind and spend the beginning of their childhood in the den, again resembling a transitional environment from the maternal uterus to the external world. In the third place are offspring that are carried by the mother. All of these offspring have grasping instincts. Finally, in the last place are the running offspring, completely developed and beginning to run almost immediately after birth and to eat plants in addition to nursing.

In the newborn human child, we see a number of movements that are undoubtedly connected phylogenetically with the grasping reflexes of the third group of mammals. When an offspring is born to an ape, it reflexively grasps the fur on the mother's body with all four extremities and hangs at her breast with his spine down. The offspring remains in this position both when he sleeps and when he is awake. When the mother moves, he, being immovably united with her, goes everywhere with her. In this case, we have a kind of functional mechanism that expresses the new dependence of the newborn on the mother that is expressed differently in marsupials.

In the human newborn, we also observe movements similar to that reflex. If we place a finger or some other long object in the hand of a newborn, he will grasp it so tightly that he can be lifted into the air and held in a hanging position for approximately a minute. The similarity between this reflex and the grasping reflex of the ape offspring is obvious. The Moro reaction, the grasping reflex that arises when the head is shaken, has the same significance; in this case, the hands and the feet are extended and then brought in again in the form of an arc. The newborn responds with the same movements to any strong and unexpected stimulus, with the same reaction of fright expressed in grasping movements. According to A. Peiper, the reaction of fright is the same grasping reflex common to man and ape. Thus, in these archaic, residual motor adaptations, we find traces common to all mammals at a unique stage of biological dependence of the newborn on the mother, dependence that continues after birth.

Finally, the primary and incontrovertible evidence of the fact that the newborn period should be considered as a transitional period between uterine and extrauterine development is the following. In the case of premature birth, the last months of embryonal development may pass under conditions of extrauterine development just as the first months after birth in cases of postmature or delayed birth may pass under conditions of uterine development.

Sometimes the child is born postmaturely. If the normal period of pregnancy is ten lunar or nine solar months (280 days), then the premature or postmature child deviates from the normal time in one direction or the other up to 40 days. The child may be born beginning with the 240th day and right up to the 320th day, counting from the last menstruation. In exceptional cases, pregnancy may continue to the 326th day. Thus, the time of birth of viable children has a range of approximately four months.

What does the study of the development of premature and postmature children show? To put it briefly, the added one to two months of extrauterine development of the premature child like the added one to two months of uterine development of the postmature child do not in themselves result in any substantial changes in subsequent development. This means that the last two months of uterine development and the first two months of extrauterine development are so closely connected with each other according to the nature of processes that occur in these periods that the periods are almost equivalent to each other. According to the data of Gesell, the postmature child undoubtedly presents a picture of general acceleration of development from the very beginning. This means that the extra month the child spends in the uterus of the mother also moves his extrauterine development forward by a corresponding period. The coefficient of mental development of such a child must be deduced with a correction for the one extra month of his uterine development.

In precisely the same way, the child is viable even if he remained in the uterus only three quarters of the time intended by nature. The behavioral mechanisms by the seventh month are already almost ready to function, and during the last two months of life as a fetus, the rate of their development slows somewhat.

In this way, survival is ensured even in case of premature birth. For this reason, the child born prematurely resembles a normal newborn to a much greater degree than we might expect. However, considering the course of development of the premature child, we must again introduce a correction into the coefficient of his mental development and take into account the circumstance that during the first two months of extrauterine development, the child was going through the unfinished embryonal period. If we ask if prematurity introduces any notable changes in mental development, then in general and on the whole, this question must be answered in the negative.[2]

We think that studies of premature and postmature children confirm without a doubt the position on the transitional character of the newborn period. However, it seems to us that the partisans of evolutionistic views of child development frequently draw the wrong conclusion from this fact, the conclusion that the act of birth, being such an undoubted and clear example of spasmodic development, must be considered as a simple stage in the evolutionary sequence of uterine and extrauterine development. The partisans of this view, while correctly seeing the continuity and connection between the two stages of development, do not note the dialectical leap the child makes in making the transition from one type of development to the other. On the basis of studies of premature and postmature children, Gesell maintains that the most general conclusion that can be drawn is that the development of behavior goes forward regularly, in ontogenetic order, regardless of the time of birth. Evidently there is a firm substrate of development which time of birth cannot especially affect. Due to this, the general character of the growth curve is the same for children born at the normal time and those born prematurely. Or, to put it more simply, the premature child, regardless of the fact that he was withdrawn from the mother's womb prematurely, continues development according to the fetal type for a certain time.

To us, such a conclusion seems unfounded. The profound continuity between the last months of uterine development and the first months of the newborn period is indisputable. We tried to illustrate this by an analysis of certain more important features of the newborn. We can also point to the undoubtedly observed movements of the fetus in the maternal uterus which also indicate that during the embryonal period of development, the life of the child is not wholly taken up by vegetative processes. But this undoubted continuity remains no more than a background against which not so much the similarity as the difference between the embryonal and postnatal state comes forward as the basic point. Like every transition, the newborn period signifies primarily a disruption of the old and the beginning of the new.

The task of the present section is not a detailed description of the genesis and dynamics of the basic neoformation that is included in the newborn period. For our purposes, it is sufficient to name this neoformation, describe it briefly, and indicate that it has all the typical traits of a neoformation of critical ages, and in this way to note the initial point that is the beginning of further development of the child's personality.

If we try to name in general terms the central and basic neoformation of the newborn period that first arises as a product of that unique stage of development and which is the initial moment of subsequent development of the personality, we might say that this neoformation will be the individual mental life of the newborn. Two points must be noted in this neoformation. The child is already alive during embryonal development. What is new that appears during the newborn period is that this life becomes individual existence separate from the organism within which it was conceived, a life that, like every individual life of man, is interwoven and involved in social life of the people around the child. This is the first point. The second point is that this individual life, being the first and most primitive form of existence of the child as social existence, is also mental life because only mental life can be a part of the social life of the people around the child.

For a long time, the question of the content of the mental life of the newborn aroused great differences of opinion and arguments in view of the fact that direct study of his mentality is completely impractical. Poets, philosophers, and psychologists were inclined to ascribe to the mentality of the newborn a somewhat complex content. Thus, Shakespeare introduces a profound, pessimistic idea into the first cry of the child through the lips of King Lear:

"When we are born, we cry that we are come
To this great stage of fools."
[King Lear, IV, vi, 187]

A. Schopenhauer introduces a similar idea into the child's cry, seeing in it an argument favoring pessimism and evidence of the fact that suffering is dominant at the very beginning of existence. I. Kant interpreted the cry of the newborn as a protest of the human spirit against sensuality being locked in chains.

Investigators who belong to the reflexological school are inclined to reject the presence of any mental life in the newborn, considering him as a living automaton that perceives and acts exclusively on the basis of certain nervous connections devoid of any traces of mentality.

However, at present, the great majority of investigators agree in admitting two basic conceptions: (1) the newborn has the rudiments of mental life in the most primitive degree, and (2) this mental life has a completely unique character. We shall consider both conceptions.

The objections to admitting a mental life in the newborn are usually based on the fact that most of the centers of the brain in the newborn are immature. Specifically, in the first place, the brain cortex, which, as we know, is most closely related to the activity of consciousness, is immature. It is noted that at least in the first days of life, a child born without a cortex does not differ from the normal child in the most obvious vital manifestations.

In itself, there is no doubt that the central nervous system of the newborn is immature. However, two points compel us to admit that this argument is insupportable. We have become accustomed to consider the brain cortex as being the site of all manifestations of consciousness. And since in the newborn, this organ is not yet functioning, we conclude that he has no consciousness. This conclusion would be mandatory only if it were established that all manifestations of our consciousness are connected with the brain cortex. But facts we have indicate that this is just not so. The brain cortex is evidently connected only with the development of higher forms of conscious activity. The life of our drives, instincts, and simpler affects is probably connected more directly with subcortical centers which to a certain degree are already functioning in the newborn.

Also, a comparison of the normal newborn with anencephalics indicates that a difference between the one and the other is noted only in the major reflex manifestations. A finer comparison shows that the child born without the higher sections of the brain does not display any kind of expressive movements. For this reason, it seems probable that the normal newborn not only is not a purely spinal-cord being, as described by R. Virchow, but, in general is not a paleencephalic being, that is, a being whose life is determined only by the ancient brain. There is a basis for assuming that the new brain participates in the behavior of the newborn in some way from the very beginning (K. Koffka). Some investigators believe that the great helplessness of the human child in comparison with the offspring of animals can be explained by the fact that ancient brain mechanisms in the human offspring are less independent in functioning due to their connections with the still not fully mature parts of the new brain (N. M. Shchelovanov).

Thus, the stage of the nervous system of the newborn does not at all exclude the possibility of mental life, but, on the contrary, compels us to assume rudiments of mentality, although completely different from the developed mentality of the adult and of an older child. Mental life connected mainly with subcortical centers and with a cortex that is structurally and functionally insufficiently mature must, naturally, differ in a major way from the mental life that is possible for a developed and mature central nervous system. The decisive argument favoring the presence of rudiments of a primitive mentality in the newborn is the fact that soon after birth, we can observe all of those basic processes of life that in older children and adults are found in connection with mental states. Such in the first place is the expressiveness of movement that shows a mental state of happiness or an elevated mood, grief or sadness, anger and fright or alarm, surprise or hesitation. Instinctive movements of the newborn connected with hunger, thirst, satiation, satisfaction, etc. can also be included here. Both groups of reactions occur in the newborn in forms which compel recognition of the presence of primitive mental manifestations at this age.

But, as has already been said, this mental life differs in a very clear way from mental life of a more developed type. We shall indicate these basic differences.

W. Stern assumes that in the newborn, together with reflexes, there must be the first traces of consciousness that develop very soon into an impressive and many sided mental life. Of course, we can speak only of the rudimentary state of mental life of the newborn from which we must exclude all strictly intellectual and volitional phenomena of consciousness. There are neither innate ideas nor actual perceptions, that is, comprehension of external objects and processes as such, nor, finally, a conscious desire or striving. The only thing that we can assume on a sure basis is an indistinct, unclear state of consciousness in which sensible and emotional parts are still inseparably merged so that we might call them the sensible, emotional states or emotionally stressed states or sensations. The presence of pleasant and unpleasant emotional states is evident from the child's general appearance, expression of the face, or character of the cry as early as in the first days of his life.

C. Bühler describes the mental life of the newborn in a similar way. The first contact of the child with the mother is so close that we might sooner speak of a merged existence than of contact. Just as the child by the act of birth separates only physically from the mother, in exactly the same way mentally, he only gradually isolates the stimuli that act on him as something coming from certain objects of the external world. At first, the child evidently more likely experiences states rather than objects if we might also formulate in this way the inadequacy of objectifying impressions from the aspect of the infant. It is difficult to say how long the child simply accepts movements, changes in place, etc. and when he begins not only to accept all of this, but also to experience that someone is spending time with him. We are inclined to think that nobody and nothing exists for the child in the first month and that he rather experiences all the stimuli and everything that surrounds him only as a subjective state.

Thus, we found two essential points that characterize the uniqueness of the mental life of the newborn. The first refers to the exclusive dominance of nondifferentiated, nonarticulated experiences representing a kind of fusion of drive, affect, and sensation. The second characterizes the mentality of the newborn as not separating himself and his experience from the perception of objective things, not yet differentiating social and physical objects. It remains for us only to indicate the third point that characterizes the mentality of the newborn in its relation to the external world.

It would be wrong to imagine the newborn's perception of the world as a chaos of segmented, unconnected, separate sensations: temperature, intraorganic, aural, optical, skin, etc. Research shows that isolating some independent and articulated perceptions is a product of much later development (K. Koffka). Still later in development, the possibility develops for isolating certain components of integral perception in the form of sensations. The initial perceptions of the child represent nonarticulated impressions of the situation as a whole where not only are separate objective moments of the situation not articulated, but elements of perception and sensation are not yet differentiated. The fact itself is remarkable that the newborn, long before he exhibits the ability to react to separately perceived, articulated elements of a situation, begins to react to intricate, complex, emotionally colored wholes. For example, the face of the mother and its expressive movements evoke a reaction in the child long before he is capable of distinct perception of form, color, or size. In the initial perception of the newborn, all external impressions appear as inseparably united with the affect or sensible tone of the perception that colors them. The child is more likely to perceive the affable or the threatening, that is, generally expressive rather than objective, elements of external activity as such.

The basic law of perception of the newborn can be formulated as follows: initially amorphous perception of the situation as a whole consists of a background against which a more or less defined and structured scene is isolated for the child, and he perceives this as a special quality against the background. The law of structure or separating figure and background is evidently the most primitive feature of mental life that forms the departure point for further development of consciousness.

Thus, we can construct for ourselves an initial and general conception on the mental life of the newborn. It remains for us to indicate what this level of mental life in the social behavior of the child will lead to subsequently. It is easy to see that the newborn does not exhibit any specific forms of social behavior. As the studies of C. Bühler and H. Hetzer show, the child's first contact with man lies beyond the limits of the newborn period. For real contact, absolutely necessary are mental processes that make the child "conscious" that someone is playing with him, and due to this the child reacts to the person differently than he does to what surrounds him. We can first speak about social impressions and reactions with any degree of confidence only with respect to the period between the second and third month, that is, beyond the limits of the newborn period. During the newborn period, the sociability of the child is characterized by complete passivity. As in his behavior, so also in his consciousness we can note nothing that would speak for social experience as such. This is a basis for identifying the newborn period, long and unanimously accepted by all biologists, as a special stage of the child's social development at that age level.

The mental life of the newborn has all the typical traits of neoformations of the critical ages. As we indicated, neoformations of this type never result in mature formations, but are transitional formations that disappear into the following stable age. What kind then is the neoformation in the newborn period? It is a unique mental life connected predominantly with subcortical sections of the brain. It is not retained as such as a stable acquisition of the child for the subsequent years. It blooms and fades in the narrow time limits that encompass the newborn stage. However, it does not disappear without a trace as a momentary episode of child development. In the subsequent course of development, it loses only its independent existence and enters as a component part, a subordinate unit, into the nervous and mental formations of a higher order.

The problem of boundaries of the newborn period is still very controversial: some authors consider this new period to be one month (K. Lashley, Troitsky, Hutinel), and others, like K. Vierordt, limit it to just a week. They frequently accept the formation of the umbilical scar or obliteration of Botallo's duct and the umbilical vein as the point at which this period ends. Finkelstein and Reis consider the time when the child gains back his initial weight after a physiological loss (ten to twenty-one days) as the limit of this period. P. P. Blonsky proposes the seventh postnatal day as the end of the newborn stage when the physiological loss of weight ends and is replaced by an increase in weight. However, we cannot but agree with M. S. Maslov that such processes as the falling away of the umbilical cord and obliteration of Botallo's duct can scarcely purposefully be considered a boundary of the newborn period since these processes have no effect on the general state of the child. Maslov assumes that if we want to identify this period, we must use the totality of the anatomic-physiological traits and features as well as metabolism. It has been established that during this period, the child is different in his unique metabolism and unique state of the blood connected with the characteristics of immunity and anaphylaxis. All of this taken together indicates that the newborn period goes far beyond the limits of the falling away of the umbilical cord and lasts no fewer than three weeks in any case and imperceptibly without a sharp boundary passes into the nursling period toward the second month.

As we see, there is every basis for assuming that the newborn period is characterized by a unique general biological picture and that the newborn lives a completely singular life. But according to the considerations we discussed in detail in the preceding chapter, the criterion for setting the boundaries for any age period must be only the basic and central neoformation that characterizes a certain stage in the social development of the child's personality. For this reason, it seems to us that in determining the boundaries of the newborn period, those data should be used which characterize the mental and social state of the newborn. Closest to this criterion are the data relating to the higher nervous activity of the child most directly connected with his mental and social life. From this point of view, the studies of M. Denisova and N. Figurin show that toward the end of the first and beginning of the second month there is a turning point in the child's development.

The authors consider the symptom of the new period to be the appearance of a smile in response to conversation, that is, the first specific reaction of the child to the human voice. The studies of C. Bühler and H. Hetzer also show that the first social reactions of the child indicating a general change in his mental life can be observed at the end of the first month and beginning of the second month of his life. They indicate that toward the end of the first month, a cry by one child evokes a responsive cry in another. Between the first and second month, the child reacts with a smile to the sound of a human voice. All of this compels the assumption that specifically this is the upper boundary of the newborn period and in crossing this, the child enters a new developmental age level.

2. The Social Situation of Development during Infancy

At first glance, it is easy to show that the infant is completely or almost completely an asocial being. He still does not have the basic means of social interaction—human speech. His life activity is confined to a significant degree to satisfying the simplest vital needs. He is much more an object than a subject, that is, an active participator in social relations. From this the impression arises easily that infancy is a period of asocial development of the child and that the infant is a purely biological being with no specific human properties, and primarily, the most basic of these—sociability. Specifically this opinion is the basis for a number of erroneous theories on the age of infancy which we shall consider subsequently.

Actually this impression and the opinion on the asocial nature of the infant based on it are a big mistake. Careful study shows that at the infancy stage, we find completely specific, most unique sociability in the infant which is based on the single and unique social situation of development that depends on two basic points. The first consists of the totality of features of the infant, apparent at first glance, which can usually be described as his complete biological helplessness. The infant cannot himself satisfy even one vital need. The most elementary and basic vital needs of the infant can be satisfied in no other way than with the help of the adults who take care of him. Feeding and changing the infant and even turning him from side to side is done only with cooperation of adults. The path through others, through adults is the basic path of the child's activity at this age. Definitely everything in the behavior of the infant is intertwined and interwoven into the sociable. Such is the objective situation of his development. It remains for us only to disclose what corresponds to the objective situation in the consciousness of the subject of development himself, that is, of the infant.

No matter what happens to the infant, he is always in a situation connected with the care giving of adults. Because of this, a completely unique form of social relations develops between the child and the adults around him. Specifically owing to the immaturity of biological functions, all of what will later be in the sphere of individual adaptation of the child and will be done by him independently now can be done in no other way than through others, in no other way than in a situation of cooperation. Thus, the first contact of the child with reality (even in carrying out the most elementary biological functions) is wholly and completely socially mediated.

Objects appear and disappear from the child's field of vision always due to the participation of adults. The child moves through space always in the arms of others. A change in his position, even a simple turning, is again intertwined in a social situation. Eliminating stimuli that bother the child and satisfying his basic needs is always done (along the same path) through others. Because of all of this, there is such a singular, unique dependence of the child on the adults that it sustains and permeates, as we have said, what would seem to be the most individual biological needs and wants of the infant. The dependence of the infant on adults creates a completely unique character of the child's relations to reality (and to himself): these relations are always mediated by others, and are always refracted through a prism of relations with another person.

Thus, the relation of the child to reality is from the very beginning a social relation. In this sense, the infant might be called a maximally social being. Every relation of the child to the outside world, even the simplest, is always a relation refracted through the relation to another person. The whole life of the infant is organized in such a way that in every situation, visibly or not, there is another person. This can be expressed in another way by saying that every relation of the child to things is a relation accomplished with the help of or through another person.

The second feature that characterizes the social situation of development in infancy is that with maximum dependence on adults, with complete interweaving and intertwining of the whole behavior of the infant into the social, the child is still without the basic means of social interaction in the form of human speech. Specifically this second trait in combination with the first is responsible for the uniqueness of the social situation in which we find the infant. By the whole organization of life, he is forced to maximum interaction with adults. But this interaction is nonverbal interaction, frequently silent interaction of a completely unique type.

The basis for all the child's development during infancy is laid down in the contradiction between maximum sociability of the infant (the situation in which the infant finds himself) and minimum capability for interaction.

3. The Genesis of the Basic Neoformation of Infancy

Before we proceed to an analytical consideration of the complex composition of the developmental processes in infancy, we want to precede it by a general and summary description of the dynamics of this age.

The beginning of infancy coincides with the end of the newborn crisis. The turning point is between the second and third month of the child's life. At this time, we can observe new manifestations in all areas. The strongest drop in the curve of daily amount of sleep has ended and the maximum daily amount of negative reactions has been left behind; food is not taken in as greedily so that the child interrupts feeding for a second and opens his eyes. All the conditions for activity besides sleeping, eating, and crying are present. The frequency of reactions to separate stimuli has diminished in comparison with that in the newborn. The internal obstacles to sleep and shuddering in response to external stimuli are much less frequent. On the other hand, the activity of the child becomes more varied and lasts longer.

The following are new forms of behavior during this time: playful experimentation, babbling, first active use of the sensory organs, first active reaction to position, first coordination of two simultaneously acting organs, first social reactions—expressive movement connected with functional satisfaction and surprise.

Everything points to the fact that the passivity with which the newborn related to the world has yielded to reciprocating interest. The latter becomes most obvious in the new manifestations of perceptive activity during the wakeful state.

As we have said, the passivity, which the child left only through the action of strong sensory stimuli, has now been replaced by the inclination to respond to stimuli. For the first time there is attention to sensory stimulation, to his own movements, his own sounds, to sound in general and attention to another person. Interest in all of this only now makes further development of every separate area possible (C. Bühler, B. Tudor-Hart, and H. Hetzer, 1931, p. 219).

H. Wallon[3] also notes that a new period in the development of the child begins with the second month; in this period, the motor system of a purely affective type gradually yields to activity approaching sensory motor activity in character. At the same time, as sensory synergies are being established (disappearance of strabismus), the face assumes an expression of attentiveness and readiness for perceiving external impressions. Visual impressions begin to absorb the child and soon he begins to listen, at first, it is true, only to sounds that he makes himself. He stretches toward objects, touches them with his hands, lips and tongue, exhibiting true activity. At this time, rudiments of hand activity begin to develop which have such a great significance for all mental development. All of these reactions properly oriented are directed toward adaptation; they are positive and if the stimulus is not too strong, they no longer drop to the negative or organic reactions that were dominant during the preceding stage.

Thus, toward the beginning of this period, the child exhibits a certain interest in the external world and the possibility of moving his activity beyond the limits of direct drives and instinctive tendencies. It is as if the external world appears for the child. This new relation to activity also signifies the onset of the infant period, or more accurately, its first stage.

The second stage of infancy is also signified by definite changes in the relations of the child to the external world. We note a turning point of similar significance between the fifth and sixth month. Beginning at this time, sleep and waking are approximately the same in duration. Between the fourth and fifth month, the daily number of neutral reactions increases incredibly as does the duration of positive expressive movements during the day. Fluctuations in preponderance of single reactions and impulsive movements on the one hand and long processes of behavior on the other continue for five months. Of new forms of behavior at this time, among others we see the first confident defensive movements, confident grasping, the first lively expressions of happiness, a cry caused by an unsuccessful deliberate movement, and possibly also the first desire, experimental acts, social reactions to care givers, and looking for removed toys. All of these forms of behavior indicate a certain activity that goes beyond the limits of response to stimulation and on to active seeking of stimuli or active pursuits, which becomes evident from the simultaneous increase in the daily number of spontaneous reactions. These facts, it seems, can no longer be explained by reciprocating interest alone. We must propose that active interest in what is around has taken its place.

To the summary description, we could add a most essential trait to the second stage of infancy: the appearance of imitation. As some authors maintain, in the first stage of infancy, there are no early forms of imitation of movement, vocal reactions, etc. The earlier imitation of actions noted by psychologists (opening the mouth—W. Preyer) or sounds (W. Stern) during the first months are only seemingly imitations. Before five months or even significantly longer, we could not get any kind of imitation. Evidently, imitation is possible only with associative reflexes.

From what has been said above with respect to periods, we can divide the first year of life into a period of passivity, a period of receptive interest, and a period of active interest, which represent a gradual transition to activity. A remarkable turning point occurs at the tenth month when, after the disappearance of purposeless movements, we can observe rudiments of further development of more complex forms of behavior: first use of a tool and use of words to express a wish. With this, the child begins a new period that ends beyond the first year of life. This period is the period of the one-year crisis, which serves as a connecting link between infancy and early childhood.

The summary description of the basic stage and the boundary periods of infancy have no purpose other than developing a most general conception of the external picture of development at the initial stage. In order to study the basic patterns of development in infancy, we must separate the process of development, which is not simple in its composition, and consider analytically its most important aspects connected with their complex internal dependence on each other and in this way elucidate the path that leads to the appearance of the basic neoformation of the given age level. We must begin with the very first most independent process, growth and development of the important organic systems that are a direct continuation of the embryonal period of development and serve as a prerequisite with respect to other higher aspects of the development of the child's personality.

At the moment of birth, the infant's brain is already formed in its basic parts (form, arrangement of separate parts, their mutual connections). However, the brain is still characterized at this time by serious immaturity from both structural and functional aspects. This immaturity is so obvious that it gave rise to the idea that the infant, according to R. Virchow, is a purely spinal-cord being in whose behavior the brain does not have any part. This theory proved to be unsustainable in light of further studies, the basic results of which we shall now present.

The first and most serious expression of immaturity of the brain we see in the fact of extremely rapid growth of brain substance in the child. According to the data of O. Pfister, the weight of the brain doubles by the fourth to fifth month. Further increase is not as rapid. According to the data of L. L. Volpin, the brain doubles in weight by eight months and at the end of a year, it is two and a half times larger. Further increase in size is slower so that after three years, it is three times the weight of the brain of a newborn. This indicates that the most rapid growth of the brain occurs during the first year of life and during the rest of life, the increase in brain substance is equal to the increase in weight during all the subsequent years taken together.

However, in itself, the total weight of the brain still says little about the internal development of the central nervous system. To elucidate this problem, we must turn to a consideration of the development of the important sections and systems of the brain. The most remarkable feature of the function of the central nervous system in infancy is that in the motor system of the child during the first months of life, primitive motor reactions predominate which are inhibited in adults and are apparent only in pathological conditions. Toward the end of the first year there are still effective mechanisms that are proper to quadrupeds. Later, the developing higher centers inhibit atavistic movements, but in pathological conditions, the inhibition may be released and these movements may appear even at a much later age. Thus, the motor systems of the newborn and the infant differ in three completely exclusive features: (1) proper to the infant are movements that completely disappear in the course of later development; (2) the character of these movements is an atavistic and ancient character in the phylogenetic sense of the word, and may be compared with ancient, phylogenetic stages of development of the central nervous system. Thus, it seems that in the development of the child's brain, we can observe as if a transitional stage of phylogenesis: from fish, in which the corpus striatum is absent and only the globus pallidus is functional, to amphibians in which the corpus striatum attains a significant stage of development (Maslov); (3) finally, the specific traits of the infant motor system that disappear in the course of development are analogous not only to the ancient phylogenetic functions, but also to pathological motor manifestations that can be observed at a more mature age in organic and functional damage to the central nervous system. All descriptions of the infant motor system are full of such similarities between the motor system of the infant and a pathological motor system in athetosis, chorea, and other nervous diseases.

These three features may be explained only in light of the basic laws of the history of development and construction of the nervous system. The three laws have prime significance for the problems in which we are interested. We will present them as E. Kretschmer formulated them.

1. Preservation of the lower centers in the form of separate stages. The lower centers and arches, older in the history of development, when acting do not simply move to the side with the gradual formation of higher centers, but continue to work jointly as subordinate units under the direction of the higher centers that are younger in such a way that in an undamaged nervous system they cannot usually be detected separately.

2. The upward transition of functions. However, the subordinate centers do not maintain their initial type of functioning in the history of development, but pass a substantial part of their former functions upward to new centers that are constructed above them (Vöster, M. Minkowski, et al.). Thus, the spinal frog, which was practically deprived of brain functions and remained exclusively with the sympathetic centers, may carry out very complex and relatively purposeful actions, for example, the rooting reflex, so that some have spoken directly of the medullar soul. Such developed functions in man are proper exclusively to the brain, especially to the cortex of the cerebrum, and after the break in the connection can no longer be done by the medulla, which functions only very primitively and fragmentarily as an isolated operative body in man.

3. Emancipation of lower centers. If the higher center is functionally weak or separated from subordinate centers as a result of shock, illness, or damage, then the general function of the nervous apparatus does not simply stop, but is transferred to a subordinate unit which becomes independent and exhibits the still remaining elements of its old type of functioning. As has been noted, even in a removed human spinal cord we still see such tonic-clonic reflex phenomena of a primitive kind. Those same patterns are then repeated in higher cortical and subcortical arches still not capable of being anatomically differentiated. We see this primarily in hysteria and catatonia: when the higher mental functions of purposeful will are disrupted, psychomotor methods of functioning that are lower from the point of view of developmental history frequently appear and assume the control of behavior; these are methods which we will later consider as hypobulic mechanisms, as a lower layer of higher volitional processes. This general neurobiological law can be formulated as follows: if within the psychomotor sphere, the action of higher units becomes functionally weak, then the closest lower unit becomes independent with its own primitive laws.

To these three basic laws, we must add still another general law first formulated by L. Edinger, who, in the process of studying animals, found that in principle the whole mechanism, beginning with the end of the medulla (to which the primary brain belongs) and ending with the olfactory nerves, is constructed in the same way in all higher and lower vertebrates and that, consequently, whether we speak of man or of fish, the basis of all simple functions is absolutely the same for the whole series.

The patterns we have presented that appear in the history of the construction of the nervous system in onto- and phylogenesis make it possible to explain the noted basic features of brain functions during infancy.

If we reject the view according to which the infant is exclusively a medullar being, then we must nevertheless admit that at this age the cortex of the brain is the most immature section of the nervous system. This is evident both in the absence over the whole course of the period of higher mental functions undoubtedly connected with the activity of the cortex and in the absence of those specific motor acts that are proper to mature and developed cortical functions. Research shows that the infant is a being whose behavior is facilitated predominantly by ancient subcortical centers of the brain, a being of the intermediate brain.

The circumstance that the lower, oldest sections of the brain mature sooner than others and are to a greater degree already mature at the moment of birth is extremely clear and is required from the point of view of development since specifically concentrated in these areas is the apparatus that plays a key role in all the economy of organic life, in all basic vital directions. The centers of instincts and of emotional life are concentrated here; they are connected, on the one hand, with the vegetative nervous system, the leading basic vital functions of the organism and on the other, with the cortex of the brain—that higher organ of human thought, will, and consciousness. However, for the age under consideration, the circumstance is characteristic that due to the immaturity of the cortex and connections between the subcortical and cortical centers, this apparatus of vegetative and primitive animal life still acts relatively independently, not being subordinate to regulation, inhibition, and control on the part of higher cortical centers.

This is why the activity of this apparatus resembles, on the one hand, the motor system of lower vertebrates in which this apparatus comprises the higher centers with no hierarchically dominating centers over them, and, on the other hand, it shows a similarity to a pathological motor system that develops due to emancipation of lower centers. Emancipation of lower centers manifested in their activity according to their own autonomous, archaic, primitive laws is normal for infancy and is due to immaturity of higher centers. From this, both the atavistic nature of the infant motor system and its remarkable similarity to pathological motor manifestations of later years become understandable. The key to the one and the other lies in the immaturity of the higher centers and the independence of lower sections of the nervous system that results from this. It is entirely natural that with the functional immaturity of the cortex there must be a motor system that is similar to, first, the motor system of animals that do not have the new brain and, second, to the pathological motor system that results from damage to the higher centers and emancipation of lower arches of action.

This is also the explanation for the third feature of the infant motor system: in the course of further development of movement, what is proper to this age almost completely disappears from the inventory of motor acts that are proper to a more mature age. Actually, the infant movements do not disappear as development progresses, but according to the first law that we cited, the centers that direct them continue to work in conjunction with higher nervous formations and enter into their composition as subordinate units and yield a part of their functions upward to younger and newer centers.

As we have said, the nervous system undergoes an extremely rapid development during the first years of life. This is expressed not only in the rapid increase in brain weight, but also in a number of qualitative changes that characterize the dynamics of construction of the nervous system during infancy. Studies have shown that at one year, three periods can be distinguished in the construction of the nerve centers and their functions that replace each other.

The first is characterized by the immaturity of the cortex and striatum and the dominant significance of the pallidum, which at this time is the highest of the independently functioning brain centers. It determines all the uniqueness of the newborn's motor system. In the initial period of development, the child is a pallidal being. That the motor acts of the newborn are controlled by the thalamopallidal system is indicated by the athetoid, slow, wormlike movements of the newborn, their mass character, and the physiological rigidity of the musculature. The motor system of the newborn very much resembles what we know from the neurological clinic about the motor system of people with damage to the striatum. In the newborn, this center is not yet covered by a myelin sheath. It guides acts of sitting, standing and walking. But its greatest significance is that it is the higher center with respect to the pallidum, assumes the task of its functions, and has a regulating and inhibiting effect on pallidal functions.

This is why the immaturity of the corpus striatum explains the independence and the inhibition-releasing functions of the pallidum. The same kind of inhibition-releasing of pallidal functions occurs in the adult when the striatum is damaged and the lower center is emancipated and begins to act according to independent laws. This is responsible for the athetoid character of the newborn's motor system. In the phylogenetic series, this motor system resembles more closely the motor system of the fish; fish have no corpus striatum, and the pallidum serves as the higher nerve center. The thalamus opticus, directly connected with the activity of the pallidum, is the organ in which all the excitations that occur in the brain cortex from external stimuli collect, where they are given an affective tone. All the apparatus that controls gestures of the body and mimicry as well as all generally expressive movements are established in the thalamus opticus. Since together with the thalamus opticus, the pallidum is connected from the very beginning with the lower spinal-brain centers, the reactions of the newborn classify him more precisely as an optopallidospinal being. These reactions are expressed by unconditioned reflexes and nondifferentiated mass movements: the first refer to the spinal activity of the newborn, the second are a pallidal function. As we have said, the striatum is the organ of sitting, standing, and walking. On the basis of this, pallidal childhood may be described as nonwalking and nonsitting, that is, lying childhood whose mobility has an automatic-mass character, phylogenetically interpreted by Vöster as the mechanism of crawling.

The second period in the development of the nervous system during infancy is the maturing of the corpus striatum. In conjunction with this, primitive mechanisms of the apparatus and synergy required for sitting, standing, and grasping appear. This period has been called the striapallidal period. The pallidal system is a lower reflex center, the striatal system is a higher reflex center with receptive-coordinating functions. The striatal system does not have direct connections with the periphery. The affective zone of the striatal system is limited exclusively to the pallidum, and it does not have a direct, associative connection with the cortex, which makes it independent if we do not consider that excitations originating from the thalamus are directed also to the corpus striatum. The most important significance of the corpus striatum is carrying out static, simultaneous functions of the brain, regulation of muscle tonus, inhibition and regulation of corpus pallidum functions, regulation of timely inhibition and release of the whole complex of agonists and antagonists; accuracy of all movements depends on the synergy of these. This same system is related to the primary automatisms such as mimicry, gesticulation, expressive movements, etc.

The transition to the third period is marked primarily by maturing of the brain cortex and the collaboration of its functions in the regulation of behavior and the motor system. This circumstance is expressed in two facts of major importance: (1) in the development of higher nervous activity, that is, a complex system of conditioned reflexes, and (2) in intellectualization and gradually acquired purposeful character of movements. In the newborn, only the so-called primary areas of the brain cortex that are connected with organs of perception and are themselves functional receptor spheres are myelinated. The development of the cortex, according to the data of P. Flechsig, consists in the fact that these primary areas gradually are connected with intermediate and terminal areas which are covered by a myelin sheath only over the course of the first half-year.

The most reliable indicator of cortical development is the development of conditioned reflex activity. The basic patterns of its development during infancy are the following: (1) the newborn has no conditioned reflexes; he displays innate reactions of the dominant type; (2) the development of conditioned reflexes occurs not chaotically, without order, and accidentally, but as subject to the process of development of dominant reactions. There is a definite dependence in the formation of a conditioned reflex on the development of dominant processes in the central nervous system. Only with this perceiving surface is it possible to form a conditioned reflex through the action of which functional interactions of a dominant kind appear in the central nervous system; (3) the time and order of the formation of genetically earliest conditioned reflexes corresponds to the time and order of the development of the dominant: since in the newborn, there is only a food dominant and position dominant, his first conditioned reflexes may be formed only within the sphere of these reactions; (4) significantly later, the visual and aural dominants develop in the child, and consequently, also the possibility of conditioned reflexes connected with these areas; (5) since the dominant reactions are connected with instinctive activity localized in the subcortical area, the formation of primary conditioned reflexes is not limited to cortical processes, but indicates the decisive role of subcortical centers and their formations and, consequently, also indicates the dependence of this process on instinctive activity.

The intellectualization of movement and its acquiring a purposeful character appear significantly later in the infant's development than the formation of the primary conditioned reflexes. This intellectualization is manifested in the child's manipulation of objects and in his first acts of instrumental thinking, that is, the simplest use of tools. The very first manifestation of this activity can be observed at the beginning of the second six months. The formation of conditioned reflexes begins to enter into the sphere of direct influence of the subcortical dominants during this period. Thus, the primary conditioned reflexes can be observed from the second month of life, and although they also evidently point to the role and participation of the cortex, they still are neither processes of accumulating systematic personal experience nor evidence of any substantial participation of cortical functions in the behavior of the infant.

The consideration of the three periods graphically confirms the basic laws of the construction of the central nervous system presented above. The pallidal motor system does not disappear as the corpus striatum matures, but is included in its function as a subordinate unit. In precisely the same way, movements proper to the time of dominance of the corpus pallidum enter as an important component part into the activity of higher psychomotor mechanisms. We found a confirmation of this in the fate of a number of reflexes that can be observed at maturity only in cases of damage to the brain. Reflexes such as the Babinski reflex and others are pathological for the adult while they are a completely normal physiological phenomenon in infancy. As the child develops, they can no longer be elicited in an independent form since they are included as subordinate units in the activity of higher centers and appear independently only in cases of pathological diseases of the brain (on the basis of the law of emancipation of lower centers).

Now we can go on to a consideration of those consequences that stem from the picture of organic and nervous development in infancy drawn above. These consequences can be found most easily in the area of sensory and motor functions of the child that basically characterize his perception and behavior, that is, two basic aspects of relation to the external world.

The first, as shown by the study of sensory and motor functions in the newborn and infant, is the initial indissoluble connectedness of perception and behavior. The connection between sensory and motor functions belongs to the number of fundamental properties of activity of the mental and nervous apparatus. Formerly it was imagined that the sensory and motor functions were initially separated and isolated from each other and an associative connection between sensory and motor processes was established only in the course of development. Actually, the relative independence of the one and the other arises only during the long process of development and is characteristic of an already high level attained by the child. The initial moment of development is characterized precisely by the indissoluble connectedness of both processes that form a subordinate unit.

Thus, in modern psychology, the problem of the relation of perceptions and actions is formulated completely opposite to the way it was stated formerly. Formerly the problem was how can the uniting of perception and action be explained. Now the problem consists of explaining how initially the single sensory motor processes acquire relative independence from each other in the course of development and develop the possibility of new, higher, more mobile and complex connections.

A study of the simple reflex of movement provides the first answer to this question. Every innate reflex is a sensory motor unit in which perception of stimulus and a response movement is a single dynamic process; its motor part is simply a dynamic continuation of the perceiving part.

From the facts of formation of conditioned reflexes, we know that the reflex arches are mobile: the perceiving segment of one arch can be connected to a single apparatus with the motor part of another, and from this it becomes understandable also that a mobile, free, and highly varied union of any perceptions with any movements is possible. For this reason, many investigators tried to explain the whole development of the sensory motor processes with the help of mechanisms of conditioned reflexes. But this attempt was unfounded because of two circumstances: (1) from this point of view, only the first part of the problem can be explained, specifically, the unity of sensory motor processes, but this can in no way explain the second part of the problem, specifically, how the relative independence and separateness of the one set of processes and the other arise and appear very distinctly during the second six months of life; (2) this explanation may be adequate only if all the behavior of the infant were actually due to reflexes; actually, separate reflex movements comprise only an insignificant and more or less accidental part in the system of behavior of the newborn and the infant. Obviously, the explanation given does not solve the whole problem but covers only that specific part of the sensory motor processes that relates to the group of unconditioned and conditioned reflexes.

For a real explanation of the connection of sensory and motor processes during the first year of life, we must take into account two other circumstances: (1) the integral, structural character that initially distinguishes each set of processes, and

(2) the more complex character of the central connection between them than that which occurs in a simple reflex arch.

Let us consider the first circumstance. Even now we sometimes encounter the opinion according to which the infant's movements are an aggregate of separate, isolated, single reflexes that only slowly and gradually unite into connected whole dynamic processes. Nothing is less true than this notion. The path of development of the motor system proceeds not from assembling separate partial movements into whole motor acts, not from the part to the whole, but from the mass, group movements that encompass the whole body, whole movements, to differentiation and isolation of separate motor acts that are later united into new units of a higher order, from the whole to the parts. In any case, such are the instinctive movements that are predominant in the infant. For this reason, the problem of the genetic relation of instincts and reflexes is a problem of very major importance for all the teaching on the age of infancy.

There are two opposing solutions to this problem. According to one, the reflex is a primary phenomenon and instinct is nothing other than a simple mechanical uniting link of reflex actions in which the final moment of one reflex serves simultaneously as a stimulus or initial moment of the next. According to another view, instinct is genetically primary and reflex is a later phylogenetic formation that arises through differentiation of instinctive movements and isolation from them of separate component parts.

All the facts known from research of instinctive activity of animals and infants compel us to admit the correctness of the second theory and reject the first as not corresponding to reality. We shall explain this using two examples. Take the feeding of the child with the mother's milk as a typical example of instinctive activity. According to the first theory, at the initial stimulation (hunger or feeling the mother's breast) the impulse is established only for the initial reflex—for the movement of finding the nipple. The feeling of contact between the nipple and the lips evokes the reflex of grasping the nipple with the lips, which as a new stimulus leads to sucking movements. The milk flowing into the mouth of the child due to the sucking movements is a new stimulus for the swallowing reflex, etc. The whole process of feeding is a simple mechanical chain of separate reflex acts.

A real study of this typical instinct shows that we have before us an integral process that has a definite sense and direction purposefully leading to satisfying a need that has arisen and not a mechanical uniting of separate reflexes of which each one taken in itself has no sense or meaning but acquires them only within the whole. The instinctive action seems to be complex, objectively purposeful, directed to satisfying a biological need and, for this reason, objectively a sensible, whole process each part of which, including the reflex movements included in it, depend on the structure of the whole. The process of feeding never occurs with a mechanical, stereotypic, repeated sequence of each separate movement. Separate elements may change but the process as a whole retains the sensible structure. Observing the infant satisfying his hunger, we can never predict that at any point he will, because of mechanical necessity, make one movement or another that is an alternating link in the reflex chain. But at each moment of the process we can confidently predict that one of the possible movements will be made that must carry out the function of the near stage in the development of this whole process.

In this way, we must admit that instincts and not reflexes are the initial form of the child's activity and that the development of the motor system of the infant is characterized more than anything by the absence of separate, disjointed, specialized movements of one organ or another and by the presence of massive, movements that involve the whole body.

The perceptions of the newborn and the infant have this kind of integral character. We have already presented the idea of K. Koffka, who describes the perceptions of the newborn as whole perception of the situation in which a quality appears against an amorphous background, inadequately defined and undifferentiated. All studies unanimously show that the initial moment in the development of perception is not a chaos of separate impressions and not a mechanical aggregate of impressions, not a mosaic of various feelings, but whole, complex situations, structures, sharply colored by affect. Thus, the perceptions of the infant, like the motor system, are characterized by initial wholeness. And the path of their development also lies from perception of the whole to perception of parts, from perception of the situation to perception of separate moments.

This structural, whole character that distinguishes the sensory and motor processes in the same way, brings us to an explanation of the connection that unites the sensory and motor processes. They are connected structurally with each other. This must be understood in this way: perceptions and action initially are a single, undifferentiated structural process where action is the dynamic continuation of perception with which it is united into a common structure. In perception and in action, as in two nonindependent parts, we find the laws of common construction of a single structure. Between them there is an internal, essential, sensible structural connection.

At the same time, we come to the second important point connected with solving this problem. We have explained that for both the sensory and the motor processes, equally essential is the development of a single structure for both of them. But the formation of structures is the function of the central apparatus. As research shows, such a central process that connects the sensory and motor functions and leads to the formation of a single central structure is, at the infant stage, stimulation, need or, more broadly speaking, affect. Perception and action are connected through affect. This explains for us what is most essential in the problem of unity of the sensory motor processes and provides the key to comprehending their development.

We will give two examples to illustrate this idea.

Experimental study of the nursling's ability to distinguish forms disclosed an extremely interesting pattern directly related to the question under consideration.[4] The nursling learned to recognize various forms—a square, a triangle, an oval, and the form of a violin, identical in plane. The child was presented with four milk bottles different in form, but absolutely the same with respect to other qualities. Only one nipple of the four that were on the bottles had a hole through which the child could get milk. The result was that almost two-thirds of the twenty-nine children studied, who were five to twelve months old, learned in the same way to select the bottle with the form that had the nipple with the hole. H. Volkelt frequently ascertained that children absolutely reliably selected their own bottle of two or even a whole series of bottles. A series of additional critical experiments made an especially strong impression; in these, a bottle of a certain form perceived by the child as his was not in his field of vision. In these cases, the behavior of the nursling changed completely, and an impression of the behavior of an adult was created: it seemed that not getting his bottle, the child looked for it (disappointed inhibition of all movements; his glance wonders; his hand does not reach out to grasp).

In Volkelt's words, an analysis of these experiments shows that the success of the method rests, obviously, on the fact that the child drinks as if "triangular" or "oval" milk. In other words, in the process of the whole experience connected with drinking from a bottle of a certain form, the nursling develops an extremely firm connection between the quality of the attractive stimulus and the experience of pleasure (that is, the most vitally important qualities, since the basic food of the nursling is milk), on the one hand, and complex qualities corresponding to that certain form of the bottle on the other hand. The one and the other form a still quite undifferentiated, diffuse feeling, regardless of the discreteness of the qualities from the point of view of an adult.

Volkelt's experiment succeeded in only three cases in which he was able to create a primitive whole of this kind. Only then were the experiences elicited in the experiment equal to the primitive consciousness. Specifically, only when the tendencies toward perception of the whole, which characterize the primitive vital being, are adequately met can we expect success in setting up the experiment. Only in this way did Volkelt's experiment, creating a kind of primitive whole of the milk and the form, result in an undoubted inclination toward the form. The same thing could be expressed differently and more precisely: Volkelt concludes that only such a mutual merging of both aspects of one and the same experience, corresponding in the primitive consciousness to getting the form and taking the milk, proves that the nursling can distinguish form.

From these experiments, we see that the development of a connection between perception of a certain form and an action of a certain kind is possible only if these processes enter into one and the same single, integral structure affectively colored by need.

Another example refers to the sphere of processes of forming the conditioned reflexes mentioned before. As we have seen, the basic pattern in the development of conditioned reflexes in the nursling consists of the fact that alternation and sequence in their development are subordinated to the order of appearance of basic dominants. In this case, at the initial stage, these dominants are dominants of a subcortical, instinctive character which determine the sphere in which a new connection between sensory and motor processes is possible in general. Consequently, the formation of conditioned reflexes also confirms the idea that only the presence of a single dominant, which is nothing other than a physiological substrate of affect, ensures the possibility of the development of a new conditional connection between perception and action.

As a result of this discussion, we can formulate a most important and essential hypothesis on the mental life of the infant: it is characterized by complete nondifferentiation of separate mental functions, exclusive dominance of primitive integral experiences, and may, in general, be described as a system of instinctive consciousness developing under the dominating action of affects and drives.

The last idea requires substantial reservations since it frequently led and leads to a completely incorrect interpretation of the whole course of the mental development of the child. Noting correctly the exclusive domination of affects and drives connected predominantly with the subcortical mechanism of consciousness and behavior of the infant, many investigators reach the conclusion from this that affects generally characterize only the primitive mentality that is lower on the developmental ladder and that as the child's development continues, the role of the affective tendencies moves further and further into the background, which results in the degree of affectivity of behavior being made the criterion of primitiveness or mental maturity of the child. This is totally incorrect. Characteristic for the initial and primitive stage is not the great significance in itself of affective tendencies that is maintained over the whole course of the child's development but two other points: (1) dominance of affects, most primitive by nature, directly connected with instinctive stimuli and drives, that is, lower affects; and (2) exclusive dominance of primitive affects with underdevelopment of the rest of the mental apparatus connected with sensory, intellectual, and motor functions.

The presence of affective stimuli is an indispensable adjunct to every new stage in the development of the child from the lowest to the highest. It might be said that affect opens the process of the child's mental development and construction of his personality and itself completes the process, concluding and crowning the development of personality as a whole. In this sense it is not accidental that affective functions disclose a direct connection both with the very old subcortical centers that develop first and are the foundation of the brain and with the new, specifically human areas of the brain (the frontal lobes) that develop last of all. This fact is an anatomical expression of the circumstance that affect is the alpha and omega, the first and last link, the prologue and epilogue of all mental development.

Participating in the process of mental development from the very beginning to the very end as an important factor, affect itself takes a complex course, changing with each new stage of constructing the personality, entering into the structure of new consciousness proper to each age, and disclosing at each new stage most profound changes in its mental nature. Specifically, affect undergoes very complex development even during the first year of life. If we compare the beginning and end stages of this period, we cannot but be impressed by the great change that occurs in the affective life of the infant.

The initial affect of the newborn confines his mental life to the narrow limits of sleeping, feeding, and crying. During the first stage of infancy, affect assumes the basic form of receptive interest in the outside world only to give way in the next stage to active interest in the environment. Finally, the conclusion of infancy directly confronts us with the one-year crisis, which, like all critical age levels, is characterized by vigorous development of affective life and is marked by the first manifestation by the child of the affect of his own personality—the first stage in the development of the child's will.

K. Bühler proposed an extremely convenient scheme which makes it possible to systematize genetically the basic forms of behavior of animals and man. Bühler gives his scheme a universal significance applying it to the animal, the child, and the adult. He attempts to place it at the base of the whole theory on infancy. Subsequently we will consider critically the possibility and justification of such an extended interpretation of the scheme.[5] As frequently happens, constructions that are unjustifiably extended far beyond their limits and, naturally, disclose their insupportability there, are from the factual aspect completely adequate for a certain limited range of phenomena. Bühler's is a scheme of this kind. It irreproachably reflects the development of behavior during infancy.

Bühler maintains that if we begin to consider all sensible methods of animal and human action, that is, objectively purposeful methods, we will see that from the bottom to the top there is a very simple and clear distinguishable three-stage construction of these, which can be termed instinct, dressage, and intellect. Instinct is the lowest stage and is also the soil in which all the higher stages grow. In man there is not one area, not one form of mental activity that is not in some way based on instinct.

These three stages, moving from the bottom to the top, as we said, truly and consistently with reality reflect development in infancy. At the first stage, an instinctive form of activity is dominant in the behavior of the infant. It differs from the same activity of animals by an inadequate readiness of these inherited forms of behavior. Actually, the pitiful helplessness of the human newborn is due to the insufficiency of ready instinctive mechanisms. Certain elementary motives and tensions that sustain life are innate in man, and in him, all higher mental organization is derived from the vague drive for existence, for activity, for well-being and happiness. But everything is very indefinite and sketchy, everything requires finishing, dressage, and intellect. In comparison with the strictly regular life of insects, the instincts of man seem to us to be diffuse, weak, ramified, and endowed with great individual differences so that in some cases, we might ask whether or not this is a natural apparatus in general.

In the incompleteness of instincts in the newborn, a certain genetic sense is clearly apparent. Human instincts, in contrast to animal instincts, do not contain almost ready and completed mechanisms of behavior. More likely, they are a certain system of stimulations, certain prerequisites and points of departure for further development. This means that in the child instinctive forms of behavior are relatively much less significant than in animals. Even such a process as walking, which the duckling and the chick have in a ready form immediately after pecking their way out of the egg, develops relatively late as the result of long development in the child, It is not a new idea that man could achieve remarkable flexibility and versatility in his capabilities if he could only discard his ready, innate mechanisms. The chick actually can walk on its own two feet immediately, but because of this, it cannot later learn to crawl, dance, walk on its knees. K. Bühler is right when he says that human instinct in its pure form can be observed in hopeless idiots, unfortunate beings who cannot benefit from training.

The second stage is characterized by the dominance of acquired personal experience added to heredity by instruction, exercise, and training. The first half-year of the child's life is essentially filled with acquiring the simple art of grasping, sitting, crawling, etc. All of this is training, self-instruction in play, which occurs with gradual exercise. The formation of conditioned reflexes, habitual movements, and habits represents similar forms that arise through instruction and training and pertain to the second stage.

The third stage in the development of infant behavior is characterized by rudiments of intellectual activity. Bühler was the first to demonstrate experimentally that toward the end of infancy, the child exhibits simple practical intelligence, visual-effective thinking absolutely similar to the actions of the chimpanzee in the famous experiments of W. Köhler. For this reason, Bühler proposed that this phase in the child's life be called the chimpanzee-like age. At this age, the child creates his first inventions, very primitive, of course, but very important in the mental sense. The essence of intellectual manifestations of the child consists in the first sensible and purposeful movements of the hand, not innate and not taught, but arising in a given situation and connected with the simplest use of detours and the use of tools. The child exhibits the ability to use a string to pull a distant object to himself, uses one object as a tool to bring another closer, etc. Bühler's experiments demonstrated that even before the rudiments of speech, the child goes through a stage of practical intellect or instrumental thinking, that is, grasping mechanical links and devising mechanical means to meet mechanical goals. Even before the appearance of speech, the child develops subjectively comprehended, that is, consciously purposeful, activity.

In Bühler's experiments, the first manifestation of practical intellect was placed at the tenth to the twelfth month. As we have said, the actual development of the first use of a tool occurs beyond the limits of infancy, but the initial manifestation of the capability undoubtedly matures during the second stage of infancy. A preparatory stage for instrumental thinking and rudiments of using objects for this purpose can be observed as early as in the six-month-old. At nine months, these manifestations can be observed in a developed form. They may be taken as the first attempts to establish mechanical relationships.

A preliminary stage in the development of this capability is the unique form of manipulating objects observed in the six-month-old. The child no longer uses only one object in play. He deals with an object as an extension of his own hand and holding it, drags it along another immobile object, pounds on it, hits it, rubs it, precisely the same thing a four-month-old does with his hands. The device of using objects is a preliminary stage to the use of tools. In the seven-month-old, we find the first hints of a principally new activity with objects, specifically, changing their form by squeezing, crumpling, stretching, and tearing. This initially destructive activity contains the first devices of forming and reconstructing. Positive forming is evident in the attempt of the eight-month-old to shove objects one into another. This manipulation of immobile objects with the help of moving objects, this action of one object on another, this change in the form of an object and rudiments of positive formation may justifiably be considered as a preliminary stage for the development of instrumental thinking. All of this leads to the simplest use of tools. The use of tools creates a new period for the child.

To conclude the consideration of the genesis of the basic neoformation, it remains for us to speak of the development of the social behavior of the infant.

We have already spoken of communication in the newborn. It is characterized by the absence of specific social reactions. The relation of the child to the adult is so merged and inseparably intertwined in his basic vital functions that no differentiated reactions can be isolated. Specifically social impressions and reactions arise when the child is two months old. It was possible to establish that a smile appears first as a social reaction. Other reactions follow, leaving no doubt that we are dealing with differentiated, specific social manifestations by the child. Between one and two months of age, the child reacts with a smile to sounds of the human voice.

As we have indicated, as early as the end of the first month, the cry of one child evokes a similar cry in another child. At two months, the cry of the child usually stops if someone comes to him. Finally, at two to three months, the child meets the glance of an adult with a smile. At the same time, a great number of forms of behavior appear which indicate that the child has entered into social interactions with the adults who care for him. The child turns to the person who speaks, listens to the human voice, is offended if the person turns away from him. The three-month-old greets an approaching person with sounds and he smiles at the person. He displays a readiness for sociability. C. Bühler notes two especially important factors that influence the development of initial forms of sociability. The first is activity initiated by the adult. The child is essentially reactive from the very beginning. The adult cares for the child and plays with him. Everything that the infant gets at this stage of life comes from the adult: not only satisfying his needs, but also all diversion and stimulation resulting from a change in position, movement, play, and conversation. The child reacts more and more to this world of experience created by the adult, but he still does not socialize with another child that is in the same room in another crib.

The second condition for experiencing sociability consists in the fact that the child must know how to control his own body. In certain positions and states when his needs are satisfied, the child is left with quite a surplus of energy. In such a state, his feelings must be active if only insignificantly. At such times, he is in a state of listening and actively looking around a little. If the comfortable and sure position the child is in is changed to another which he has not yet mastered, all his energy will be directed to eliminating his discomfort. The child no longer has energy for smiling at the speaker or exchanging glances with him. For example, a child in a sitting position who cannot yet wholly manage his body will exhibit less activity when sitting. The limits of his activity increase when he is learning to sit, stand, and walk. In a prone position, the infant enters into communication with others much more easily than he does when sitting. In this case, the obstacle to communication is a lack of activity on the part of the child.

In this respect, at five months, there is usually a change: successes which children make in controlling their bodies, its position and movement, lead to the five- or six-month-old seeking contact with his peers. During the second half-year, all the basic social interrelations characteristic for two children of this age are developing. They smile and chatter at each other, give and take toys alternately, they play with each other and play together. During the second half-year, specific needs for sociability develop in the child. With complete confidence, we can say that a positive interest in people is elicited by the fact that all the needs of the child are met by adults. Active endeavors at socializing are expressed during the second half-year by the fact that the child seeks the glance of another person, smiles at him, chatters, draws toward the person, grasps him, and is dissatisfied when the person moves away.

In general outline, an inventory of social forms of behavior during the first year is presented in the work of C. Bühler and her colleagues. It is apparent that the first phase of social manifestations on the part of the child is marked by passivity, reactivity, and dominance of negative emotions (crying and dissatisfaction when an adult leaves). The second phase is marked by active seeking of contact not only with adults, but also with peers, common activity of children, and the appearance of the most primitive relations of dominance and subordination, protest, despotism, compliance, etc.

In the first place, we must, of course, be interested in two circumstances that are closely connected with each other and directly affect the genesis of social developments at this age. The first consists of that common root from which social development of the infant originates. The second consists of the unique character that social intercourse acquires during infancy which distinguishes the sociability of the infant from that of the older child.

The common root of all social manifestations during infancy is the unique situation of development of which we have already spoken. From the very beginning, the infant is confronted only by situations in which his whole behavior is intertwined and interwoven into sociability. His path to things and to the satisfaction of his own needs is always channeled through relations with another person. Specifically for this reason, the relations of the newborn cannot be differentiated and isolated from the common, merged situation into which they are interwoven. Later, when they begin to differentiate, they continue to retain the initial character in the sense that communication with an adult serves as a basic way for the child to manifest his own activity. Almost all personal activity of the infant pours into the stream of his social relations. His relation to the external world is always a relation through another person. For this reason, if we can say that in the individual behavior of the infant, everything is intertwined and interwoven into the social, then the opposite also seems true: all social manifestations of the infant are intertwined and interwoven in his concrete, actual situation, forming with it a merged and indissoluble whole.

The specific, unique, infantile sociability that results from this is evident primarily in the fact that the social intercourse of the child has not yet been separated from the whole process of his intercourse with the external world, with things and processes of satisfying his vital needs. This intercourse still lacks the most basic means: human speech. In the wordless, pre-speech, visual-acting communication, interrelations that are no longer seen in subsequent development of the child move to the forefront. This is not so much communication based on mutual understanding as emotional expression, a transfer of affect, a negative or positive reaction to a change in the central point of any infant situation—the appearance of another person.

The adult is the center of every situation during infancy. It is natural for this reason that the simple closeness or distancing of the person signifies for the child a sharp and radical change in the situation in which he finds himself. If we were not afraid to use a graphic expression, we might say that a simple approach and distancing of an adult arms and disarms the activity of the child. In the absence of the adult, the infant falls into a situation of helplessness. His activity with respect to the external world is seemingly paralyzed or at least limited and narrowed to a high degree. It is as if his hands and feet were suddenly taken away from him: the possibility of moving, changing his position, grasping a needed object. For the child's activity, the most usual and natural way through another person is opened by the presence of an adult. This is why another person is always the psychological center of every situation for the infant. This is why, for the infant, the sense of every situation is determined in the first place by this center, that is, its social content, or, to put it more broadly, the relation of the child to the world depends on and is largely derived from his most direct and concrete relations with an adult.

4. The Basic Neoformation in Infancy

Now after a separate consideration of the most important lines of development in infancy, we can answer the main question relative to the basic neoformation of infancy and in this way, approach the analysis of the most important theories on the initial period of child development. So what is there that is new that arises as a result of the very complex process of development during infancy?

We have seen that the main aspects of child development exhibit an internal unity so that each of them has its own sense, its own significance, and only in the future is included in the single and whole process of development of the basic neoformation of the age. The helplessness of the infant is connected with the still unfinished formation of the skeleton, with undeveloped musculature, with the dominance of the more mature vegetative organic functions, with the dominance of ancient sections of the brain and immaturity of all the centers that determine specifically human forms of activity, with instinctive consciousness centered on the most important vital needs—this helplessness is not only the initial moment for determining the social situation of development of the infant, but also directly affects two circumstances that are directly related to the basic neoformation: (1) the progressive increase in energy resources of the infant as a necessary prerequisite of all higher lines of development and (2) the dynamic change of the initial relation to the world in the course of infant development.

P. P. Blonsky distinguishes three basic stages in infant development from the point of view of the interrelation of his energy resources and his intercourse with his environment. The helplessness of the child determines his place in the environment. At the stage of absolute toothless childhood, the child is a weak being lying in bed and requiring care. On the part of the child, the social stimulus is mainly a cry as a reaction to pain, hunger, and discomfort. Interrelations between him and the environment are based mainly on food. It is completely clear that at this time he is connected most of all with the mother as one who feeds and cares for him.

At the stage when incisors come through, when the child can move in his crib, the interrelation between him and the environment becomes immeasurably more complex. On the one hand, the child endeavors to use the power of adults for changing position and getting the objects he wants. On the other hand, he begins to understand the behavior of the adults, and his psychological, though elementary, socializing with them is established.

In the second year of life, the child is equal to the adult in a room in the situation where little movement is required, and between them a relation of cooperation, though elementary and simple, is established.

Describing the higher social development of the child, we have already indicated that, on the one hand, the energy factor that more or less determines the potentials of activity of the child is the basic prerequisite for the development of his social manifestations and communication with adults. Thus, the genesis of the basic neoformation has very deep roots, in the most intimate internal processes of organic growth and maturation.

On the other hand, the social situation of development that is created by the infant's helplessness determines the direction in which the activity of the infant is realized, the direction toward objects of the surrounding world through another person. But if the child were not a growing, maturing, and developing being, if he were not changing over the course of infancy but remained in the initial state in which we find the newborn, from day to day the social situation of development would determine the life of the child as a turning in one and the same circle with no possibility of moving forward. Then the life of the infant would be reduced only to an endless reproduction of one and the same situation that occurs in pathological forms of development. Actually, the infant is a growing and developing, that is, a changing being, and for that reason his life from day to day resembles not so much a turning in a circle and reproducing one and the same situation as it does a movement up along a spiral related to a qualitative change in the situation of development itself.

In the course of development, the infant's activity increases, his energy supply increases, his movements are improved, his hands and feet grow stronger, new, younger and higher sections of the brain mature, and new forms of behavior and new forms of dealing with the environment develop. Because of all of this, the circle of his relations to reality is extended and, consequently, his making use of the path through an adult becomes broader and more varied, but on the other hand, there is a heightened basic contradiction between the increased complexity and variety of social relations of the child and the impossibility of verbal communication. All of this cannot but lead to a situation in which the basic neoformation of the newborn period—instinctive mental life—changes in a most decisive and radical way. It is very easy to understand the change if we take into account two basic features that distinguish the mentality of the newborn: first, the child does not yet separate not only himself, but also other people from the merged situation that develops on the basis of his instinctive needs; second, for the child there is still nothing and no one at this period; more likely, he experiences states rather than specific objective content. Both of these features disappear in the neoformation of infancy.

The neoformation can be determined if we take into account the basic direction which the infant's development is taking. As we have seen, this direction consists in that only one path to the external world is open to the child's activity—the path that lies through another person. It is completely natural for this reason to expect that in the experience of the infant, his mutual activity with another person in a concrete situation must be differented, isolated, and formed first of all. It is natural to expect that the infant in his consciousness has not yet separated himself from his mother.

If the child is physically separated from the mother at the moment of birth, then biologically, he does not separate from her until the very end of infancy as long as he does not learn to walk by himself, and his psychological emancipation from the mother, separating himself from initial communication with her, usually occurs only outside the limits of infancy, in early childhood. For this reason, the basic neoformations of infancy may best of all be designated by the term introduced in German literature as a name for the initially appearing mental commonality of the infant and the mother, a communication that serves as the point of departure for further development of consciousness. First, what arises in the consciousness of the infant may be termed most precisely as "Ur-wir," that is, "great-we" ["great" as in "great-grandfather"]. This initial consciousness of mental commonality which precedes the development of consciousness of his own personality (that is, consciousness of a differentiated and separated "I") is a consciousness of "we," but not the mobile, complex consciousness of "we" that includes the "I," the consciousness that appears when the child is older. This initial "we" relates to the later "we" as an ancestor to a descendant.

That this consciousness of "great-we," develops in the infant and dominates that whole age we can see from two facts of fundamental importance. The first was elucidated in the research of H. Wallon on the child's development of a conception of his own body. As the study shows, the child at first does not separate even his body from the surrounding world of things. He comes to consciousness of external objects earlier than he recognizes his own body. Initially the child looks at the members of his own body as peripheral objects, and long before he recognizes them as his, he unconsciously learns to coordinate the movements of his hand and eye or both hands. Thus, the infant not knowing his own body relates to his own members as to peripheral things and cannot, of course, have any kind of conception of himself.

G. Compayré defines perfectly this feature of the mental life devoid of its center of consciousness or personality. Strictly speaking, this mental life cannot even be called consciousness. Compayré says that actually we cannot even say that the child has consciousness in the true sense of the word during the first days of his life, that is, consciousness that makes it possible for us to judge our own existence. About the child, we may say: he lives, but is not conscious of his life himself. But if there is no self-consciousness, then from the first days of life, there undoubtedly are vaguely felt and, consequently, conscious impressions. Compayré is completely right when he describes the initial consciousness of the infant as passive. If we understand that word in the meaning that Spinoza used in differentiating passive and active, passive or effective mental states, then we can with complete justification maintain that the initial consciousness of the infant still completely lacks active mental states, that is, mental states internally determined by the personality. In this sense, we might say that the child passes in this period an animal-like stage of development that is marked by absence of consciousness of his own activity, his own personality.

If the first fact characterizes the inability of the infant to separate his own body and his own independent existence from what surrounds it and to be conscious of it, then the second fact indicates more than anything the extent to which his social relations and his relations to external objects are still directly merged. We find an illustration of this fact in the studies of S. Fajans on the effect of spatial separation of an object on its affective attraction for the infant and the preschool child. The studies show that optical distancing of the object also means mental distancing proportional to the distance of the infant from the object: there is a decrease in the affective attraction of the object. Together with spatial distancing, the contact between the infant and the goal is broken. For him, the world at a distance seems not to exist. His goals in the physical sense also are directly near.

The data presented by Fajans show that in 75% of the cases, the infant's affect to an object is significantly stronger if the object is placed nearby. In only 25% of the cases, distancing the object produced no noticeable changes in affect and never was there an increase in affect when the distance of the object increased. In young children, in 10% of the cases, affect increased with distance; in 85%, affect did not depend on whether the object was nearby or far away, and in only 5% of the cases, the affect to the nearby object was stronger than to the object at a distance. This can, of course, be explained by the narrow limits of the infant's living space.

However, the observations of Fajans require two notes: As grasping develops, it is easy to see that at first the child grasps an object that touches his hand. When he is older, he grasps an object even when it does not. The first and directly acting stimulus is now replaced by a specific reaction to the perception of the object itself. C. Bühler correctly connects this fact with the fact that the child develops a new relation to the object at a distance because all his needs are satisfied by adults and because of increased social interaction.

Thus, we see that the social development of the child is evident not only in the direct and immediate growth of his social manifestations, but also in the change and increasing complexity of his relation to things, primarily to the world at a distance. A distant object now elicits an affective need to get it (regardless of whether it is beyond his reach) because the object is included in the social situation of grasping through others.

We have confirmation of this in another factual observation with which we wanted to supplement the data presented above. We saw that the infant sets only physically close goals, but for the child, optical distance of objects is equal to mental distance and disappearance of the affective stimulation that attracts him to the object. This distinguishes the infant from the small child. The second very important difference is that when the object moves away and is out of his reach, for a young child, the situation changes easily: the object situation between the child and the goal is turned into a personal social situation between him and the experimenter. For the young child, the social aspect and the object in the situation are already adequately differentiated. For this reason, we see in him the following interesting phenomenon: when he is unsuccessful and cannot reach his goal, the object situation turns into a social situation.

For the infant, this is still impossible. For the infant, the social and the object situation are still not separated. When the object moves away, as we have seen, in most cases, affective attraction is lost for the infant. But when the infant stops reaching for the distant object, it is very easy to renew his attempts and elicit a lively affect and a lively turning toward the object if the adult moves very close to the object. It is remarkable that renewing the attempts toward the object is directed not toward the adult, but toward the object itself. This new turning to the object is apparent to the same degree whether the object is nearby or farther away. The experimenter says that we might think that the approach of an adult to the object signifies a new hope for the child or that the simple spatial closeness of the adult significantly reinforces the intensity of the field around the object.

The young child reacts in the same way or even more strongly to a person in the situation of his own helplessness, but his reaction has a differentiated character. When he is unable to get the object himself, he turns not to the object which remains unattainable, but to the director of the experiment. The infant reacts completely differently. He continues to turn as before toward the unattainable object although nothing has changed in the object situation.

It is difficult to imagine clearer experimental evidence for the fact that, first, for the infant, the center of every object situation is another person who changes its significance and sense and, second, that the relation to the object and the relation to the person have not yet been separated in the infant. In itself, the object loses affective attractive force for the child the farther away it is, but this force regains its former intensity as soon as a person appears together with the object and is close to it and in a single optical field with it. From a number of experiments, we know the effect of the structure of the optical field on the perception of an object by an animal and by an infant. We know that the perceived object changes its properties for the infant depending on what kind of structure the object is a part of, depending on what lies together with it.

Here we meet with a completely new phenomenon: in the object situation nothing has changed. The child perceives the object just as far away and as unattainable as before. He still does not in the least recognize that he must turn for help to an adult in order to reach the goal that is unattainable for him. But the affective attraction of the object lying at a distance depends on whether or not this object lies in the same field in which the child perceives the person. The object beside the person even if unattainable and at a distance, has the same affective stimulating force as an object that is close to the child and which he can grasp himself. This could not be demonstrated more clearly than in the experiments of Fajans: for the child, the relation to the external world depends wholly on the relation through another person, and in the psychological situation of the infant, the object and the social content are still merged.

Both considerations: (1) the infant's not knowing his own body and (2) the dependence of his affective attraction to things on the possibility of experiencing the situation together with another person wholly and completely confirm the dominance of "great-we" in the consciousness of the infant. The first consideration is evidence from the negative aspect in a direct and immediate way that the child still is not conscious even of his own physical "I." The second consideration indicates from the positive aspect that the simplest affective desire is renewed in the child not otherwise but by contiguity of the object and another person, not otherwise but under conditions of consciousness of "great-we."

Usually the course of social development of the child is sketched in an opposite way. The infant is presented as a purely biological being who knows nothing except himself, is wholly submerged in the world of his own internal experiences and is not capable of any kind of contact with his environment. Only slowly and gradually does the infant become a social being, socializing his desires, thought, and acts. This conception is mistaken. According to it, the undeveloped mentality of the child is maximally isolated, minimally capable of social relation, and reacting to the environment only to the most primitive stimulation of the external world.

Everything we know about the mentality of the infant compels rejecting such a conception categorically. The mentality of the infant from the first moment of his life is locked into common life with other people. The child initially reacts not to separate feelings, but to the people around him. The child reacts differently to a loud sound and to temperature stimulation or a prick. Even at this time, the child reacts differently to the different affective color of the human voice and to changes in facial expression. A loud sound, if considered purely energetically, is much more impressive than the human voice; nevertheless the child is initially seemingly deaf with respect to a simple and strong stimulus, but reacts sensibly and in a differentiated way to stimuli much weaker and more difficult to perceive that come from the people around him. The child initially reacts not to stimuli as such but to the expression of the faces of living people he sees. At the first stages of mental development, children show a preference for those impressions that refer to their mental connection with living people. The child is not so much in contact with a world of lifeless external stimuli as across and through it to a much more internal, although primitive, communication with the personalities that surround him.

W. Peters defines very well the unique experiences proper to this stage. He says that the child perceives the world not in its objective categorical quality, as something separate from his "I," but initially knows only his own kind of "we," within which "I" and the other form a single connected structure and seem to mutually support each other. Since the child at first does not know his "I," in the expression of F. Schiller, objectively speaking, he lives more in another than in himself. But what is most important, in the other, the child specifically lives in the way in which we live in our "I." Even at a later age, there is still a trace in the child of the insufficient separation of his personality from the social whole and from the surrounding world. We shall return to discuss this when we consider the theory of infancy.

Peters, it seems to us, quite correctly explains imitation in infancy and in early childhood by the unique consciousness of mental intercourse. The child is capable much earlier of real imitation than of repeating movements that arise through a purely associative path. Intercourse as a mental fact is internal motivation, imitative action on the part of the child. He merges in his activity directly with the one he imitates. The child never imitates the movements of nonliving objects, for example, the swing of a pendulum. Obviously, his imitative actions arise only when there is personal communication between the infant and the person whom he imitates. This is why imitation is so little developed in animals and so closely connected with understanding and with intellectual processes.

With Peters, we may accept the graphic comparison of the activity of a child who is at this stage of development of consciousness with that of any small children playing ball: in playing ball, we have a complete merging of "I" and "you" in a single action of the internal "we."

Actually, imitation must evidently be referred to a number of specifically human features. The studies of W. Köhler showed that imitation of the ape is limited to the narrow range of its own intellectual potentials. Imitation of a complex, sensible, and purposeful action never is successful without an understanding of the structure of the situation. Thus, the chimpanzee may imitate only such actions as lie within the zone of his own intellectual potentials. All studies of imitation in apes show that apes are very poor at aping. Not only do we not observe the exceptional effort to imitate, famous in fables, but the potential for imitation even in the higher apes is immeasurably poorer than in man. Imitation in the animal is distinguished by being limited to the zone of his own potentials. For this reason the animal cannot learn anything new through imitation. In the child, on the contrary, with the help of imitation, new behavior develops which had never existed before in his experience.

Having explained the basic neoformation of infancy, we can move to a condensed and concise consideration of the basic theories of this age.

5. Basic Theories on Infancy

Reflexological theory.[6] According to this theory, in the initial moment of development, the infant is a being of unconditioned reflexes. The whole content and development of the personality in infancy, including mental and social aspects, occurs by the process of forming conditioned reflexes, their differentiation, their complex interweaving and combining with each other, and the construction of ever higher super-reflexes over the first conditioned reflexes. With this explanation, the reflexological theory attempts to account for all the real complexity of the process.

The development of higher nervous activity, specifically the process of forming conditioned reflexes, is undoubtedly one of the most important aspects of development in infancy, and the foundation for personal experience of the child is established here. But this process is in the middle in the sense that it is itself facilitated by other, more complex processes of development that act as prerequisites for the development of conditioned reflex activity. In its turn, it serves as a prerequisite for more complex and higher forms of mental and social development of the child. For this reason, the reflexological theory may be an adequate conception for explaining one intermediate aspect of development, but it inevitably leads to simplifying all development and to ignoring the independent mechanisms of higher processes of mental and social development. It cannot explain these aspects of development by its existence alone since, on the one hand, it ignores the development of the child's mentality and, on the other, treats the development of social interrelations of the child from the point of view of the law of the relation of an organism to the physical environment. In this way, it inevitably allows the higher patterns to be reduced to the lower and development to be interpreted mechanistically. Mechanism is most clearly apparent in the fact that this theory is not capable of perceiving the main difference between the social development of the child and the development of the animal.

The three-stage theory.[7] This theory, which we expounded previously, is characterized by the same defect as the one above: it also tries to encompass the development of animals and man in one law. It is really and truly the reflexological theory changed in form and augmented since, on the one hand, it is not limited to a purely objective consideration of behavior, but introduces internal mental activity connected with instincts and habits into the sphere of analysis, and on the other hand, it introduces a third stage above the dressage stage—intellect, qualitatively different from the stage of habit formation.

This theory also is adequate only when applied to the narrow range of developing reactions during infancy. Of necessity, it places at the same level the intellectual activity of apes and all higher manifestations of human thinking that develop in the child over the course of childhood. Its tendency to identify human intellect with the intellect of animals finds a clear expression in designating the last stage of infancy the chimpanzee-like age. Ignoring the social nature of man is the root and source of this error.

We have just seen that what takes place in infants is impossible in the world of animals, and the relation to a situation is essentially impossible for the chimpanzee. As we attempted to show with the experiments of Fajans, for the infant even the simplest relation to an object is determined and mediated by the social content of a situation. Ignoring this, the three-stage theory closes for itself any possibility for explaining the existing and profound, principal differences between the intellect of the child and the intellect of the chimpanzee regardless of their external similarity. The differences are due to the unique socially mediated relation of the infant to the situation.

The structural theory.[8] The structural theory on infancy, as we have seen, notes correctly the initial point and certain very important features of infant development. But it disarms itself when it confronts the problems of development as such. Even at the outset the initial moments of development are structural. In the further course of development, the structures become more complex, more and more differentiated and penetrate into each other. From this point of view, however, it is impossible to explain how anything new can arise in development at all. From the point of view of the structural theory, the initial and end point of development, like all intermediate points, is subject to the law of structure to the same extent. As the French proverb says, the more it changes, the more it stays the same.

The structural principle in itself cannot give us the key to understanding the course of development. It is not surprising therefore that the structural theory is more productive and can provide a scientific explanation when it pertains to more elementary, primitive, and initial moments. The structural theory, like the two preceding theories, attempts to explain the development of animals and man on the same principle which, in light of this conception, seems to be structurally identical. For this reason, although the theory is most productive when applied to infancy, it displays its inadequacy as soon as an attempt is made to apply it to the development of higher, specifically human properties of the child. Even within the first age of infancy, it cannot explain the central problem of the formation of man, which is, on the whole, inexplicable from the point of view of a theory that encompasses the development of animals and man in one principle.

The theory that understands infancy as a subjectivistic stage of development. According to this theory, the newborn is a being closed within himself, wholly immersed in his own subjectivity who turns only slowly and gradually to the objective world. The content of the development of the first year of life can be reduced to a transition from the stage of complete immersion in subjective experiences to intensive directedness to the object and to the first perception of objective connections. The dynamics of this period is a movement from the "I" to the external world. It is natural that, from the point of view of this theory, objective relations are perceived by the child initially as relations of doing and not relations of being. For this reason, in speaking of this period, we must speak not so much of perceiving dependencies as of establishing relations between objects.

The basic idea of the theory on complete subjectivism in infancy, of the developmental path during this period from an internal nucleus of personality, from the "I" to the external world, as we shall see, is presented even more clearly in the following theory, which we shall consider last. Critical notes on it will refer also to the present theory.

The theory of solipsism characteristic of infancy.[9] This theory is connected on the one hand with the idea of the preceding theory brought to an extreme, and on the other, with theories of infancy developed by the psychoanalytic school (S. Bernfeld). This theory is a kind of synthesis of the two conceptions. In its most complete and consistent form, it was developed by Piaget, who maintains that the infant's consciousness is a riddle for us. One path for penetrating it is the regressive path. Piaget states that we know that the most significant feature that distinguishes the behavior and thinking of the child from that of the adult is its egocentrism. This increases as we go down the age levels. In an eighteen-year-old, egocentrism is expressed differently from the way it is expressed in the ten-year-old or in the six-year-old, etc. At age four, egocentrism occupies all the thought of the child. If we consider this egocentrism overall, then we may assume, as Piaget does, that an infant is characterized by absolute egocentrism, which may be defined as the solipsism of the first year.

According to Piaget, logical thinking develops late in the child. It always includes something of the social in it. It is connected with speech. Without words, we would think as if in a dream: in images united with feeling and having a confused, wholly individual and affective meaning. This kind of thinking, unlike socialized, logically mature thinking, we observe in dreams and in some patients. It has been termed autistic thinking. Autism and logical thinking are two poles: one is purely individual, the other, purely social. Our normal, mature thinking fluctuates constantly between these two poles. In dreams and in certain mental illnesses, man loses all interest in objective activity. He is immersed in a world of his own affects that find their expression in graphic, emotionally colored thinking.

According to this theory, the infant also lives seemingly in dreams. S. Freud speaks of the narcissism of the infant thus: he literally has no interest in anything except himself. The infant, like a solipsist, accepts everything that surrounds him as himself, identifying the world with his own idea of it. Further development of the infant consists in a gradual disappearance of solipsism and a gradual socialization of thinking and consciousness of the child turning toward external reality. Egocentrism natural to the child of a much later age is a compromise between the initial solipsism and gradual socialization of thought. The degree of egocentrism may for this reason be a measure of the child's progress along the developmental path. From this point of view, Piaget touches on a number of children's reactions which he observed in an experiment and which are close to the type of behavior that frequently appears in infancy, for example, a magical relation to things.

Even from a simple presentation of the theory, it is easy to see that it is an attempt to present the infant development in a form turned inside out. This theory is a direct and polar opposite of the conception of infant development we presented. We saw that the initial point of infant development is characterized by the fact that all vital manifestations of the infant are intertwined and interwoven in the social, that through long development, the child develops a consciousness of the "great-we," and that consciousness of an indivisible mental communication and absence of the possibility of self-observation are the most distinctive properties of the infant's consciousness. The theory of solipsism confirms that the child is a presocial being wholly immersed in the world of dream thinking and subject to affective interest in himself. The error at the base of this theory, as well as of Freud's theory, consists in the incorrect contrasting of the two tendencies: (1) the tendency to satisfy needs and (2) the tendency to adapt to reality, that is, the pleasure principle and the reality principle and autistic thinking and logical thinking. Actually, neither represent polar opposites, but are very closely united with each other. The tendency to satisfy needs is essentially only the other side of the tendency toward adaptation. Neither does pleasure contradict reality. They not only do not exclude each other, but almost coincide in infancy.

In precisely the same way, logical and autistic thinking, affect and intellect, are not two mutually exclusive poles, but two mental functions, closely connected with each other and inseparable, that appear at each age as an undifferentiated unity although they contain ever newer relations between affective and intellectual functions. The genetic problem is solved from this point of view since autistic thinking can be accepted as primary and primitive. As we know, Freud defended this point of view. E. Bleuler demonstrated that autistic thinking is a function that develops late. He speaks against Freud's idea that in the course of development, the mechanisms of pleasure are primary and that the child is separated by a shell from the external world and lives an autistic life and hallucinates about satisfying his internal needs. Bleuler maintains that he does not see a hallucinatory satisfaction in the infant; he sees satisfaction only after actual taking in of food. In observing an older child, he did not see the child preferring an imagined apple to a real one.

In all his drives, the newborn reacts to reality and in the spirit of reality. Never can we find or even imagine a viable being that would not react to reality in the first place, that would not act regardless of how low its stage of development was.

Bleuler demonstrates that the autistic function requires a maturation of complex prerequisites in the form of speech, concepts, and ability to remember. The autistic function is not as primitive as simple forms of a real function.

Thus, animal psychology, like infant psychology, knows only real function. Autistic thinking of the child makes great strides immediately after the development of speech and major steps in the development of concepts. Thus, autistic thinking not only does not coincide with unconscious and wordless thinking, but itself depends on the development of speech. It is not an initial, but a derivative form. Autistic thinking is not a primitive form of thinking; it can only develop after thinking, operating with the help of pictures in the memory alone, becomes dominant in the immediate mental reaction to actual external situations. Ordinary thinking—a function of what is real—is primary and is as necessary to every viable being endowed with a mind as are actions corresponding to reality.

Attempts have been made to limit the theory of solipsism by applying it only to the newborn period. Partisans of this view explain that the stage of solipsism does not last long and loses its absolute character within two months. The first breach occurs when the child begins to respond to the voice or smile of the adult with general animation or a responsive smile. In general, in light of data on the sociability of the infant, it is difficult to subscribe to the conception of solipsism relative to a child older than two months. According to our determinations, it is fully applicable only to children who are profoundly retarded or to idiots.

Another of Piaget's statements regarding infantile autism is also more applicable to the mentally deficient than to the normal child. This compromising point of view does not essentially refute, but confirms Piaget, reinforcing his idea on the primacy of autistic thinking. Moreover, we cannot but agree with Bleuler who showed that specifically at primitive stages of development all possibility of nonrealistic thinking is excluded. Beginning with a certain stage of development, an autistic function joins the initial realistic functions and develops together with it from that point on. Bleuler says that an imbecile is a genuine and real politician. His autistic thinking is simplified just as his realistic thinking is. Recently, K. Lewin demonstrated that the imagination—one of the most clear manifestations of autistic thinking—is extremely underdeveloped in retarded children. From the development of the normal child, we know that this function begins to develop in him to a noticeable extent only during the preschool age.

We think for this reason that the theory of solipsism must be not simply limited, but replaced by an opposite theory since all facts presented in its defense receive a real explanation from the opposite point of view.

Thus, Peters showed that the basis for egocentric speech and egocentric thinking of the child is not autism and not a deliberate isolation from communication, but something opposite to that in mental structure. Piaget, who in Peter's opinion emphasizes egocentrism of children and makes it the cornerstone of the explanation of the unique in children's mentality, must nevertheless establish that children speak with each other and one does not hear the other. Of course, externally they seem not to consider each other, but it is specifically because they still preserve to a certain degree traces of the direct communication that characterized their consciousness as a dominant trait.

In conclusion, we would only like to say that facts presented by Piaget are really explained in the light of the teaching given above on the basic neoformation of infancy. Piaget, analyzing the logical actions of the infant, foresees objections that his theory may evoke. He writes: we might think that the infant uses any action to obtain any result since he simply assumes that parents will carry out his wishes. According to this hypothesis, the device the child uses for affecting things is simply a unique language that he uses in communicating with the people around him. This will be not magic, but a request. Thus, we can state that a one-and-a-half- or two-year-old child communicates with his parents when he needs something and simply says, "please," not bothering to say precisely what he wants; that is how convinced he is that his parents know all his wishes. But if this hypothesis is true for the child who is already beginning to speak, then prior to that time, it is completely unfounded according to the words of Piaget. Piaget considers the following circumstance to be one of the principal arguments against this hypothesis and the best evidence that primitive behavior is not social and the behavior of the first year cannot be considered social: the child does not distinguish between people and things. For this reason Piaget believes that at this age we can speak only of solipsistic, and not at all of social behavior.

However, as we have seen, even at two months of age, the child exhibits all the developing specific reactions of a social nature which are increasing in complexity (reactions to the human voice, to the expression on a person's face); the active seeking of contact with another person and other symptoms show indisputably that even in infancy, the child distinguishes people from things.

We have seen from the experiments of Fajans that the relation of the child to an object is determined entirely by the social content of the situation in which the object is presented. As to the behavior of the child in these experiments, could we say that he does not distinguish a person from a thing? The only correct part of Piaget's idea is that for the infant, the social content and the object content of a situation are still not differentiated. In contrast with the child of two who can speak, the infant cannot differentiate between a request to the adult for help and direct action on a thing. As we have seen in the experiments with an object at a distance from the child, the child, having given up reaching for the unreachable goal, renews his attempts with his former animation when a person appears near the goal. True, in this case, the child does not turn to the experimenter for help, but continues to reach directly for the object, which creates the impression of magical behavior. But the experiment demonstrates with undoubted clarity that these actions that seem magical in external appearance in the situation with the unreachable goal, arise in the child under the influence of the path through another person, which is normal for the child, and that suddenly makes reaching the goal possible. The child is not yet conscious of this path and cannot use it deliberately, but only in the presence of this path are his quasimagical actions realized. Careful analysis of Piaget's experiments would also show that the child reacts with magical actions not to the situation with the missing object but to the situation whose center is the path to the object that lies through relations to another person. Thus, the infant's solipsistic behavior is actually social behavior characteristic of the infant's "great-we" consciousness.

Chapter 8
THE CRISIS OF THE FIRST YEAR[1]

The empirical content of the crisis of the first year of life is extremely simple and easy. It was studied earlier than all the other ages, but its crisis character was not emphasized. We are speaking of walking, of the period when one cannot say whether the child is or is not walking, about the establishment of walking, when, using a highly dialectical formula, we might say about walking what we say about the unity of being and nonbeing, that is, when it is and is not. Everyone knows that it is a rare child who starts to walk instantly, although there are such children. A more careful study of a child who began to walk instantly shows that in such a case, we are usually dealing with a latent period of development and establishment and a relatively late manifestation of walking. But frequently even after walking begins, we observe its loss. This indicates that a complete maturing of walking has not yet happened.

In early childhood, the child is already walking: poorly, with difficulty, but nevertheless it is a child for whom walking has become the basic form of moving through space.

Establishment of walking is the first point in the content of this crisis.

The second point refers to speech. Here again, we have a process in development where we cannot say whether the child is or is not talking, when speech is and is not. This process too is not completed in a day, although cases have been described in which a child started speaking instantly. Here too, we have a latent period of establishing speech which lasts approximately three months.

The third point pertains to the aspect of affect and will. E. Kretschmer called these reactions hypobulic. What we have in mind here is that in connection with the crisis, the child makes his first acts of protest, opposition, standing up to others, "uncontrollability" in the language of familial authoritarian rearing. Kretschmer also termed these phenomena hypobulic in the sense that they pertain to volitional reaction, represent a qualitatively completely different stage in the development of volitional actions, and are not differentiated with respect to will and affect.

Such reactions of the child at the crisis age are sometimes manifested with great force and sharpness, especially in cases of improper rearing, and acquire a character of regular hypobulic incidents which is described in connection with teaching on the difficult childhood. Usually, the child who has been denied something or who was not understood displays a sharp increase in affect that frequently ends with the child lying on the floor, screaming furiously, refusing to walk, and if he walks, he stomps, but there is no loss of consciousness nor is there salivation or enuresis or any other trait that characterizes epileptic seizures. There is only an inclination (which also makes the reaction hypobulic) sometimes directed against certain prohibitions, refusals, etc., and expressed as it is usually described, in a certain regression; the child seemingly returns to an earlier period (when he throws himself on the floor, flounders, refuses to walk, etc.), but, of course, he uses this in a completely different way.

These are the three points that are usually described as the content of the crisis of the first year of life.

We will approach the crisis mainly from the aspect of speech and put aside the other two points. I chose speech in view of the fact that it is evidently connected most of all with the appearance of childhood consciousness and with the child's social relations.

The first question pertains to the process of genesis of speech. How does the genesis of speech itself occur? Here we are dealing with two or three opposite, mutually exclusive points of view or theories.

The first is the theory of gradual development of speech on an associative basis. To a certain degree, this theory is already dead and to fight against it would mean to fight with the dead, which is only of historical interest. We must, however, say something about it since, as always happens, theories die, but leave certain conclusions as a legacy and these, like children, outlive their parents. Some followers of the indicated theory even now impede the teaching on the development of speech in children, and without overcoming their errors, we cannot properly approach this problem.

The associative theory presents the matter exceptionally directly and clearly: the connection between the word and its meaning is a straight associative connection between two members. The child sees an object, a clock for example, hears the complex of sounds "k-l-ah-k," and between the one and the other a certain connection is established that is enough for the child on hearing the word "clock," to remember the object that is connected with the word. In the graphic expression of a student of H. Ebbinghaus, the word recalls its meaning along the associative connection the way a coat recalls its wearer. We see a hat, we know that the hat belongs to a certain person and the hat reminds us of the person.

From this point of view, consequently, all problems are solved. First, in itself, the relation between the meaning of the word and the word is drawn as something very elementary and simple. Second, all possibility of further development of children's speech is eliminated: if an associative dependence is established, it can subsequently be made more precise, enriched, in place of one dependence, there may be twenty, but an associative connection in itself is not a base for development in the true sense of the word if we understand development to be the process in which something new arises at a subsequent stage, something that was not there before. From this point of view, the development of children's speech is reduced exclusively to developing vocabulary, that is, it is a quantitative increase, an enrichment and elaboration of the associative connections, but development in the true sense of that word is denied completely.

The student of Ebbinghaus formulates this position very clearly when he says that children's words acquire meaning once and for all. This is capital that undergoes no change, no development over the whole duration of life, that is, the child acquires knowledge and develops, but the word remains unchanged over the whole course of his development. From this point of view, the problem of the appearance of children's speech is also solved because, on the one hand, everything is reduced to a slow accumulation of articulation and phonation movements, and on the other hand, it is reduced to preserving the connections between the object and the word that represents the object.

The associative point of view died and was buried a long time ago, and it would be useless even to criticize it now: its unacceptability is so clear that we might leave it at that. But, although it has long been buried, nevertheless the idea that the word acquires meaning *once and for all*, that this is the child's only property, has been retained in later theories also. It seems to me that we must begin with a discussion of this in order to construct a correct theory of children's speech. Research that came after the associative theory excluded the problem on the development of the meanings of words from its field of vision. The associative theory was taken on faith, but it was understood that associative psychology incorrectly explains the mechanism of the origin of verbal designations and sets itself the task of explaining the origin of words, but by a method that would satisfy the requirement *once and for all*. The second group of theories goes further historically; W. Stern is a typical representative of this group.

According to Stern's theory, the first word is a fundamental step in the child's development. This step also is taken once and for all. However, it consists not in a simple associative connection between the sound and the object because such an associative connection occurs in animals also (it is very easy to teach a dog to turn its eyes and look at an object that you name). Stern maintains that the child essentially makes the greatest discovery of his life: he learns that everything has its own name or (another formulation of this law) the child discovers the connection between sign and meaning, that is, he discovers the symbolizing function of speech, the fact that every thing can be designated by a sign, by a symbol.

This point of view was very productive for factual studies; it discovered facts that the associative theory could not discover. It indicated that there is no slow and gradual accumulation of associative connections in the development of speech, but that soon after the discovery, there is a spasmodic increase in the child's vocabulary.

The second symptom that Stern points to is the child's transition from a passive to an active increase in vocabulary. No one has ever seen an animal that learned to understand human words and would ask for the name of an object that had not been named. Stern says that it is typical for a child to know as many words as he has been taught; then he begins to ask for the names of things, that is, he behaves as if he understood that each thing is called something. Stern believes that this discovery by the child must be termed the child's first general concept.

Finally, the third symptom consists in the following: the child asks his first questions on names, that is, active increase in vocabulary leads to the child's asking about each new thing: "What is that?" Actually, all three symptoms belong to early childhood, but are derived from the discovery of which Stern speaks.

What Supports Stern's theory?

First, it is supported by the three symptoms of major importance which always indicate whether or not a fundamental turning point in the development of the child's speech has occurred. Second, this theory sheds penetrating light from the point of view of specific features of human thinking on the act of formation of the child's first deliberate word, that is, it rejects the associative character of the connection between sign and meaning. Third, the change in development of speech that occurs has a seemingly catastrophic, almost an instantaneous character.

Thus, there are data that indicate that Stern's theory has grasped something real that actually occurs in the child's life. What speaks against it is that it interprets the points indicated completely incorrectly. I had occasion to express my ideas to Stern himself. In response, I heard that a number of the ideas had excited him even from the time he set out the theory, that is, from the time when he wrote the book, "Die Kindersprache" ("Children's Speech"). Some objections were expressed by other critics also. For this reason, Stern is working on changing his theory, but not in the direction that was indicated in my objections, but in another direction of which I shall speak later. We find traces of this revision in Stern's latest work.

What speaks against this theory? In my opinion, certain facts of major significance that must be specified in order to clear the ground for a correct solution of the problem.

First, it is improbable that a child who is a year old or a year and three months old would be so intellectually developed and could himself make such a fundamental discovery of the connection between sign and meaning, and form for himself the first general concept, a child who would thus be a theoretician capable of making the great generalization that every thing has its own name. This, as Stern maintains, is the essence of speech. Of course, for us adults, the idea of speech is the fact that every thing has its own name. It is difficult to admit that an eighteen-month-old child can discover the idea of speech. This is so inconsistent with the intellectual level of development of the child who cannot even open a matchbox, this is so contrary to the syncretic thinking of the child!

Stern admits that this objection is entirely valid.

Second, experimental studies show: not only does a child of eighteen months not discover the logical nature of speech, but even a schoolchild still does not fully understand what a word means, does not take into account what the connection between object and word is, and many adults, especially those who are retarded in cultural development, even to the end of their lives do not know this.

As the studies of J. Piaget, H. Wallon, and others have shown, even during school age, the child has a tendency not to understand the conditionality of speech but to *consider the name of a thing as one of its attributes*. For example, when one asks a child of three why a cow is called a cow, he will answer: "Because it has horns," or "Because it gives milk," that is, to the question as to reasons for a name, he never answers that that is simply its name, that people contrived this arbitrary designation. He will always look for an explanation for the name in properties of the thing itself: a herring is called a herring because it is salted or because it swims in the sea; a cow is called a cow because it gives milk and a calf is called a calf because it is still small and does not give milk.

Children of preschool age were tested. A number of objects were named and the children were asked why these objects were named as they were: according to indications of sound, arbitrarily, etc. The objects are called as they are because it matches their properties — this was the sense of the responses. The young child always uses the properties of the things as a base. This caused Wallon to be the first to say that the child even later does not understand this arbitrariness but retains a notion about the word as one of the attributes of the thing, one of the properties of the thing.

Later Piaget and other authors demonstrated the same thing.

H. Wallon recalls Humboldt's well-known linguistic anecdote (by the way, in the last imperialistic war similar facts were published by linguists of various countries). In the Humboldt anecdote, a Russian soldier is discussing why in German water is called "Wasser" and in French, something else, and in English, something else. "But you know, water is water and not Wasser." The soldier believes that his language is correct and all the other languages name water incorrectly. For Humboldt (and for me too), this is the essential trait, the symptom of the following: in itself, the name of a thing is so closely ingrown into the thing that it is difficult even to imagine that the name could be something else.

Consequently, experimental work also demonstrates that a child at this age does not make such "discoveries."

I will not present all the objections to Stern's theory, I will note only that experimental analysis of children's first questions showed the following: the child never asks about a name, but he asks about the purpose or sense of a thing.

In my opinion, the main defect of Stern's theory is the logical error it contains, an error that has been called "petitio principii" in logic. This may be crudely translated as "ass backward" or "putting the cart before the horse." The essence of the matter is as follows: instead of saying how a general concept of speech develops in the child, it is assumed that from the very beginning, it is generated by the child. This is the same kind of mistake as in the case where it was thought that language appeared by mutual agreement, that people lived apart, could not reach an understanding, and then gathered together and agreed: "Let's call this by this name and that, by that name." What is the defect in this theory? It assumes that the meaning of language existed before language, that the idea of language and advantages that it provides existed before the beginning of language.

Stern does the same thing. Moreover, in order to explain how an understanding of the connection between sign and meaning arises in the child, how this understanding is different at different stages of life, he assumes that the discovery is made first, that is, the child who cannot use speech already has the concept of what speech is. According to this theory, speech originates with the concept of it, but the actual course of development lies in the fact that in the process of speech, the child develops a certain idea about it.

Finally, Stern's point of view completely excludes the question of the development of children's speech, its sense aspect, because if at age one and half, I made a discovery, the greatest in all my life, then there would be nothing left for me to do but reach the conclusions that I would need.

In a parody paper, K. Bühler stated it very well: Stern presents the child and his speech development as a rentier who acquires capital and then clips coupons.

On this basis, Stern arrives at positions that are in scandalous contradiction to all the data of actual studies. As we know, the basic idea of Stern's monograph, "Die Kindersprache," is that speech development ends at age five and only small changes occur after that, but current studies show that some new concepts become possible only when the child is of school age. It seems to me that the basic defect in Stern's conception is in the attempt to move what is most important in development back to the beginning. Stern's central idea is specifically this: everything develops like a leaf from a bud. On this path, Stern enters into personalistics.[2] For this reason, there is a tendency to put the development back to the very beginning, that is, to bring to the forefront the initial stages of development and confirm their controlling significance. This can be seen also in other authors, in K. Bühler and A. Gesell, who state that essentially all of the development revolves around the first years of life.

All of this leads us to reject Stern's point of view. It must be said that at present it has already been abandoned in psychology. In its place, we have a number of new points of view. I will discuss these briefly.

The Bühler point of view. What Stern considers an instantaneous discovery is the result of microscopic movement growing day by day and spreading over the course of several months, that is, we have here an attempt to show that this is a discovery of a molecular formation. Bühler supports his theory with observations of deaf-mute children in Viennese schools.

The point of view of H. Wallon. The child actually makes a discovery at this age. Whether accidentally or not is another question. Wallon is also inclined to admit such a "Eureka" in the child's consciousness. He believes that the child does not make the discovery accidentally. However, the child discovers not the general concept and rule that every thing has its own name, but only the method of dealing with things. If the child finds that some things can be opened (for example, if you took off the lid of a box for him), he will try to open all objects, even those that do not have a lid. Wallon assumes that the whole history of the development of speech is based on the fact that the possibility of naming things, the possibility that a thing could be named, was opened for the child. This is a seemingly new activity with things, and since the child discovered it in relation to one thing, he will then transfer it to a relation with a number of other things. Thus, for Wallon, the child discovers not the logical sense, not the connection between sign and meaning, but a new method of playing with things, a new method of dealing with them.

From the point of view of K. Koffka and all of structural psychology, this first discovery of the child is presented in the form of a structural act. The child discovers the unique structure, "thing—name," just as the ape discovers the function of the stick in the situation when the fruit is far away and cannot be reached except with the help of a stick. Koffka's theory has now merged with Wallon's theory.

The theories of Bühler, Koffka, and Wallon are more consistent with facts than Stern's theory because they grew out of criticism of this theory, but they all include the defect of Stern's theory which came from associative theory, that is, the assumption that everything here happens once and for all; the child discovers structure, a method of dealing with things, he discovers that as far as the meaning of these words is concerned, it is not subject to change and development.

Thus, although these theories ameliorate the intellectualism of Stern's theory, they oppose its most important idealistic thesis — deriving speech from the concept of speech—they are as much in error with respect to the origin of speech as the Stern theory because they tolerate immutability in origin and development of children's words. Let us try in a few words to show what is most essential in modern teaching on the point of origin of speech in order to note in this way the central point of the crisis of the first year.

I shall begin with the facts. Whoever attentively observes the beginning of children's speech cannot bypass a very important period in its development which has become the subject of intense attention during the last decade and is still little elucidated in textbooks. Moreover, it is very important for understanding the development of speech in the child.

Thus far we have spoken of two periods of development of speech in children. We tried to establish that even at infancy when the child has no language in the true sense of the word, the social situation of development leads to the child's developing a very great, complex, and multifaceted need to communicate with adults. Because the infant himself does not walk and cannot move an object closer to himself or farther away, he must act through others. No level of childhood requires as great a number of forms of cooperation, most elementary cooperation, as does infancy. Acting through others is the basic form of activity of the child. This age is characterized by the fact that the child lacks the most basic means of communication — speech. In this is contained the extremely peculiar contradiction in the development of the infant. The child creates a number of surrogates of speech. We have already discussed gestures that the child develops which, from the point of view of development of speech, result in a gesture as important as the pointing gesture. Thus, communication with those around him is established.

We have indicated a number of forms that replace speech, that is, means of communication which, while they are not means of speech, are a kind of preparatory stage for the development of speech. Then we spoke of the development of speech in early childhood when the child basically adopts the language of the adults. Between the first period, called the mute period in the child's development, and the second, when the basic facts of his native language take shape for the child, there is a period of development that W. Eliasberg proposed calling children's autonomous speech (1928). Eliasberg says that before a child begins to speak in our language, he compels us to speak in his language. This period helps us understand how the transition occurs that takes the child from the mute period, when he only prattles, to the period when he can speak in the true sense of the word. The transition from the mute to the speaking period of development is accomplished through children's autonomous speech.

What kind of period is this? In order to answer the question better, we must briefly explain the history of this problem, the history of introducing this concept into science.

Strange as this may seem, the first to describe children's autonomous speech and understand and evaluate its great significance was Charles Darwin (1881), who was not directly concerned with the problems of child development, but being a brilliant observer, in following the development of his grandson, was able to notice that before going on to the speaking period, the child spoke an original language. The originality consisted of the fact that, *first*, the sound composition of the words used by the child differed sharply from the sound composition of our words. In its motor aspects, that is, from articulation and phonetic aspects, that speech did not coincide with our speech. Usually it consisted of such words as "poo-foo" and "bo-bo," and sometimes of fragments of our words. These are words that differ according to the external or sound form from words of our language. Sometimes they are similar to our words and sometimes they are very different, sometimes they resemble our distorted words.

The *second* difference, more essential and more important, to which Darwin called attention is that the words of autonomous speech *differ from our words in meaning also.* Darwin's famous example is often cited in textbooks. Once, on seeing a duck swimming in a pond, his grandson, whether imitating its sounds or what the adults called it, began to call it, "ooah." These sounds were pronounced by the child when he was at a pond and saw a duck swimming in the water. Then the boy began to use the same sounds for milk spilled on the table, for any liquid, wine in a glass, even milk in a bottle, obviously transferring this name because there was water or a liquid. Once the child was playing with old coins with pictures of birds. He began to call them "ooah" also. Finally, all small, round, shiny objects that resembled coins (buttons, medals) began to be called "ooah."

Thus, if we were to record the child's meaning of the word, "ooah," we would find some kind of initial meaning from which all the other meanings are derived (a duck on water). This meaning is almost always very complex. It is not separated into isolated qualities like the meaning of separate words; such a meaning represents the whole picture.

From the initial meaning, the child makes a transition to a number of other meanings that are derived from separate parts of the picture. From water, the word went to a puddle, to any liquid, and later to a bottle. From the duck, the word went to coins with a picture of an eagle and from this to buttons, medals, etc.

Many examples can be given for the meaning of the autonomous word, "poo-foo." It stands for a bottle with iodine, iodine itself, a bottle over which people blow to produce a whistle, a cigarette which produces smoke, tobacco, the process of quenching because that also requires blowing, etc. The word and its meaning encompass a whole complex of things that we can in no way designate in one word.

From the aspect of meaning, these words do not coincide with our words and not one of them can be fully translated into our language.

From autonomous speech, it never happens that the child knows how to say *iodine, bottle, cigarette*, that he knows not only to say and distinguish constant properties of objects (iodine, bottle, etc.), but only whimsically continues to say, "poo-foo." Actually neither our words nor our concepts are accessible to the child.

We shall return to an analysis of children's meanings. Now we shall limit ourselves to establishing this fact. Everyone now agrees that the meaning of such a word is constructed differently from the way we construct words.

Thus, we found two traits that distinguish children's autonomous speech from the general course of development of children's language. The first difference is the *phonetic* structure of speech, the second, the *sense aspect* of children's speech.

This is the source of the third feature of children's autonomous speech which Darwin properly appreciated; if in sound and sense respects this speech differs from ours, then communication with the help of this speech must differ sharply from communication with the help of our speech. Communication is possible only between the child and the people who understand the meaning of his words. Is it not true that you and I, not knowing the whole history of the word, "ooah," would not understand what it meant for Darwin's grandson.

It is not communication that is, on the whole, possible with all people as it is with our words. Communication is possible only with people initiated into the code of children's speech. For this reason, German authors have long disdainfully called this language *Ammensprache*, that is, the language of wet nurses and nannies, which the investigators assumed was artificially created by the adults for the children and differed in that it was understandable only by people who were caring for the given child.

Adults trying to adapt to children's language actually tolerate distortion of common words which they are teaching the child. When the nanny says "bo-bo" to the child instead of "bol'no" [it hurts], then of course, we are dealing with distortion of speech which the adults tolerate in communicating with the child. With respect to older children, we always tolerate another error: since, from our point of view, the child is small, it seems to us that everything must seem small to him. For this reason, to a very young child, pointing to a skyscraper, we say, "domik" [little house], pointing to a big horse, we say, "little horse," losing sight of the fact that a large building and a large horse must seem enormous to a small child and that it would be more correct to say, "big building," and "huge horse." Such distortions actually have their place, but it would be incorrect to say that all of the children's autonomous language is the language of wet nurses and nannies. The fact is that before he masters our articulation and phonetics, the child masters some kind of rudiments of words and rudiments of meanings that do not coincide with ours.

Even if we were initiated into the meaning of children's words, we would be able to understand the child in no other way than in some kind of concrete situation. If the child says "ooah," then it might be a button, milk, a duck in the water, a coin. You would not know what he has in mind. If, on a walk through the garden, the child shouts, "ooah," and pulls forward, this means that he wants to be taken to the pond. If he is in a room and says, "ooah," this means that he wants to play with buttons.

Communication with children at this period is possible only in a concrete situation. The word may be used in communication only when the object is in sight. If the object is in sight, then the word becomes understandable.

We can see that the difficulties of understanding are very great. According to my conceptions, *one of the most necessary hypotheses is the one that proves that all hypobulic manifestations of the child are the result of the difficulty of mutual understanding.*

This means that we have come to the third feature of autonomous speech: it allows communication, but in other forms and with a different character than the communication that becomes possible for the child later.

Finally, the last, the fourth of the basic distinctive features of autonomous language is that the possible connection between separate words is also extremely original. This language usually is agrammatical, does not have a subject method of combining separate words and meanings into communicating speech (for us, this is done through syntax and etymology). Here completely different laws of connecting and uniting words dominate — laws of uniting interjections that trip all over each other, resembling a number of unconnected exclamations that we utter sometimes under strong affect and agitation.

These are the four basic features which confront us in the study of children's autonomous speech. I believe that they were all more or less clearly recognized by Darwin, who was the first to describe the speech of his grandson. Despite the fact that it was Darwin who did this, his observations were not properly valued or understood. Many examples were cited from his observations, but no one knew how to correlate them or could understand that what was involved was a unique period in the development of children's speech. For this reason, the teaching on children's autonomous speech immediately after Darwin's paper appeared faded away to some extent, although a number of investigators in a careful recording of children's first words accumulated much factual material that characterizes autonomous speech. No one understood that the matter concerned a special period in the development of children's speech.

The study of this question was revived due to the observations of the famous German academic, K. Stumpf. He made observations of his own child, who was developing in a very unique way. Unlike the usual child who explains himself with the help of this speech only toward the end of the first and beginning of the second year, Stumpf's son used children's autonomous speech for the first several years (three or four). The boy understood the language of the people around him, but always responded in his own language. Since this was a developed language (it was developed by the child over several years), he had complex rules for joining and constructing separate words. The child used his own language and refused to speak in German until one beautiful day, the parents, upon returning home in the evening, were told by the nanny (or governess) that the child suddenly made a transition to ordinary German and abandoned autonomous speech. This story is the exception and not the rule. It is an anomaly of child development if the child remains at the stage of autonomous speech for several years. But because of the delay of several years, autonomous speech was splendidly developed and its rules could be studied with a completeness as they could not have been explained if the period lasted several months between the end of the first and third quarter of the second year, as usually happens in normal development.

However, Stumpf's information was regarded as a curious case. Several decades of scientific work were required to note two basic facts that now form the base for the teaching on children's autonomous speech.

The first fact is that autonomous speech is not a rare case, not an exception, but the rule, the law, which is observed in the speech development of every child. The law may be formed as follows: before the child makes the transition from the mute period to the language of the adults, he exhibits children's autonomous speech in his development. I have indicated the features that distinguish it. Now the term *autonomous* is not quite apt, but is more or less fixed in science and in current literature and must be understood. Speech is termed autonomous because it is constructed seemingly according to its own laws different from the laws of construction of real speech. This speech has another sound system, another sense aspect, other forms of communication, and other forms of connection. For this reason, it was called autonomous.

Thus, the first rule is that children's autonomous speech is a necessary period in the development of every normal child.

The second rule: in many forms of underdevelopment of speech, in disruption of speech development, children's autonomous speech appears very often and determines the features of the anomalous forms of speech development. For example, retardation is often expressed primarily in the lingering on of the child's autonomous speech. Other speech disruptions in childhood also result in autonomous speech continuing sometimes for several years but nevertheless fulfilling the basic genetic function, that is, serving as a bridge across which the child makes the transition from the mute period to language. In the development of the normal and the anomalous child, autonomous speech plays an essential role.

We must not say that this child gets this speech from nannies and wet nurses, that this is the language of wet nurses. This is the language of the child himself because all the meanings are established not by the wet nurse, but by the child himself, because frequently, the child creates his "bo-bo" from fragments of normally pronounced words. For example, the mother says "tumbler," a complete word, but the child gets "ler" or something else.

In all normally occurring child development, we can observe autonomous speech for which three points are typical. *The first point.* Speech is a motor action, that is, from the articulation and phonetic aspects it does not coincide with our speech. Usually words such as "poo-foo" and "bo-bo" are fragments of our words; sometimes, as investigators are now saying, this resembles a radical language, that is, a language in which only roots exist and not formed words. In meaning, they do not coincide with any of our words, and not one meaning of "poo-foo" or "bo-bo" can be fully translated into our language. We see the same thing when we consider Darwin's famous example where "oo-ah" first signified a duck swimming in water and then any round object. There are many examples of how a child's word, its sensible meaning, encompasses a complex of things that we do not designate with one word.

The *second* feature. The meaning of autonomous speech does not coincide with the meaning of our words.

The *third* feature. Together with his own words, the child has an understanding of our words, that is, before he begins to speak, the child understands a number of words. He understands the words we form: "stand," "sit," "bread," "milk," "hot," etc., and this does not interfere with the other speech. For this reason, H. Idelberger and others are inclined to think that children's autonomous speech exists together with or in a certain connection with our speech.

Finally, the *last.*

Children's autonomous speech and its meanings are developed with the active participation of the child.

It is a fact that in the development of each child there is a period of children's autonomous speech. Its beginning and end signify the beginning and end of the crisis of the first year of life. Of a child who practices autonomous speech, we cannot really say whether or not he has speech because he does not have speech in our sense of the word; nor is it a mute period since he does talk, that is, we are dealing with a required transitional formation that signifies the boundaries of the crisis.

Some authors were so extreme in criticizing this theory that they maintained that this language is created exclusively by the child himself. For example, Eliasberg believes that the child really compels people to speak with him in his language. But it would be wrong to say that it is the language of the child himself. This is true in isolated cases, for example, when Stumpf's five-year-old did not want to converse in another language, although he understood very well what was said to him. But this language can in no way be considered as *Ammensprache* nor as strictly autonomous[3] language — it is always the result of interaction of the child with the people around him.

Having become familiar with certain basic features of children's autonomous speech, we shall move to the facts that are derived from observing the development of normal and anomalous children which will help us see more clearly some features of this period in order to reach conclusions on the development of speech in the child. I shall give examples from children's vocabulary (day nursery or home) during the second year of life at the stage of children's autonomous speech.

Nona is one year three months old. She is a girl in a day nursery group. She has seventeen words of autonomous speech. Among these is "kkh-kh," which signifies cat, fur, and all furry objects, then hair and especially long hair. We are dealing with a word that in the phonetic aspect is constructed differently and whose meaning, it is true, is not as rich as the "ooah" in Darwin's example, but which is not constructed like the meanings of our words. Initially, "kkh-kh" signified a cat according to similarity in sound, then, according to the similarity of feeling the fur of the cat, it was transferred to all fur and then to hair.

We find a more interesting and complex formation of a word in children when autonomous speech was somewhat delayed or when we have journals that were kept for a long time.

Angelina is one year three months old. Her word, "ka," had eleven meanings over the whole course of its development. Initially (at eleven months) it was a yellow stone with which the girl played. Then it signified egg soap, then all stones of any color and any form. Then until she was one year one month old, it also signified kasha, then large grains of sugar, then everything sweet, kissel, a cutlet, a bobbin, a pencil, and a soap dish with soap. Here the meaning spread from a yellow stone to yellow soap. This is understandable. Later this was what any stone was called, which is also understandable. Later everything sweet like kissel acquired this meaning, once this word was used to designate sugar. But a pencil or a bobbin has no relation or similarity of traits to those objects. "Ka" in this case represents the beginning of the words, "karandash" [pencil] and "katushka" [bobbin] in the language of the adults. The child catches only the initial "ka."

Some objects are included in the structure of the meaning of this word according to one trait, others, according to another. For example, the yellow soap was included because of the color, kissel, according to sweetness, the stone, according to hardness, but the bobbin and the pencil, according to similarity of sound [in Russian]. All of these meanings form a family of objects that are designated by the one word, "ka."

Is it possible to understand this "ka?" This girl's father, a physiologist who kept a journal, wrote that the word was a riddle because it was excruciatingly difficult to guess what the child had in mind in saying "ka," and understanding was always reached with the help of the *visual* situation. Here we clearly see an illustration of situational understanding and the impossibility of understanding the meaning of words when they are removed from the concrete situation.

Our words can replace the situation but the words of autonomous speech cannot serve this function but have only the purpose of isolating some one thing in a situation. They have an indicative function and a function of naming, but not the function of meaning that can represent absent objects and meanings.

This pertains to the basic properties of children's autonomous speech. The words of autonomous speech have an indicative and nominative function, but do not have a significative function. They have no possibility of replacing absent objects, but can in a visual situation indicate its separate aspects or parts and give these parts names. For this reason, using autonomous speech, the child can converse only about what he sees, as distinct from using developed speech with which we can converse about objects that are not before us.

The next difference between children's autonomous speech and ours is the relation that exists between separate meanings of words. Essential for the development of children's concepts and children's words is the development of a system of common relations between the meanings of individual words. In the speech clinic of the Experimental Defectology Institute (EDI)[4] there was at one time a child who knew the words *table, chair,* and *cupboard*, but not the word *furniture*. Meanwhile, development of relations between meanings is an essential factor for development of children's speech. The word *furniture* is not simply an alternative word in a series of such words as *table* or *cupboard*. The word *furniture* is a higher concept that includes all of the foregoing words. It is a most essential factor not proper to children's autonomous speech. A trait according to which children's autonomous speech can always be distinguished from speech that has already passed to a higher level is the absence of common relations between separate meanings of words.

What are common relations? We will call relations in meaning of words like, let us say, *furniture* and *chair* common relations. One is a higher concept, the other, a lower. The relation of *table* and *chair* is not a relation of coordination.

In children's autonomous speech, there is no relation of coordination. From the child's vocabulary, it is obvious that his speech consists of words that lie, so to speak, together with each other but are not related to each other in the form of a certain hierarchy. Conversely, more specific meanings appear within one word, for example, "ka" is a yellow stone, and all stones of any color, or a soap dish with soap in general and specifically yellow soap. A different degree of commonality exists within the meaning of one and the same word, and these words themselves have no common relation to each other.

If you take any vocabulary of autonomous speech, you will not find words there that would be in the same relation to each other as *furniture* and *table and chair* or *flower and rose*, that is, in a relation in which the meanings of words are different with respect to commonality, but are in a certain relation to each other. The impression is that in children's autonomous speech, the meanings of a word still reflect one object or another, one situation or another, but do not reflect the connection of objects with each other, except for the situational connection that is given in the visual picture that makes up the content of the initial meaning of the word in autonomous speech. From this, it follows that the meaning of a word in autonomous speech is not constant, but situational. One and the same word means one thing now and another in a different situation. As we have seen, the word "ka" in this vocabulary may mean eleven different things, and in each new situation, the word will stand for something new. The meaning of the words is not constant, but changes depending on the concrete situation. We repeat, this meaning is not objective, but situational. For us, every object has a name regardless of the situation it finds itself in, but in children's autonomous speech, an object has various names depending on the situation.

Let us take an example of anomalous development. One of the children in the clinic was being studied. The child used the words *zelenina* for light colors and *sinina* for dark colors. If the child was given two leaves, bright yellow and dark yellow, he would call the first *zelenina* and the second, *sinina*. If, however, he was given the same dark yellow leaf and a brown one at the same time, then the yellow was called *zelenina* and the brown one, *sinina*. One and the same color was called something else depending on what lay next to it. The child designated light and dark, but for him there was no absolute color quality. There was a comparative degree: lighter or darker. The meaning of the word did not yet have an objective constancy.

We have a similar example from observations of Stumpf's son, who called one and the same color by different names. Green against a white background and green against a black background had different names depending on the structure in which the color was perceived.

A boy, Zhenya, age five years six months, belonged to the group of children who hear, but begin to speak late and who develop independence with difficulty. His parents came to the clinic with a complaint that the child was not developing speech properly and that he understood the speech of others poorly. The complaint about poor understanding is common for children who use autonomous speech. In pathology, autonomous speech differs in sound and sense characteristics from ordinary speech, and for this reason presents great difficulty for the child in communicating with other children and with adults. Frequently a translator is needed who knows the meaning of the words said and can translate them into our language. An example in Zhenya's vocabulary: there were words whose meaning was made clear in a conversation with him that involved naming pictures. *Narrow glasses* meant *eyes, kon* meant *horse*, etc. In his words, we see first phrases.

When autonomous speech lingers too long in a child who understands adults' speech very well, the need arises for a cohesive transmission, and even in autonomous speech, the child starts on the path to forming sentences. But because this speech lacks syntactic unity, these *sentences* show little resemblance to ours. They resemble more closely the simple stringing along of words or distorted sentences of our language: "You me take," etc.

And two more cases that may serve as a concrete illustration:

The child used the word *trua* for *to stroll, go for a walk*, then he used this word for all the equipment for taking a walk: boots, galoshes, cap. Later *trua* signified that the milk had been drunk, that is, it went for a walk.

F. A. Rau[5] told of a girl whose autonomous speech was very well developed and exhibited a special type of word formation that exists in a number of languages. For example, "f-f" signified *fire*, "din'" signified *an object that moves*, and from this "fadin'" was a *train* and "tpru-din'" signified a *cat*. This is complex word formation from separate root words in children's autonomous speech which does not turn into ordinary speech in a timely fashion. Here we are dealing with hyperbolic forms.

One boy used such general categories as *insects* and *birds*. For him, "roster" (rooster) signified our common word, *bird*. Such more stable designations refer to traits of a richly developed autonomous speech and provide good possibilities for a transition from autonomous speech to real speech.

I would still like to show the meaning of children's autonomous speech for one level of the child's development or another, to show how the development of children's speech is reflected in the features of the thinking of the child and what kind of features of his thinking must result from features of autonomous speech. It seems to me that there are several such features that can be established very easily after the explanation of the nature of children's autonomous speech.

First, as has been said, the meaning of words in children's autonomous speech is always situational, that is, it is realized when the thing that is signified by the word is in sight. Consequently, at the stage of autonomous speech there is still no possibility of verbal thinking separate from the visual situation. As soon as the word is separated from the visual situation, it cannot realize its meaning. The child cannot think with the help of words outside the visual situation. Consequently, at the stage of children's autonomous speech, the child's thinking acquires some initial traits of the thinking of oral speech but of the kind that cannot yet be separated from the visual. The connection of oral thinking with visual thinking was most clearly apparent in the fact that the words could have only such relations as would reflect direct relations of things to each other where the meaning of the words of autonomous speech were not in common relation with each other, that is, one meaning had no relation to another meaning as, let us say, *furniture* has a common relation to *chair*.

Second, owing to this, how can words be combined with each other? Only as objects that the child can see are combined. Let us say, *the train is running (sweat is running)*. They can be combined only in a way as to reflect the connection of direct impressions. Connections of things established through thinking at this stage of development of autonomous speech are still not accessible to thinking. For this reason, thinking still has an extremely nonindependent character. It comprises a kind of subordinate part of the child's perception, his orientation in what surrounds him, and a number of affective-volitional thoughts he expresses in which the intellectual content is secondary.

What does affective-volitional content of children's words mean? It means that what the child expresses in speech corresponds to our judgments, and, more likely, to our exclamations, which we use to convey an affective coloring, an affective attitude, emotional reaction, or volitional tendency.

If we analyze the content of children's autonomous speech, and the level of thinking that corresponds to it, we will find that since children's autonomous speech transmits an affective content, it is still not uncoupled from perception. It transmits perceived impressions and it ascertains, but does not deduce and does not reach conclusions. It is full of the volitive, but not the intellectual points connected with thinking in the true sense of the word.

Thus, we believe that children's autonomous speech not only represents an extremely original stage in the development of children's speech, but that this stage corresponds to a unique stage in the development of thinking. Depending on the stage of development at which speech is, thinking exhibits certain features. Before the child's speech reaches a certain level of development, his thinking too cannot go beyond that certain level. The level which confronts us is characterized in the same way by both the unique period in the development of speech and the unique period in development of the child's thinking.

When does a normal child go through a period of autonomous speech? We said that he does so in the crisis of the first year of life, that is, at that turning point when the child passes from infancy to early childhood. This usually begins at the end of the first year and ends in the second year. During the crisis of the first year of life, the normal child uses autonomous speech. Its beginning and end signify the beginning and end of the crisis of the first year of life.

Does this mean that we consider children's autonomous speech as a central neoformation of the critical age? It seems so to me. But this point of view is insufficiently developed, and for this reason it will be necessary to be very careful about reaching conclusions about the nature of the neoformations of one critical age or another. In any case, the appearance of children's autonomous speech as a transitional form from the mute to the verbal is one of the most important facts.

We have seen two other factors in the crisis: the establishment of walking and hypobulic and affective outbursts of the child, etc., but, of course, the task is always not in matching a number of neoformations with this, but in finding their central methods. Of course, it is important to understand neoformations from the point of view of that whole which occurs in growth that signifies a new stage in development and the structure of all the new changes.

Can we believe that children's autonomous speech is simply the first phase of development of speech, that it does not differ from it in any significant way and that, consequently, there is no difference between studying children's autonomous speech and the theory of Stern's discovery? Can we pose the question in such a way that autonomous speech in its essence is our speech? Perhaps it coincides with it not in the structure of words or in meanings, but their "core" is identical?

I would respond thus: the "core" — the essence of children's autonomous speech — is and is not ours, and in this lies all its originality as a transitional formation between mute and verbal communication. In what is it ours, and what can come from it? That it is ours is so clear that we need not stop to consider this. It is much more important to say how it is not ours. It seems to me that it is not ours not only in the sense that the word does not sound like ours and has a different meaning, but it is not ours in a deeper sense: its principle of structure is completely different from that of our speech since it does not have constant meanings in general. I will present parallel analogues of the differences. Let us take the behavior of apes in Köhler's experiments. The animal, as we know, uses a box or a stick as a tool in certain cases. From an external aspect, the essence of this operation is the same as it is in man when he uses a tool, and this led Köhler to maintain that the use of the stick by the chimpanzee is actually and typically similar to the action of man.

Critics say: but what kind of use of tools is this if another ape sits on the box which the ape used as a stand and the box stops being a tool and is converted into a thing for sitting on or lying on, and the ape in this situation wanders about the area, attempts to jump for the fruit, sits down on the box on which the other ape is lying, and wipes away perspiration? Consequently, she sees the box but cannot use it as a tool in this situation. What kind of a tool is it if it loses the properties of a tool outside the working situation? Köhler himself says that primitive man using a stick for digging in the earth prepares the stick ahead of time. While in the situation of the ape there is something new, it is not the same thing as in the primitive man; although there is something new from which the use of a tool might come, the use itself of a tool is not yet there.

Something similar to this can be observed also in children's autonomous speech. Imagine speech in which words have no constant meaning but in each new situation, they mean something different than in the preceding situation. In the example I gave, the word, "poo-foo," meant a bottle with iodine in one situation, and in another, the iodine itself, etc. Consequently, such a word differs from words of the stage in which they have a constant meaning. At this point, there is still no symbolization at all. Words of children's autonomous speech differ from words at the stage where in the consciousness some communicative meanings are formed that are more or less firm and constant. In autonomous speech, the word itself signifies everything and therefore nothing.

What is at the beginning of every symbol? With all the fantastic quality and all the debatability of the whole array of ideas in the theory of N. Ya. Marr, one idea seems to me to be indisputable: the initial words of human language, how man expresses himself — the first words designated everything or very much. And the first words of the child designate almost everything. But what kind of words are these? Words of the type "this" or "that"; they are applied to any object. Can we say that these are real words? No, this is only an indicative function of the word itself; from it something that symbolizes will arise later, but so far the word that designates everything is simply a vocal indicative gesture, and it is preserved in all words because every word of man points to a certain object.

Finally, the last difference.

If we can take the matter to be as Stern indicates it (the meaning of the word, the connection of the meaning of the word with the word is a very simple thing organized in an elementary way), then, of course, the "core" is either this kind or it is not, but this makes the study of children's autonomous speech ever more valuable because it makes it possible to disclose the "core" of the word and a number of its functions, for example, the indicative function. Further, we will see that in childhood a nominative function of the word also develops. This is an important transition (in "poo-foo" there is still no significative function).

Speaking of children's autonomous speech, we have in mind not a one-layer, but a multilayer structure of the "core." We might think of children's autonomous speech only as a transitional stage of development which in relation to real speech is simultaneously our speech and not our speech, that is, it contains something of our speech, but much in it is not of our speech. We know that children who do not move up through autonomous speech, that is, idiots and aphasics, in essence remain without speech, although from our point of view, their autonomous speech seems to be a symbol. For example, the aphasic says "poo-foo" instead of *bottle*. With the word "poo-foo," he can signify a number of concepts.

For the child, speech does not yet exist in his consciousness as a recognized principle of symbolization and for this reason, the disparity with Stern's "discovery" is colossal. It is another matter to show how a phenomenon such as the initial stage of children's speech arises through transitional formations. In this sense, we see a number of jumps in the development of children's speech not only at the border of autonomous and nonautonomous speech, but also in its subsequent development.

Understanding the period of appearance and establishment of children's speech allows penetrating so deeply into the course of its development that it becomes possible to approach correct theories of speech development and to disclose the inadequacies of the constructs of bourgeois science pertaining to this problem.

We must not lose sight of other neoformations: walking, hypobulic incidents, etc.

Just as I remind myself to be careful, I have decided not to let myself go into theoretical discussion now and am forced to limit myself to showing where, from my point of view, and in which direction we should look for the general change in which we are interested in the critical age we are describing. It seems to me that speech pertains to the central neoformation of that age.

I think that the child's development considered from the point of view of stages in the development of the personality, from the point of view of the child's relations with his environment, from the point of view of basic activity at each stage is closely connected with the history of the development of the child's consciousness. If I would want to answer this question formally, I might indicate the famous words of Marx that "consciousness is relation to the environment."[6] But essentially, it is true that the relation of the personality to the environment characterizes in the most intimate way the structure of consciousness and, consequently, it seems to me that studying the age levels and their neoformations from the point of view of consciousness is a legitimate approach to a correct answer to this question. And the advantage here is no small thing because contemporary science still does not know how to study facts that characterize consciousness. There is no doubt that speech is closely connected with consciousness. I do not want to make a mistake and, in pointing to the relation to the environment, to consciousness, to speech, I do not want to reduce everything to speech. Of course, I must proceed from both the top and the bottom, from such symptoms as teeth, walking, and the child's speech; I must be interested in the first and second actors in this drama. It seems to me that the study of changes in the child's consciousness and the study of speech is theoretically central to understanding all the other changes which concern us here.

To consider age level theoretically means to find such changes in the child's personality as a whole within which all of these points would become clear to us, some as prerequisites and others as certain factors, etc.

It is difficult to understand directly what the relation is between the change in structure of consciousness and acquisition of speech. Ordinarily, all investigators limited themselves to indicating that they are related, or that the one and the other distinguishes man from the animal and is a specific human property; or, to turn to an analogy for help (as I did earlier), they maintained that in relation to the child's social space, speech plays a role similar to the role of walking in his relation to physical space. This analogy has little value. None of the works I know answers the simple question as to what is the relation between these neoformations. From the genetic point of view, we spoke of what distinguishes the child's basic acquisitions during the critical period. Does the child make the new acquisitions during the critical age or does development do the destructive work? We would answer this question positively. We have seen many times that during the critical age, as during the whole period of development, the child makes new acquisitions, otherwise development would not be development.

But how are the child's acquisitions during a critical age different? They have a transitional character. The acquisition during a critical age never remains in subsequent life, whereas acquisitions that the child makes during a stable age are retained. During a stable age, the child learns to walk, talk, write, etc. During a transitional age, the child acquires autonomous speech. If it is retained for the whole of life, that is not normal.

In children's autonomous speech, we find various forms typical for the crisis of the first year. The beginning of this form and the end of children's [autonomous] speech may be considered as a symptom of the beginning and end of the critical age.

True speech arises and autonomous speech disappears together with the end of the critical age; although a feature of the acquisition of these critical ages is their transitional character, they have a very great genetic significance: they are seemingly a transitional bridge. Without the formation of autonomous speech, the child would never make the transition from the mute to the verbal period of development. Properly, the acquisition of critical age levels is not destroyed but is only transformed into a more complex formation. It fulfills a specific genetic function in the transition from one stage of development to another.

The transitions that arise during critical age levels, specifically children's autonomous speech, are infinitely interesting because they represent segments of the child's development in which we see displayed the dialectical pattern of development.

Chapter 9
Early Childhood[1]

It seems to me that in approaching the study of each age level, including early childhood, we need to ask what kind of neoformations appear at the given age, that is, what new thing that was not present in preceding stages is produced in the process of development at the given stage because the process of development itself obviously consists primarily of the appearance of new formations at each stage. Neoformations appear at the end of each age level and represent the result of the development that occurred during that period. The task of analysis is, first, to trace the paths and the genesis of the neoformation, second, to describe the neoformation, and third, to establish the connection between the neoformation and the subsequent levels of development.

What is the central neoformation of early childhood, that is, what is produced in development and what is established in this way as a foundation for future development? This is the central question. In order to approach a solution to the question, I would like first of all to gather some material and to review certain important problems of this question in order to reach conclusions based on them. It is necessary to consider them separately and then to proceed to certain generalizations.

We shall first consider the relation of the child to external reality, to the external environment. Here we have a number of points that we must describe in order to develop an idea regarding the relation of the child to external reality at this level of development. It seems to me that we might consider the unique relation of the child to the situation in the sense of his behavior and his acting within the situation, which has been well demonstrated experimentally.

I believe that K. Lewin, the famous German scientist and structural psychologist, has demonstrated this experimentally best of all. To him we owe the best of the works that elucidate this aspect. He tried to construct a theory on the child's unique behavior in an external situation in early childhood.

What are the principal traits that characterize the child's behavior? I will indicate the more important traits graphically. This is the *Situationsgebundheit* and *Feldmassigkeit*, that is, a connectedness of the situation itself. The child enters into the situation and his behavior is wholly determined by the situation, he enters into it as some dynamic part of it. And as *Feldmassigkeit*, Lewin has in mind any situation that structural psychology regards as a field of human action, and human activity is considered in connection with the structure of this field. According to Lewin, the child's actions at this stage of development are wholly and absolutely "field" actions, that is, exclusively adapted to the structure of the field in which the present action occurs in the perception of the child.

The experiment shows what this consists of: each object has a seeming affect, attracting or repelling, that arouses motivation in the child. Each object "draws" the child to touch it, pick it up, to feel it, or, conversely, not to touch it; the object acquires what Lewin terms *Aufforderungscharakter* — a certain imperative character. Everything has some affect so arousing that for the child, it acquires a character of a "compulsory" affect and for this reason, at this age, the child finds in the world of things and objects a kind of force field in which he is always affected by things that attract or repel. For him there is no neutral or "disinterested" relation to the things around him. As Lewin graphically expresses it, a ladder lures the child to climb, a door, to be opened or closed, a bell, to be rung, a box to be covered or uncovered, a ball to be rolled. In a word, for the child in this situation, each thing is charged with this affective attracting or repelling force and has an affective valence which provokes him correspondingly to action, that is, leads him.

In order to understand how the child acts in one situation or another in early childhood, we can provide a somewhat remote analogy to how we behave if we find ourselves at the mercy of some situation. This rarely happens to us. In Lewin's experiment, this was the procedure: the subject was invited to the laboratory, then the experimenter left for several minutes with the excuse that he had to prepare something for the experiment, and he left the subjects alone in the new environment. He waited ten to fifteen minutes. In this situation, the subject frequently began to look around the room. If there was a clock, he would check the time; if there was an envelope, he would check to see if there was something in it or if it was empty. In this state, every action of the person is determined by what he sees, which is a remote analogy to the behavior of the child in early childhood.

This is the source of the child's connectedness solely to a present situation. In contrast to later age levels, in early childhood, the child does not bring knowledge of other possible things into the situation; in general, as Lewin expresses it, the child is not attracted by anything that is in the wings of the situation, anything that might change the situation. This is why things themselves, concrete objects within a situation, play such a major role.

Lewin describes an experiment that demonstrated how difficult it is for a child before he is two years old to sit on an object that is not in his visual field. This was an experiment with a large rock that the child walked around, looked at from all sides, etc. Then the child turned his back to the rock to sit down, but as soon as he turned, he lost sight of the rock. Then the child held on to the rock and turned to sit. Finally, one child, recorded on film (which is presented in Lewin's book, 1926), solved the difficulty in a unique way: he bent down and looked between his legs so that he had the rock in his visual field even when his back was turned to it. Then he could sit down. Some children help themselves by keeping a hand on the rock. In another case, the experimenter himself placed the child's hand on the rock and the child sat down on his own hand because he had no feeling that there was a whole rock behind the piece of rock that his hand was covering. This kind of connectedness of the child to the visual field evidently indicates the unique activity of the child's consciousness in this situation.

To illustrate, I will give an example from our experiments. My colleague, L. S. Slavina,[2] had the job of observing if in a free situation, a child can verbally, if I may say so, "fly away," leave the situation and say something that he does not see before him. For this we used a technique, highly developed in the clinic, of repeating sentences. Two-year-olds repeat without any difficulty sentences such as: "The chicken is walking," "Koko is walking," or "The dog is running." But the child cannot say "Tanya is walking," when Tanya is sitting on a chair before him. This sentence gets the reaction, "Tanya is sitting." In all three series, all forty children responded incorrectly when the attention of the child was drawn in by the situation. Looking at Tanya sitting there, it was difficult for the child to say, "Tanya is walking." What he sees affects him much more, and for this reason, his words cannot be inconsistent with reality. This explains one of the facts to which investigators called attention long ago: in early childhood, the child almost cannot lie. Only toward the end of early childhood does the child develop a very elementary capacity to say something that is actually not so. Thus far he is not capable of invention. A simple example thoroughly studied recently indicates this. The child is sick; when the pain is sharp, he reacts affectively — he cries and is capricious. But he cannot be dangerously sick, however, since he does not experience direct pain but is upset by the consciousness of illness. Thus, a child at this age cannot speak of anything but what is happening before his eyes or what he hears.

What is responsible for this kind of behavior?

First, what characterizes the consciousness of the child is the development of unity between sensory and motor functions. Everything the child sees, he wants to touch. Observing a two-year-old left to himself, we see that the child is constantly active, constantly bustling, but he is active exclusively in the concrete situation, that is, he does only what surrounding things nudge him to do.

Earlier it was assumed that sensory-motor unity develops from a simple physiological reflex, but this is not so even at a very young age. A swaddled child may sometimes peacefully look around, but for early childhood, it is characteristic that every perception is unfailingly followed by action. This does not happen in infancy until its last phase when sensory-motor unity specific to that age develops.

The Leipzig school[3] called attention to the fact that the very first perception of the child is an affectively colored perception, that is, the child sees every object with a different affective coloration. In other words, perception and feeling are an indivisible unity. We learn to look at things abstracting ourselves from any direct emotion that they evoke and not exhibiting any great interest in a number of things. But for the young child, this is impossible. Perception and affect are still not differentiated, they are directly and closely connected with each other. The experiments of F. Krueger and H. Volkelt showed that in us and in animals, the sensory tone of perception is always retained. For example, blue and yellow evoke in us a sensory tone of cold and heat. A certain sensory tone of perception accompanies our ideas, and this indicates that genetically they are connected with each other.

The unity of affective-receptive factors produces a third factor for characterizing consciousness in early childhood — for acting in a situation. We are dealing with this kind of unique system of consciousness when perception is directly connected with action. Consequently, if we characterize the system of consciousness from the point of view of leading functions that work jointly in early childhood, then we must say that this is a unity of affective perception or affect and action. Lewin's experiments elucidate these circumstances splendidly for us.

It is specifically the attractive force of things, the affective charge of every object, that conceals in itself the source of attraction for the child. In other words, the uniqueness of the sensory-motor unity (it can be considered as established by the experimental works of Lewin), characteristic specifically for this age, consists in the fact that it is not a primary reflex connection, but a connection through affect. Specifically the affective nature of perception results in this unity. Thus, we are dealing here with a completely unique relation to reality.

For the child in early childhood to be conscious in general still does not mean to perceive and process what is perceived with the help of attention, memory, and thinking. All of these functions have not yet been differentiated, they act as a whole in consciousness and are subordinated to perception to the extent that they participate in the process of perception.

Everyone knows from simple observation that memory in early childhood always appears in active perception, in recognizing. Everyone knows that thinking at this age is strictly visual thinking, as being able to reestablish a connection, but in a visually presented situation. Everyone knows that in early childhood affects also appear predominantly at the time of visual perception of the object to which the affect is directed. For a child at this age, as far as he exhibits intellectual activity, thinking does not mean remembering. Only for a child of school age does thinking mean to remember, that is, to depend on his own past experience.

There is one fact that is called the fact of amnesia. None of us remember infancy. If individual people who are geniuses, as, for example, L. Tolstoy, maintain that they remember a feeling of constraint in being swaddled, sensing warm water and soap in being bathed, then evidently we are dealing in this case with complex reminiscence. As far as consciousness of each of us is concerned, as a rule, we forget infancy and we forget early childhood. Hardly anyone remembers distinctly (not from accounts of those nearby) anything of his childhood before the age of three, except isolated, exceptional impressions, except fragments, frequently incomprehensible.

Connected recollections from the time of early childhood are usually not retained in consciousness, so memory is organized uniquely and it participates very little in all the activity of consciousness. Memory comes to the forefront in subsequent years; it would be correct to say that in early childhood, thinking means investigating given, affectively colored connections and to undertaking original actions corresponding to the external perceived situation. At this age, visual, affectively colored perception directly transferred into action is dominant.

Perception itself differs in two respects which should be considered. The first feature of perception is its affective character. I. M. Sechenov[4] believed that the most important feature of the very young child is the intensity of his perception. At an early age, every perception is manic. Whoever sees a child look at a new thing sees the essential difference between his perception and ours.

The second feature (which is a general law for subsequent development also): when perception is the dominant function of consciousness, this means that perception is placed in the maximally favorable conditions of development. Since all consciousness acts only on the basis of perception, perception develops earlier than the other functions. This is connected with two basic laws of child development, which I will recall. The first says that functions, like parts of the body, develop not proportionally and evenly, but at each age there is a dominant function.

The second law says that the most fundamental functions that are needed from the beginning, which facilitate the others, develop earlier. For this reason, it is not surprising that development of mental functions of the child begins with the development of perception. If all consciousness works for perception, if perception is created as something new at a given age, then it is obvious that the child attains the greatest success not in the area of memory, but in the area of perception.

In this connection, there is still the problem of childhood autism. There are two points of view. (And it seems to me that these two now no longer enjoy equal rights from the point of view of identical probability. Facts indicate that one of these points of view is closer to the truth.) According to one point of view, the logic of dreams is the initial point in the development of children's thinking. Thinking is autistic and wholly directed to satisfying desires; it is not the realistic thinking that, according to the point of view we are considering, develops at relatively late stages of development. This is the *Lustprinzip* — Freud's pleasure principle.

However, E. Bleuler showed that this is not so. In the animal world, we simply do not meet with autistic functions of thinking, that is, thinking separated from action. To ascribe to the infant such states of consciousness in which he would realize his desires, drives, tendencies, in general, for consciousness to serve the pleasure principle exclusively is a purely logical construct. Pleasure that an infant gets at an early age is connected with the real obtaining of food, with real stimuli, etc.

Bleuler called attention to the following. If Freud's point of view were correct, then the autistic character of thinking would have to decline as the child developed. Bleuler was the first to call attention to the increase in autistic thinking after the age of one and a half, that is, after the first acquisition of speech.

Now we have the work of Gabriel which demonstrates that autistic thinking increases as thinking rises to a higher level—at the age of three and at the age of thirteen in connection with the formation of concepts. This is understandable. Of course, speech is one of the powerful means for the development of thinking that is not connected directly to a situation. Speech always makes it possible to introduce something into a situation that the situation does not directly contain, and we can always say in words something that is not pertinent to a given situation. For this reason, verbal thinking is connected with the development of children's autistic thinking.

Autistic thinking at early stages of development as an important factor for describing the relation of the child to reality is almost nonexistent. Over almost the whole course of three years of life, it remains in an embryonic state. As Gabriel showed, we are dealing here only with rudiments of autistic thinking.

In terms of the old psychology, we could say that a child of this age has no imagination, that is, he has no possibility of constructing in thought and in the imagination a visual situation that differs from that which is presented to him directly. If we consider the child's relation to external reality, we will see that the child appears before us very much as a realistic being who differs from an older child by his connectedness to the situation and in the fact that he is wholly at the mercy of the things that are before him at the time. In this case, we still do not see a break away from reality, which is the basis for autistic thinking.

Now let us consider the relations of the child to other people. The external aspect of this is now being studied very broadly. A number of papers have appeared which through experiment and systematic observation show the presence at infancy of relatively developed forms of the child's relations to other people, relations that seem primitive only from the point of view of adults. These relations become more complex over time to the extent that some investigators speak directly of early childhood as an age in which the central neoformation is the development of bases for person-to-person relations, that is, the bases for social relations.

Attempts have been made to construct a theory in this respect, and it seems to me that one of the theories that is also being developed more and more experimentally is correct. According to this theory, the uniqueness of the child's social relations consists in the following: the child at the moment of birth and in infancy is separated physiologically from the mother (according to the old expression), but is not separated from her biologically — he cannot change position and cannot feed himself. The child who begins to walk is separated from the mother biologically, but is still not separated psychologically—he still has no conception of himself as a particular, separate being except for those situations in which he is always involved with other people.

The first conception the child has of his being is a conception of separateness or particularity (not in the sense of contrasting himself to others, but in the sense of separating himself from things with which he operates and in contrasting himself to things in a social situation, himself merged with other people).

German investigators believe that two stages into which early childhood can be divided can be set apart in the following way. The first stage "Ur-wir" is a "great-we" consciousness that precedes the concept "I" and from which the "I" is extracted. Actually, a number of facts show that the child takes no account of what he understands and what others understand. As Piaget correctly noted, to the child it seems that adults know his every wish. There is a study on the child's development of two-word sentences when one-word sentences no longer are satisfactory, specifically due to their ambiguity. For the child, the word signifies the most varied things, and in each situation it is understood differently. Gabriel described these constant misunderstandings very well. In his opinion, investigators did not turn their attention in vain to the adults' difficulties in understanding a child who is just beginning to speak.

Allow me to present an example from Gabriel's experiments which I cited in another connection. For the child in an experimental situation involved in broad clinical observations, a situation was created in which adults did not understand the child's words. He wants something, the adults do not understand him, he begins to be angry and the situation ends in the adults' asking him questions in order to understand what he wants.

What is of interest here with respect to the topic that interests us? It seems to me that the child does not know that what he is thinking is known only to him and that the adults may not understand it. For the child, the problem of the adults not understanding him does not yet exist. He says "poo-foo" and it seems to him that he must be given what he is asking for. This happens because the adults continuously interpret the behavior of the child in order to guess what he wants. For this reason, as Piaget correctly maintains, the child has a feeling that adults must understand his wishes correctly, and he does not separate what is in his consciousness from what is in the consciousness of the adult. For this reason, primary also is the consciousness of "great-we" from which only gradually the child's conception of himself is extracted.

The very expression "I myself" appears in the second stage of early childhood. Authors call the second stage the "stage of the external 'I' in the 'we,'" and this is the stage in which the child opposes his independent actions to cooperative actions with adults. For example, he takes a spoon and wants to feed himself, protesting against being fed. But when we consider his consciousness, his being understood by adults and the external aspect of the process, he still remains merged in the "great-we" state.

Whether this theory resolves the problem correctly or not, it seems to me that, in any case, it indicates correctly the uniqueness of the relation of the child to the people around him and the extraction from the unity, child—adult, of a personal "I." The child's "I myself" appears comparatively late. One of the studies describes very well this stage when the child understands more than he can say. The child himself cannot yet put his thoughts and ideas into motion. I would say that where we are dealing with an external situation, things are controlling the child, and when the child is active in the situation, this is connected with the involvement of others, with turning to adults.

Now we shall consider the basic types of activity[5] of the child at the stage of early childhood. This is one of the most difficult problems and it seems to me the least developed theoretically. The old definition of play as every activity of the child that does not pursue getting results regards all types of children's activity as being equivalent. From the point of view of the adult, whether the child opens and closes a door or plays with a hobby-horse, he does both for pleasure, for play, not seriously, not in order to get something. All of this is called play.

We must say that many authors wanted to bring some clarity to the problem. The first was K. Groos, who tried to declassify children's play and find a different approach to it. He showed that experimental play has a different relationship to the child's thinking and to his future goal-directed nonplay actions than symbolic play in which the child imagines that he is a horse, a hunter, etc. One of Groos's students, A. Weiss, tried to show that various types of play activity are very different from each other or, as he expressed it, they have little in common from the psychological aspect. The question arose in his mind as to whether all the different types of similar activity can be called "play."

P. P. Blonsky assumes that play is only a common name for the most varied activities of the child. As far as I know, Blonsky evidently approaches the extreme in this statement. He is inclined to think that "play in general" does not exist, that there is no type of activity which would fit this concept because the concept of play itself is a concept of adults, and for the child, everything is serious. So this concept must also be eliminated from psychology. Blonsky describes the following episode. When it was necessary to ask a psychologist to write a paper on "play" for an encyclopedia, he announced that "play" is a word with nothing behind it which should be eliminated from psychology.

The idea pertaining to breaking up the concept "play," which I heard in Leningrad from D. B. Elkonin, seems to me to be most productive. Play must be considered as a completely original activity and not as a mixed concept that unites all types of children's activities, particularly those that Groos called experimental play. For example, the child closes and opens a box, doing this many times in a row, knocks, carries things from place to place. None of this is play in the true sense of the word. We might say that these types of activity are related to each other as prattling is related to speech, but in any case, this is not play.

It seems to me that most productive and pertinent to the essence of the matter would be the positive definition of play which is indicated by this idea, specifically, that play is a unique relation to reality that is characterized by creating imaginary situations or transferring the properties of some objects to others. This makes it possible to solve the problem of play in early childhood.[6] Here we do not have the complete absence of play which, from this point of view, characterizes infancy. We come upon games in early childhood. Everyone agrees that a child of this age eats, tends to a doll, can drink from an empty cup, etc. However, it would be dangerous, it seems to me, not to see a substantial difference between this "play" and play in the true sense of the word during preschool age — with the creation of imaginary situations. Studies show that play in the figurative sense, with imaginary situations, appears in a rudimentary form only toward the end of early childhood. Games connected with introducing elements of imagination into a situation appear only in the third year. It is another matter that these "play" manifestations are quite meager and sink in the broad sea of activities that Lewin described which come directly from the situation itself.

Lewin already had the idea that the definition of child behavior that he gave has little resemblance to creation of a play situation in the true sense of the word. Of course, the child who must look between his legs to sit on a rock is so closely tied to present objects that creation of an imaginary situation is difficult for him.

Finally, last and most important. Study has shown that the creation of an imaginary situation in the true sense of the word does not yet exist in early childhood. At two years, the child quite freely tends to a doll and does with it approximately what the mother or nurse does with her: she tucks the doll in, feeds it, even puts it on the potty. But it is interesting that the child has no conception of the doll being her daughter, that she is the doll's nurse or mother. She tends to a teddy bear as if it were a bear, a doll as if it were a doll, that is, this is play from the point of view of the adult, but it differs greatly from the play of an older child when the child himself plays a role and things play a role. In this play, a doll is actually a small girl, and the child is one of the parents, although the doll just as affectively insists on being put on the potty, being fed, as, let us say, a round ball insists that it be rolled. There is no extended imaginary situation where the child himself clearly plays some role and noticeably changes the property of a thing. For example, experiment has shown that for the very young child, not everything can be a doll. At age two, the child who freely tends to a doll or a bear, has difficulty in doing this with a bottle and does it completely differently. For this reason, if, as they say, characteristic for play is the fact that everything can be anything, this is not characteristic for the play of the very young child. Thus, in this case, we have *seeming* play, but for the child himself, it is not deliberate play.

This theory always seemed to me to be extremely attractive, and now it acquires a special meaning. W. Stern introduced into psychology the concept of *Ernstspiel* (serious play) and applied it to adolescence, pointing to the fact that such play has a transitional character between play and a serious relation to reality and is a specific type of activity. As A. Homburger and his students have shown, the concept of *serious play* is much closer to what is observed in early childhood: we are dealing with play in which the play situation is not yet differentiated in the consciousness of the child from the real situation. When preschoolers play mother and father or train, they clearly know how to conduct themselves in the play situation, that is, they behave the whole time in conformity with the logic of the situation that is developing. In analogy to Lewin's expression, for the preschooler, a certain closed field develops in which he moves, but at the same time, he does not lose his conception of the real meaning of things. If in the game, a chair is a horse and the chair must be moved to a different place, it does not disturb the child to carry the chair although a horse is not carried in one's arms. Characteristic for the play of an older child is the presence of the field of ideas and the visible field.

In early childhood, there is quasi-play or "playing itself." Objectively this is play, but it is not yet play for the child; specifically, the experiment of Dohme is extremely interesting in that he shows how the very young child repeats a series of actions with respect, let us say, to a doll, but this is not yet connected into a single situation in which he goes somewhere with the doll, asks the doctor to come to see her, etc. There is no connected story or conversion of it into action, dramatization in the true sense of the word, and there is no specific movement in the plan of this situation created by the child himself.

Turning to the neoformations, which we considered in detail with speech, we see that the very fact of acquiring speech is in sharp contradiction to everything of which I spoke thus far that characterizes early childhood. In other words, speech instantly starts to shatter sensory-motor unity and to break up the situational connectedness of the child. As the child develops, his relation changes not only to the new, but also to the old elements of the environment because the nature of their effect on the child changes. There is a change in the social situation of development that prevailed at the beginning of this age. Suddenly, the child becomes entirely different — the old social situation of development is destroyed and a new age-level begins.

We can understand what is new in the relations of the child to the environment in early childhood in light of the analysis of the development of children's speech because the development of speech as a means of personal contact, as a means of understanding the speech of those around him, is the central line of development of the child of this age and essentially changes the relations of the child to the environment.

A study deaf-mute children shows that the central neoformation — speech as a communicative function — does not develop in them.

Speech plays a role in the function of personal contact, plays a role like activity connected with people, that is, it is external and cooperative — in the form of a dialogue. Where speech plays a role in the communicative function, it is connected with pronunciation and talking and is manifested in vocalization.

The study of the vocalized, that is, the external aspect of speech, began long ago. The material is very rich. Certain theories have also been developed. However, now that investigators began to study speech in all its complexity from the aspect of meaning, the points of view of its external aspect have changed. The development of the vocal aspect of speech was usually thought of as follows: speech consists of individual sound elements very easily symbolized in writing. In a certain sense, this idea is irrefutable because all vocal speech is constructed from a certain number of elements. Initially the child masters a limited number of elements, is not able to use all the elements of vocal speech and distorts them, that is, here we have in mind the so-called physiological ankyloglossia and underdevelopment of the articulation apparatus that is age-related in contrast to pathological ankyloglossia. Further development consists in differentiation of elements, and by two and a half years of age, toward the end of early childhood, the child is able to use all the sound baggage. As elements are mastered, sound combinations are mastered. It seems that knowing how to pronounce individual sounds, the child subsequently masters certain sound combinations (the work of W. and K. Stern).

This view of the development of speech was subjected to doubt since it results in a number of contradictory positions. We will present some of these.

1. If the child masters all sounds, he must then master all combinations, that is, mastering certain sounds, the child must without difficulty also master new words — therefore development consists only in a quantitative increase in vocabulary.

A comparison was made between the development of the sound aspect of speech and assimilation of written speech. It actually is facilitated by mastery of elements, but is mastery not of separate words, but of the very principle of writing. In oral speech, the picture is different. Speaking against the analogy between oral and written speech, old authors said that oral speech can properly be equated to mastery of elements and their combinations in learning a foreign language. The child masters the word as a complex of sounds because he needs to relearn it every time anew just the way we do when dealing with learning a foreign language.

But if I master the English alphabet, that still does not mean that I know the English language. It seems that the child does not master words in his own language in this way. Assimilating one's native language occupies a middle position between what happens in the development of written language and what happens in learning a foreign language. If mastery of the sound aspect of speech proceeded from elements, from the alphabet, then there might be only two paths to learning it: through gradual learning of each new combination as in a foreign language or through mastering the elements that make producing any combinations possible and mastering speech instantly as this occurs in the development of written speech. In the development of oral speech, we find, on the one hand, elements of what occurs in written speech: having mastered instantly one set of words or another, that is, having mastered the structure, the child seems able to master all words; on the other hand, it is like mastering foreign words, where each word must pass through the sensory into the active plane through memorizing. Having mastered the sound aspect of speech, the child does not have to memorize words, but he must master each new word separately.

2. In written speech, it is easier to isolate an element when the child has assimilated the alphabet and is learning to write. It is easier for him to write a letter than to write a word, but in oral speech, isolating the elements is more difficult. The child pronounces a whole sentence or a word very well, but cannot name a syllable that is a part of it, let alone individual letters.

If the analogy between the development of the vocal aspect of speech and written speech were correct, this would not be so.

3. If the path of speech development went from the sound to the complex, then the child would have very great difficulty with the analytical work. In actual speech, the child hears not separate sounds, but connected speech.

Consequently, from the point of view of these opinions, the child plays the role of an analyst and must capture and isolate separate sounds — letters, alphabets — and he must create an alphabet himself, that is, carry out the supreme effort of generalizing that factually contradicts the real level of his development. To imagine all of this in a child who is a year and a half old — is nonsense. Also, in treating the problem in this way, we lose the connection between the sound and semantic aspects of speech because in itself sound is meaningless.

Thus, the old theory not only resulted in a complete break between the sound aspect and the semantic aspect of speech, but also in an absurd idea: in order to study a word phonetically, the child must make it meaningless, and from the point of view of the semantic aspect, conversely, he must work over a complex that is formless from the point of view of sounds, that is, in order to elucidate the development of the semantic aspect, a breakdown of the sound aspect was proposed and vice versa. The old theory ignored the real conditions that determine the development of speech, specifically, speech interaction.

New points of view on this problem appeared in approximately 1928 as a result of the intersection of research from various areas. The attempt to review the old teaching on the development of the sound aspect of speech encompassed linguistics, pedagogy, speech psychology, the area studying speech pathology, etc.

From the point of view of the old conception, the sound aspect of speech consists of a series of elements and their combination. The old phonetics was based on the physiological nature of speech, on articulation, etc. The development of speech was considered through the prism of the development of the motor system of fine articulation movements: explanations were given of what kind of fine movements were necessary for mastering one sound or another. Let us say, in order to master the sound "r," a finer articulation of the motor system was required than for the sound "b." The development of the motor system was considered to be the only source of development.

The new theory (phonology[7] — in contrast to the old — phonetics) began with indicating that the real functional meaning of separate sounds of human speech is not directly connected to their physiological properties. Neither is there a proportionality between their physical (acoustic) properties and functional meaning. At the end of the second half year, the development of the sound aspect of the child's speech does not proceed in parallel with the physical properties of sound, but depends on the degree of functional meaning of the sound in human speech. In the sounds, "b—p," "v—f," and "g—k," the physical voiced and voiceless quality are the common properties for this whole series of sounds. Their functional meaning in speech does not correspond with their physical properties.

We have three orders of phenomena: (1) development of the sound aspect of children's speech, (2) the physical and physiological difficulties, and (3) the development of functional meanings.

We might say that the development of children's speech displays a dependence not on increasing complexity of physiological and physical difficulties, but is connected with the development of functional meanings in speech. If, however, there is a dependence on physiological features also, then this is because physiological properties themselves are connected with the functional meaning.

How can we determine the functional meaning of a sound in the development of speech? The question is based on the methodological problem, on how analysis should be applied in sciences that study integral formations. Analysis is indispensable here also, but analysis breaks things down, while it is necessary to study the whole as a whole.[8]

Two types of analysis must be distinguished. The first, separation into elements, is an unsuccessful type that destroys the properties of the whole; the second type is a breakdown of the whole into indivisible units and the study of the cell that has retained all the properties of the whole. In studying speech, it must be the analysis of units (precisely as in the study of the problem of the effect of the environment on the child). This type of analysis rejects the possibility of breaking speech down to separate sound elements. The sounds of human speech have a definite meaning. This is the first and basic factor that characterizes human speech. In breaking speech down into elements, the elements lose meaning and in this way, analysis of speech loses the properties of analysis; it no longer is breaking it down into parts, but raising it to the general. In the new phonetics — phonology — the unit of analysis of speech has changed, the phoneme has been advanced as the unit of human speech and the unit of the development of children's speech. From the point of view of this new phonetics, the development of children's speech occurs through development of a system of phonemes and not through an accumulation of separate sounds.

The phoneme is not just a sound, it is a sound that has meaning, a sound that has not lost meaning, a certain unit that has a primary property to a minimal degree, which belongs to speech as a whole. Sounds develop not in themselves, but from the point of view of their meaning. Functional meaning depends on the development of sensible meaning. We can speak of the development of human speech only when the unity of sound and meaning is preserved.

In language development, there is no phoneme in the absolute sense, there is only a relative consideration of the phoneme against a background of other phonemes. Mastering the phoneme occurs under conditions of perceiving other phonemes and in correlation with them. The basic law of perception of phonemes is the law of perception of the sound aspect of speech, and like all other perceptions, it is a perception of something against a background of something (figure and background). Every phoneme is perceived and reproduced as a phoneme against a background of phonemes, that is, the perception of a phoneme occurs only against a background of human speech.

In characterizing the development of children's oral speech, we must point out that it occurs not like written speech, not like the study of a foreign language, but seemingly along a midline between these two types, a line that now becomes apparent. Because he hears the speech of adults, the child has a much broader background of speech than those "figures" that are at his disposal. As soon as a phoneme appears with its phone, analogous structures also appear, that is, perception proceeds structurally.

Mastering the structure of the relation of the phoneme and the phone in one particular case, the child masters the structure as a whole. For example, conjugating any one verb leads to mastery of conjugation rules. K. I. Chukovsky and Markhlevskaya emphasize most strongly the influence of the speech phone and the influence of the semantic aspect of speech on the development of oral speech.

We will summarize.

1. The sound aspect of children's speech develops in direct functional dependence on the semantic aspect of children's speech, that is, it is subordinate to it.

2. The sound aspect of speech functions according to laws of phonological relations, that is, the word may be recognized against a background of other words. For the child in early childhood, sensory speech is the background, that is, the speech of the people around him.

3. Growth and development of speech are connected with differentiation of meanings.

4. The path of development is not the path of development of elements of speech. Each language has different systems according to which types of relations of sound units that have meaning are constructed. The child assimilates the system of their construction. Within it, he masters various types of relations and instantly masters the structure. This explains the spasmodic development of children's speech. The problem of being multilingual may also be considered in this light. The old conviction that if the child assimilates two languages simultaneously, the development of one will interfere with the development of the other has a new elucidation and refutation. It seems that as long as the two languages are assimilated by the child as closed structures and the course of their development does not intersect, they will not interfere with each other. The experiments of Pavlovich and Ilyasevich, in which one language was taught by the mother and another by the father, and neither parent spoke with the child in the language of the other, showed that closed language structures were formed under conditions of a certain type of cooperation, but had no mutual influence that would inhibit all development. This leads to the hypothesis on development of language under conditions of cooperation which are a decisive factor here.

Thus, the subordination of the development of oral speech to the semantic aspect of speech is stressed yet again.

What is the path of development of the semantic aspect of speech? It was believed that the connection "thing—name" was the path, and the fact of personal contact was ignored. Thus, according to Stern, a child at the age of one and a half years discovers the word while a seven-year-old cannot. Criticizing this hypothesis, Bernfeld points to the fact that, according to Stern, the concept arises of itself and we have a closed circle—this is Stern's mistake.

In order to explain how the first syncretic communication is constructed, we must not ignore the real situation of development, the situation of cooperation. K. Bühler and K. Koffka believe the hypothesis that the child discovers the word to be incorrect — he discovers the structural relation. And here is the error. It consists of the rejection of social intercourse, and, of course, in dealing with a thing, its name is irrelevant, the name is a function of communication.

Speech is a means of social intercourse. It arises from the need for means of communication. For the child, only prattling occurs spontaneously. The whole special quality of intercourse is that it is impossible without communication. The only method of intercourse without communication is the indicative (pointing) gesture that precedes speech. Any element of language that the child shares with the adult or obtains from the adult is communication, even if primitive and incomplete, but still communication. At the first stages, it is possible only if the child has a visual image. The child is not in a position to communicate about absent objects and is not in a position to speak about absent objects.

Communication is brought into development by an act of personal contact. The prevalence of passive speech over active is retained over the whole course of childhood. The child learns to understand speech sooner than he learns to communicate. Thus, in assimilating speech, the question is not one of the child's interpreting the word, but of distorted, deformed words from the speech of the adults, that is, of the child's deformed understanding of the adult's speech. This means that the child develops as a social whole, as a social being. But at each age, the meaning of children's words is different, and for this reason, the degree of adequacy of the child's intercourse with the adult changes at each age level. The type of communication in its turn determines the type of intercourse that is possible between the child and the adult. The social situation gives rise to various meanings of words, and these meanings develop. This is the "Ur-wir" of early childhood. Nondifferentiated personal contact breaks up and types of communication change so that the old situation of intercourse comes to an end. The new type of communication requires a new type of intercourse also. The examples of communication in children's autonomous speech, which we gave earlier ("poo-foo") as an example of the indicative functions of communication, shows the limited nature of the circle of possible personal contact with this kind of speech. When communication reaches a certain level of development, the old situation of personal contact abolishes itself, and then we are dealing with a critical age. The conceptions we presented lead to a deeper understanding of the interrelations of the environment and the child in the development of the child's speech. During stable age levels, the social situation (personal contact) does not change, there are only small, molecular changes in *communication*, fine and invisible, which accumulate and result in displacements and crises. Reproduction of the former situation of development from day to day is impossible. The need arises and is realized in a new type of intercourse.

The basic neoformation in early childhood is connected with speech, and because of this, the child is evidently involved in the social environment differently than is the infant, that is, his relation to the social unity of which he himself is a part changes.

In recent years, there has been a reconsideration of the teaching on the development of children's speech. The basic principle according to which the analysis of development of children's speech has been reconstructed is analysis connected with ideal forms, against a background of and in close dependence on ideal forms, that is, on the developed speech of adults. The old teaching on language considered the meaning of the word, overlooking its function as a means of personal contact. Speech was considered outside its social function, as an individual activity of the child. Rich material was accumulated which made extended speech diagnostics possible, but a causal explanation of development remained completely obscure.

Children's speech is not a personal activity of the child, and its disjunction from ideal forms — the speech of the adult— is a major mistake. Only consideration of individual speech as a part of a dialogue, cooperation and communication, provides the key to understanding its changes. Not one problem (grammatization, two-word sentences, etc.) can be explained outside this aspect. Every word of the child, even the most primitive, is part of the whole within which it interacts with the ideal form. The ideal form is the source of the child's speech development.

Such is the genesis of the development of children's speech. We see that the source of the neoformation is closely connected with the relations between the child and adults — in cooperation with them. This, specifically, is what nudges the child onto a new path of communication, to mastering speech, etc. Mastering speech leads to a reconstruction of the whole structure of consciousness.

In order to create yet another point of support for the conclusions, we will now turn to the problem of the relation between perception and a thing.

Human perception is organized according to very complex principles. The first principle consists of constancy, that is, in stability of perception. If you study features of human perception, you will see that the same characteristic traits appear in the development of a number of its aspects. If I look at a match at a certain distance from my eyes, then move it ten times farther away, it would seem that the match must be ten times smaller because its reflection on the retina changes in direct proportion to increase in distance of the object from the eye. Why do I know that a tumbler is smaller than a decanter? Only because these objects are reflected differently on the retina.

An object that is farther away by more than ten times, the match for example, seems to me to be the same size as before. Thus we say that this object preserves constancy of size regardless of the distance to which it is moved, regardless of the different character of the retinal excitation. The biological significance of constancy is extremely great. A mother moving ten steps away melts in the infant's eyes and increases in size by a factor of ten when she comes close again. You understand what that would mean if we retained that kind of perception. Moving about the room, we would see objects becoming larger, then smaller.

The same thing pertains to the position of an object in space. How do I distinguish between a moving object and an object that is immobile? The moving object produces a series of traces at different points on the retina. In this way I realize movement of one object or another. On this basis, when looking out the window of a train, we experience the illusion that everything is moving past us. From the point of view of elementary physics laws, it would have to happen in this way: I turn my head to the right and all the objects that are on my right are also displaced on my retina. If I turned my head to the left, the same thing would happen with the objects that are to my left. The process itself, strictly speaking, occurs in this way. But we perceive it differently.

The same thing might be said with respect to color. E. Hering determined that a piece of coal at midday reflects white rays to the same extent that a piece of chalk does in the evening. This is a very interesting point. But the perception of the color of the coal or the chalk does not depend on the conditions of perception — here we are dealing with constancy of color.

Finally, the constancy of form. We always look at a thing at a certain angle. I do not now see the surface of the table as a rectangle. Every time I look at the table from different points of view, completely different geometric forms will be reflected on the retina; meanwhile I will always perceive the thing from the point of view of a stable form. I can provide a whole series of examples, but they will mainly indicate one and the same thing.

The perception of the size of an object, its color, form, position in space — in the course of development, all of this becomes constant regardless of the conditions of observation. Some investigators try to explain constancy on the basis of properties of perception itself: nerve bundles from the retina to the cortex have both centripetal and centrifugal paths, and the centripetal and centrifugal paths are not motor paths, but participate in the act of perception, that is, the retina is illuminated both externally and internally (O. Pötzl), excitation enters the brain and from there finds its way again to the retina.

Some disturbances in perception can be explained by the fact that centripetal paths are preserved, but centrifugal paths are disrupted, the regulation in the nervous system suffers and the patient begins to perceive as if the perception were done only by the peripheral organs.

This also explains constancy: the retina is illuminated internally — we experience as perceptions the central excitations. Centrifugal paths are myelinated later than the centripetal, and this concludes the development of the process of perception. But the process does not occur in such a way that we perceive colored surfaces and geometric figures separately and then add knowledge to this — and I see that this is a person and that, an object. I see a person and the shape of objects instantly. In a room, I see a lamp, a door, people. This is, of course, interpreted perception. The assumption that interpreted perception is a given from the very beginning is a mistake. The infant does not see, does not perceive instantly the way we do. Only by the age of three does the child's perception approach most closely to the perception of the adult. This approach is produced in all sensible or objective perception. This conception has several meanings. I will allow myself to consider each of them separately, since we will encounter them again, especially when we move on to the preschool age, to play, etc.

I will give an example. There are patients who suffer from a certain disease of the brain — agnosia, that is, loss of meaningful perception. They see objects, but do not recognize them and cannot name them. The patients say: white, cold, slippery, round, but do not know that it is a clock. In contrast to this, our perception cannot see a part of the whole, but always sees the general purpose of the object.

For me, this room breaks down to the perception of separate objects. I see separate objects, but what do I see initially? Their general or their individual characteristics? I say that this is a lamp, this is a cabinet, and at the same time, the perception develops that this is a lamp, etc. This means that perception became a generalized perception. When you see that something is a clock, that means that you perceive not simply the color, the light, the form, but you identify the general traits that are characteristic for the given object. This is a meaningful perception, a generalized perception. It is a classifying of the given object as a certain type of object.

Long before the work of structural psychology, this act itself was not fully understood, but now it seems extremely simple and clear. The basic law of human perception says that our perception is not made up of some elements or others that are later summarized, but is integral. From the points of view of this law, we are speaking of generalized perceptions. The general law of perception says: not one objectively perceived property is isolated, but is always perceived as a part of some kind of whole. Perception of the whole is determined by the nature of that whole of which it is a part.

What does it mean to see only the general? It means to perceive something not as a part of a given structure, but only as a meaningful structure. If we study the perception of the infant, when he is shown two similar things together, it seems that his perception of them is determined as the whole of the structure to which they belong. The following is an experiment of H. Volkelt: you put down a small ring and a large ring; the perception of the infant will change each time depending on what the ring is next to. From this, it is obvious that everything is perceived depending on the visible structure.

Constant perception develops in connection with a number of activities of the child. As the experiment shows, the period to age three is an age of the development of a stable perception of meaning independent of external situations. In this connection, for example, it is necessary to understand the first questions of the child. Most remarkable is the fact that the child suddenly begins to ask. *Suddenly*

— that means that actually, more or less, a turning point occurs. The child begins to ask questions: "What is that? Who is that?"

Meaningful perception is a generalized perception, that is, perception that makes up a part of a more complex structure that is subject to all the basic structural laws. But together with the fact that it makes up a part of a directly visible structure, it simultaneously makes up a part of another structure, a meaningful structure and, for this reason, it is very easy to paralyze this structure of meaning or impede it.

I will give an example. We have before us a puzzle picture. We must find the tiger or the lion, but cannot see it because parts of the body that make up the body of the tiger are at the same time parts of other images in the picture. This is why it is difficult for us to see the tiger. This law was later successfully applied in military camouflage. A German scientist created a whole system of camouflage based on the fact that for military purposes it is important not only to color one piece of armament the color of the locale, but also to place it in such a way that it is a part of another structure. This is one of the best examples of camouflage. I am presenting this as an example of how things may be perceived in various structures depending on how they appear at different visual angles.

A generalized structure is a structure that enters into the structure of generalization. You have a meaningful perception because you recognize the visible structure (that is, you perceive it as a meaningful whole).

As new research shows, the first questions of children evidently are directly connected to the development of meaningful perception of reality, with the development that the world is becoming for the child a world of things that have a certain meaning. How does it become possible to interpret things with the help of human speech, how does interpreted perception develop? It seems to me that the problem has been solved very well in modern psychology in connection with the development of the meaning of the word.

What is the meaning of a word? We have spoken at one time of the various solutions of this problem in associative psychology, in structural psychology, and in the psychology of personalism. Now psychology also solves this problem in different ways, but two positions can be considered as established. The first is that the meaning of a word develops, that the semantic aspect of speech develops, and, second, that there is no simple associative connection, that behind the meaning of the word there are more complex mental processes. What are they? We can name them, saying that every meaning of a word is a generalization, behind every meaning of a word lies a generalization and abstraction. Why? T. Hobbs said that we use the same word to designate different things, that if there were as many words as there things in the world, then everything would have its own name. Since there are more things than words, the child will, willy-nilly, designate various things with one and the same word. In other words, every meaning of a word hides behind itself a generalization, an abstraction. To say this is to solve the problem of the development of the meaning of words in advance. Of course, it is clear in advance that generalization in a child of one and a half and in an adult cannot be the same thing, and for this reason, although a word has acquired meaning to the child and he calls a thing by the same name we do, he generalizes the thing in ways that are different, that is, the structure of his generalization is different.

The development of generalization in mastering speech also leads to the fact that things begin to be seen not only in their situational relation to each other, but also in a generalization that lies behind the word. Here, among other things, the correctness of the dialectical understanding of the process of abstraction is splendidly confirmed. In itself, the process of abstraction and generalization is not an isolation of traits and an impoverishment of the thing, but in generalization, connections of the given object with a number of other objects are established. Because of this, abstraction is richer, that is, the word includes a greater number of connections and ideas of the object than simple perception of the object.

Investigators say: from the history of the development of children's perceptions, we can see that the process of abstraction is a process of enrichment and not of emaciation of traits and properties. What is interpreted perception? In interpreted perception, I see in the object something more than is contained in the direct visual act, and perception of the object is to a certain degree an abstraction; traces of generalizations are contained in the perception.

I have already touched on the idea that every generalization is directly connected with intercourse, that intercourse is possible to the extent that we generalize. In contemporary psychology, the position has been quite clearly noted that was expressed by K. Marx[9] when he said that for man an object exists as a social object. When I speak of one object or another, this means that I not only see the physical properties of the object, but I also generalize the object according to its social purpose.

Finally, the very last: to the extent that the child develops an interest in the people around him, his sociability develops. A very interesting phenomenon develops. If we return to an explanation of the example I gave with respect to the ability of the child to become oriented in a given environment, we said the following. When the child has to sit down on a rock, he cannot do it independently because he does not see the rock. This is due to the fact that the child is capable of acting only with respect to things that he has before him. Hegel cites a similar situation, the sense of which is that animals, unlike people, are slaves to their visual field; they can look only at what catches their eye. They cannot isolate any detail or part if it does not catch their eye. A child in early childhood also is seemingly a slave to his visual field. If you turn on a very strong lamp in one corner of the room and a small lamp in another corner, so that both lamps are in the child's visual field, and try to turn his attention to the small lamp, the infant will not be able to respond to your request. In early childhood, the child cannot look at the small lamp. Thus, at this age, the child perceives visual structures, but not meaningful structures.

It is interesting that only at this age does the child form a stable picture of the world, ordered with respect to objects, for the first time broken up with the help of speech. In early childhood for the first time, there is before the child not the blind play of certain structural fields that was before the infant, but a structurally, objectively formed world; things acquire a certain meaning. This is a period when an objectively formed world has just appeared before the child, this is the source of the child's questions about the meaning of what he sees, and this is why the child finds it so difficult to understand words figuratively. In early childhood, words are not yet very separate from the objects they represent, and the child calls one and the same thing with different words: chair—horse, etc.

I will cite the study of my colleague, N. G. Morozova,[10] who showed that experiments with a child up to three years of age which required changing names of objects were not successful. Let us say that a child of three is given a clock, a bottle, and a pencil and the names of these objects are changed; then, using the new name, the experimenter asks the child to point to or take the object named. What is a fascinating game for the preschooler is not successful with the child in early childhood, since the experimenter is confronted by the child's failure to understand the instructions, and even when the experimenter demonstrates the instruction, the experiment is still unsuccessful.

We studied the ability of the child to understand the symbolic game played out for him and his ability to play out and describe this kind of game. We agreed with the child that the pencil is sick, that this is a house, a garden, a cab, etc. (arbitrarily assigning these names to other objects), and without saying anything, showed the corresponding situation. For a child younger than three, this experiment was not successful. Noticeable success with the most elementary series began at age three years eight months, with the understanding that an easier series may possibly be accessible earlier, but not in early childhood.

As a rule, the active involvement of a child in experimentally renaming objects (which is an easier task for the preschooler) is not possible in early childhood. Thus, this is the age during which the interpreted, objective shaping of the world appears and is fixed, but not the age at which the child can play with meanings and shift them as a preschooler can.

What I am talking about now shows that in early childhood, together with the development of speech, what seems to me to be a most essential positive trait of human consciousness at later stages of development appears, specifically, the interpreted and systemic structure of consciousness. For the child, together with speech, the beginning of interpretation and consciousness of activity around him develops. What I said about perception illustrates this idea well. Perception of geometric figures, on the one hand, and pictures of certain objects, on the other, have different roots. Perception of *Sinn* (meaning) develops not from further development of purely structural qualities, but is in a direct connection with speech and is impossible outside speech.

As systemic construction of consciousness, it seems to me, we should understand the unique relation of separate functions to each other, that is, that at each age level, certain functions are in a certain relation to each other and form a certain system of consciousness.

For early childhood, such an interrelation of separate functions is characteristic so that affectively colored perception is dominant and is at the center of the structure, and all the other functions of consciousness operate around it, leading through affect to action.

Systemic construction of consciousness might arbitrarily be called external construction of consciousness, whereas meaningful construction, the character of generalization, is its internal structure. In connecting generalization with personal contact, we see that generalization acts as a function of consciousness as a whole and not only of thinking alone. All the acts of consciousness are generalization. Such is the microscopic structure of consciousness. In the form of a general thesis, I will say that the change in the system of relations of functions to each other consists of a direct and very close connection with the meaning of words and, specifically, with the result that the meaning of words begins to mediate mental processes. If we consider the meaning of the word that a child of this age uses, we can see that behind the meaning of the child's word is a generalized perception, that is, a structure of that group of objects to which the given object belongs (in contrast to the pointing gesture, which pertains to any or almost any object). The child thinks mainly in generalized perceptions, that is, a general perception is the first active form of the structure of the meaning of the child's word. The generalized perception of objects also makes up the structure of the meaning of the child's word in the first place, which brings us to a very important conclusion: at this age, the child is already talking, and toward the end of the third year, the child speaks well. Material with enormous content is at his disposal, and the child is now no longer dependent only on the visible situation. However, this material still remains concrete material. The vocabulary of the child has few words that do not have a concrete meaning. For this reason, in different situations, the child's word refers to one and the same thing, to a similarly perceived thing or object.

I can give a simple example borrowed from Piaget's observations and experiments.

What does the word mean for the child?

Piaget shows that for the child of this age, different types of meanings for one and the same word are insufficiently differentiated. For example, the word, "nel'zya" [it is impossible, must not, ought not]: it is impossible to light a lamp a second time; that one ought not talk at dinner, that one must not tell mother a lie, that is, all the physical, moral, and other "nel'zya" merge for the child into one and refer to a group of forbidden actions. This means that internally the meaning of these "nel'zya" did not become differentiated. This example shows the extent to which the child interprets the perception of one object or another. The organization of thinking within speech remains meager. The child has no feeling for the separate word. The organization within verbal thinking is fettered by things that are represented by the words and for this reason, for the child, words are not connected with anything except those concrete objects to which they refer. When you ask a child of this age why a cow is called a cow, he replies: "Because it has horns" or "Because it gives milk." If he is asked if a cow could be called something else, he answers that it's impossible. If he is asked if the sun could be called a cow, he will say that this is impossible because the sun is yellow and the cow has horns.

Thus, for the child, the word is a designation either for the object or for a property of the object, which the child has difficulty in separating. This is why from this age to the third year, children's word formations appear that are distortions of words. This occurs not because the child has difficulty with pronouncing or repeating one word or another, but because that is how he interprets the words. Children's words such as "Maselin" (instead of "Vaseline,") "mocress" (instead of "compress") have as their base the indicative feature of children's speech. The word is interpreted together with another leading word ("mokryi + kompress" [wet + compress] or "vazelin + mazat'" [Vaseline + rub]) because it refers to one and the same object. It is natural that although the child is talking at this time, he does not know the word itself. For him, the word itself is a transparent glass through which he looks at what is hidden behind this glass, but does not see the glass itself. Therefore, the organization of the word is extremely difficult. All of the child's speech at this age is completely unconscious. The child speaks, but is not conscious of how he speaks, is not conscious of the process itself, and does not know how to select arbitrarily those words or those sounds that he needs. For example, he pronounces such words as *Moscow* and *Leningrad* easily, but if he is asked to make the sound *sk* or *gr* before the age of three, he cannot do so, although these sounds are not difficult for him because they are a part of a structure of words that he systematically pronounces.

If we try to determine to what extent a child is conscious of a word as such, then we are convinced that only the thing about which we are speaking stands behind the word, and the differentiation between the word and the object has not yet been made the way it is at later age levels.

What is the result of the change in the structure of consciousness? In early childhood, primary generalizations develop that result in a specific type of generalization signifying a certain correlation of functions. How does the child perceive the external world and act in it? Perception is a basic function of this age and matures early. Most important changes in perception occur at this time; it is differentiated from internal experiences, and a relative stability of sizes, forms, etc. appears. The general law of mental development says that the functions that are dominant at this age are in the most favorable conditions. This explains all the changes in perception that occur.

The most essential is the interrelation of meaning and systemic structure of consciousness. The dominance of perception implies a certain nonindependence, a certain dependence, of all other functions on perception.

In light of what has been said, the relation of functions which we indicated previously is understandable. Memory is realized in active perception (in recognizing). It acts as a certain factor in the act of perception itself, being its continuation and development. Attention also occurs through the prism of perception.

Thinking represents a visual-practical restructuring of the situation, of the perceived field. Thinking is developed most strongly in generalization. During this period, the child talks and people talk with him about what he sees. Confronted by things, he names them, and here the connection between these things and the relationship of objects develops. Thus, all functions work within perception. What does this mean for perception itself? We have shown that an interpreted perception does not mean simply combining perception with the activity of thinking, the activity of making generalizations. Perception, turned into a new relationship with thinking, is no longer on the affective-motor plane as Lewin describes it.

It changes in subsequent development. To perceive at an older age will mean to remember, generalize, etc. At this point, memory will correct perception (its orthoscopic quality), and there will be a possibility of movement of structure and background through the function of attention and the categorizing quality of perception, that is, its interpretation. Perception is converted from a function into a complex system that changes subsequently, but its basic traits are acquired at this point. The systemic structure of consciousness elucidates the development of a constant picture of the world. The categorizing quality of perception, perception of an object as a representative of a group of objects, is the second feature, the feature of generalization.

Nonverbal perception gradually is replaced by verbal perception. Objective perception develops in conjunction with naming an object. The infant and the child perceive objects in the room differently. The fact that the child makes a transition from mute perception to verbal perception introduces substantial changes into perception itself. Earlier it was assumed that the function of speech was substitution for an object. Studies have shown that this is a function that develops late, and that the appearance of speech has a different significance. After speech develops, another method of seeing appears — isolating the figure from the background. Speech changes the structure of perception due to generalization. It analyzes what is perceived and categorizes it, signifying a complex logical processing, that is, dividing the object, action, quality, etc. into parts.

What does this system of consciousness mean for internal perception, for introspection? The child's generalization is a generalization of perception. In the internal world, the child is aware of his own perception most of all. He has a quite rich introspection on the plane of visual and aural perception ("I see," "I don't hear very well"). This characterizes his internal activity ("I'll have a look"). Active direction and spontaneous arousal to action of perception — this is the voluntary form of his internal activity. Spontaneous memory and thinking do not yet appear.

The systemic structure of consciousness casts light also on perception of reality, on activity in it, and on relation to oneself. By age three, the child also controls affect, the old social situation of development is inadequate, the child enters the crisis of the third year and a new situation in personal contact is created.

I am inclined to consider the appearance of systemic consciousness, of which I spoke, as a central, characteristic factor in consciousness since specifically for man it is essential that he not simply perceive, but interpret the world, and his consciousness always moves in the plane of something interpreted.

To say that man acts consciously and deliberately is not one and the same thing. For me, this is the basis for proposing that the central neoformation of early childhood is specifically the development of consciousness in the true sense of the word. I think that here for the first time we are definitely confronted by consciousness and those characteristic factors in it that distinguish man from the mental life of animals and from the mental states of man that are not fully conscious and developed. I could recall the words of K. Marx regarding consciousness and its connection with speech[11] not to confirm this point of view, but to introduce a broader theoretical understanding into the context. The aspect of consciousness that Marx has in mind when he calls language practical consciousness, consciousness that exists for others and is meaningful for me — this consciousness itself that he calls a historical product—actually appears together with speech, that is, in any case, when the child begins to interpret in speech both objects and his own activity, when conscious contact with others, not that direct social connection of infancy, is possible.

In other words, it seems to me that early childhood is that stage when meaning and systemic construction of consciousness appear, when historical human consciousness appears, existing for others and, of course, for the child himself. It is that center on the basis of which it is possible to understand all the qualitative features of the relations of the child to the external situation, the relation of the child to connections with other people, and the uniqueness of types of activity which we find here. In other words, it seems to me that this hypothesis, which also has a factual basis in the establishment of meaning and systemic consciousness, elucidates very well all the problems that I tried to present.

In conclusion, I will allow myself to say that since a differentiated system of separate functions first arises in a given structure, the center of which is perception, and since the basis of perception is generalization, objectively we are dealing with the appearance of the very basic features of human consciousness, and this must be considered as one of the neoformations that first arise at this age.

Chapter 10
THE CRISIS AT AGE THREE[1]

We have three points of view which we will use to analyze the crisis at age three.

First we must assume that all changes and all events that happen during the period of this crisis are grouped around some neoformation of a transitional type. Consequently, when we analyze the symptoms of the crisis, we must answer, albeit conditionally, the question as to what it is that is new that appears during the indicated time and what is the fate of the neoformation that disappears after it. Then we must consider what change is occurring in the central and peripheral lines of development. Finally, we must evaluate the critical age from the point of view of the zone of its proximal development, that is, the relation to subsequent growth.

In considering the crisis at age three, we must not proceed only from a theoretical plan. We have no other way than the analysis of factual materials to realize in the process of analysis the basic theories that were developed for elucidating this material. In order to interpret what occurs during the period at age three, we must first of all consider the situation of development—internal and external—in which the crisis is occurring. The consideration must start with the symptoms of the age. The symptoms of crisis that come to the forefront in the literature have been called the first zone of symptoms, or the seven experiences, of the crisis at age three. They are all described as communal concepts and require analysis in order to give them a precise, scientific definition.

The first symptom, which characterizes the onset of the crisis, is the development of *negativism*. We must clearly see what we are talking about here. When people speak of children's negativism, it must be distinguished from ordinary disobedience. In negativism, all of the child's behavior goes contrary to what adults require of him. If the child does not want to do something because it is unpleasant for him (for example, he is playing and is told to go to bed, but he doesn't want to), this is not negativism. The child wants to do what attracts him, for which there is a drive, but he is forbidden to do it; if he does it anyway, this would not be negativism. This would be an act of refusing to acquiesce to the demand of the adults, a reaction that is motivated by the strong wish of the child.

As negativism, we will consider such manifestations in the behavior of the child when he does not want to do something only because an adult told him to, that is, this reaction is not a reaction to the content of an action, but only to the request of adults. As a distinguishing mark from ordinary disobedience, negativism consists in the fact that the child *does not do something because he was asked to*. The child is playing outside and he doesn't want to go in. He is told to go to bed, but he doesn't do it regardless of the fact that his mother asks him to. And if she asked him to do something else, he would do as he pleased. In a reaction of negativism,

283

the child does not do what he is asked to do specifically because he is asked to. What happens here is a unique shift in motivation.

Let me give a typical example of behavior from observations in our clinic. A four-year-old girl with a lingering age-three crisis and clearly expressed negativism wants to be taken to a conference at which children are evaluated. The girl even prepares to go there. I invite the girl. But because I ask her, she will not go at all. She resists with all her might. "Well, then go home." She does not go. "Well, come here." She doesn't come. When she is left in the room, she begins to cry. She is hurt because she was not taken. Thus, negativism forces the child to act *against* her affective wishes. The girl wanted to go, but because she was asked to do so, she would never do it.

In a severe form of negativism, the matter comes to a point where one can get a contrary response to any proposal presented in an authoritative tone. Some authors describe similar experiments beautifully. For example, an adult approaches a child and says in an authoritative tone: "This coat is black," and gets the answer, "No, it's white." And when the statement is: "It's white," the child answers: "No, it's black." The drive to contradict, the drive to do the opposite of what he is asked to do, is negativism in the true sense of the word.

A negative reaction differs from ordinary disobedience in two essential points. First, in this case, *social relations*, relations to another person, are at the forefront. With this kind of action of the child, the reaction is not motivated by the content of the situation itself: does the child want to do what he is asked to do or not. Negativism is an act with a social character: it is addressed primarily to the person and not to the content of what the child is asked to do. The second essential point is the new relation of the child to his own affect. The child does not act directly under the influence of the affect, but acts counter to his tendency. Apropos the relation to affect, I will recall early childhood before the crisis at age three. From the point of view of all studies, most characteristic for early childhood is the complete unity of affect and activity. The child is entirely under the control of affect, entirely within the situation. During preschool age, motive develops as well with respect to other people, which comes directly from affect and is connected with other situations. If the refusal of the child, if the motivation for the refusal is within the situation, if he does not act because he does not want to do what he is asked or wants to do something else, then this still is not negativism. Negativism is the reaction, the tendency, in which the motive is outside the given situation.

The second symptom of the crisis at age three is stubbornness. If we must be able to distinguish negativism from ordinary stubbornness, then we must be able to distinguish stubbornness from persistence. For example, the child wants something and persistently insists that it be done. This is not stubbornness, this occurs even before the crisis at age three. For example, the child wants to have something, but cannot get it immediately. He tries persistently to be given the thing. This is not stubbornness. Stubbornness is the reaction of the child when he insists on something not because he wants it very much, but *because he demands it.* He persists in his demands. Let us say that the child is called to come in from outside; he refuses, he is given reasons that are convincing, but because he has already refused, he does not go in. The motive for stubbornness is the fact that the child is bound by his initial decision. Only this is stubbornness.

Two points distinguish stubbornness from ordinary persistence. The first, like negativism, is related to motivation. If the child insists on what he finds desirable at the time, this will not be stubbornness. For example, he likes to go sledding and for this reason will try to spend the whole day outside.

The second point: if a social tendency is characteristic for negativism, that is, if the child does something contrary to what adults tell him, then in stubbornness, the characteristic tendency is toward himself. We cannot say that the child freely makes a transition from one affect to another; no, he does so only because *he said so* and he sticks by what he said. We have a different relation of motives to the child's own personality than before the onset of the crisis.

A third point is referred to by the German word "Trotz." The symptom is considered to be so central for this age that the whole critical age has been called, "trotz alter," or in Russian, the age of obstinacy.

How does this symptom differ from the first two? Obstinacy differs from negativism in that it is impersonal. Negativism is always directed against an adult who is urging the child to do something or other. Obstinacy is more apt to be directed against norms of rearing established for the child, against the way of life; it is expressed in a unique childish dissatisfaction that evokes a *"da nu!"* [not really!], with which the child responds to everything that he is asked to do. Here an obstinate attitude is apparent not with respect to the person, but with respect to the whole way of life that developed up to the age of three, with respect to norms that are proposed, toward toys that interested him previously. Obstinacy differs from stubbornness in that it is directed outward, with respect to the external, and is evoked by the child's drive to insist on his own way.

It is fully understandable why obstinacy appears as the main symptom of the crisis at age three in authoritarian bourgeois family rearing. Before that, the child was petted and obedient, he was led by the hand, and suddenly, he becomes an obstinate being with whom no one is satisfied. This is contrary to the good, smooth, soft child, this is a being that is always opposed to what is being done with him.

Obstinacy differs from ordinary inadequate complaisance by its tendentiousness. The child rebels and his discontented attitude that evokes the "da nu!" is tendentious in the sense that it actually is permeated with a cryptic revolt against what the child was doing earlier.

Then there is the fourth symptom, which the Germans call "Eigensinn" or *self-will*, willfulness. It consists of a tendency of the child toward independence. This did not exist previously. Now the child wants to do everything himself.

Of the symptoms of the crisis we are analyzing, there are three more, but they are secondary in importance. The first is *protest-rebellion*. Everything in the child's behavior begins to have a protesting character in a number of different manifestations, something that could not exist earlier. The whole behavior of the child acquires traits of protest as if the child found himself in a state of war with those around him, in a constant conflict with them. Frequent, childish arguments with parents are an ordinary matter. Connected with this symptom is devaluation. For example, in a very good family, the child begins to curse. C. Bühler graphically described the horror of a family when the mother heard the child say that she is a fool, something he could not say earlier.

The child tries to devalue a toy, rejects it, and words and terms appear in his vocabulary that represent everything bad, negative, and all of this pertains to things which in themselves cause no unpleasantness. Finally, there is a symptom with two aspects that is manifested differently in different families. In a family with a single child, it occurs as a drive toward *despotism*. The child exhibits a desire to exercise despotic power over those around him. Mother must not leave home, she must sit in the room as he wants her to. He must be given everything he wants: not what he does not want, but what he wants. The child finds a thousand ways to exercise power over those around him. At this point, the child tries to reestablish the state that existed in early childhood when actually all of his wishes were carried out and to become the master of the situation. In a family with several children, this symptom is called the symptom of *jealousy*—with respect to the younger or the older if there are other children in the family. In this case, the same tendency toward control, toward despotism, toward power, appears as the source of a jealous attitude toward the other children.

These are the basic symptoms that color the descriptions of the crisis at age three. Considering these symptoms, it is easy to see that the crisis is manifested mainly in traits that make it possible to recognize in it a kind of rebellion against authoritarian rearing, and it is a kind of protest by the child who wants independence, who has outgrown the norms and form of care that obtained in early childhood. In its typical symptoms, the crisis has such an obvious character of revolt against the care-giver that this strikes all investigators.

In the symptoms indicated, the child acts as a difficult child. The child who caused no worry or difficulty earlier now appears as a being that has become difficult for the adults. Because of this, an impression is created that the child has changed greatly over a short period of time. From the "bebi" carried in arms, he has turned into an obstinate, stubborn, negative, rejecting, jealous, or despotic being so that suddenly his whole appearance in the family is changed.

It is not difficult to see that in all of the symptoms described, there are also some changes in social relations of the child to the people close to him. All of this was established mainly on the basis of material on family rearing, since rearing in early childhood in bourgeois countries exists almost exclusively as a form of individual family rearing. True, we now have various preschool institutions, and in different countries, there are institutions for community care with abnormal forms of philanthropic rearing, but actually the mass experiment of bourgeois rearing in early childhood—in contrast to school—is individual, family rearing. All the symptoms indicate one and the same thing: something changes abruptly in the child's relations with the close, family environment with which he is bound by affective ties, outside which his existence would, up to this point, be unthinkable.

In early childhood, the child is a being who is always under the control of direct, affective relations with those around him to whom he is related. In the crisis at age three, something happens that is called division into two: conflicts can occur here, the child may abuse his mother and may break toys in anger if they are given to him at a bad time; there is a change in the affective-volitional sphere that indicates increased independence and activity of the child. All the symptoms develop around the axis "I" and the people around him. These symptoms indicate that the relations of the child to people around him or to his own personality are changing.

In general, the symptoms taken together create the impression of emancipation of the child: it is as if adults led him by the hand before, but now he has developed a tendency to walk independently. This has been noted by some investigators as the characteristic trait of the crisis. Many times, I have called attention to the idea of Charles Darwin that at the moment the child is born, he is separated from the mother, but neither his feeding nor moving about is possible without the mother. Darwin believes that this is an expression of the child's biological dependence, his biological inseparability (in marsupials, there is a morphological adaptation—the pouch in which offspring are placed after birth). Continuing Darwin's idea, we must say that in early childhood, the child is separated biologically, but psychologically, he is still not separated from the people around him. Beringer provides a basis for saying that up to the age of three, the child is not separated socially from those around him, and during the crisis at age three, we are dealing with a new stage of emancipation.

Now I must, even if briefly, talk about the so-called second layer of symptoms, that is, about the consequences of the basic symptoms, and about their further development. The second layer of symptoms is, in its turn, divided into two groups One group includes the symptoms that are the result of the child's goal of independence. Due to changes in the child's social relations, in his affective sphere, in everything that is most dear and of value to him that affects his strongest, deepest experiences, he is confronted by a series of external and internal conflicts, and we deal very often with neurotic reactions of children. These reactions have the nature of a disease. In neuropathic children, specifically at the crisis at age three, we frequently see the manifestation of neurotic reactions, for example, enuresis, that is, bedwetting. The child, having become accustomed to neatness, in an unfavorable course of the crisis, frequently regresses in this respect to an earlier stage. There are nighttime fears, disturbed sleep, and other neuropathic symptoms and sometimes severe speech impediments, stuttering, sharply increased negativism, stubbornness, so-called hypobulic incidents, that is, unique types of fits that externally resemble accidents, but are actually not painful accidents in the true sense of the word (the child shakes, throws himself on the floor, pounds with his hands and feet), and these are extremely severe traits of negativism, stubbornness, devaluation, and protest, of which we have already spoken.

Allow me to present an example from my own observations of a completely normal child with a very difficult course through the crisis at age three. The child was four years old, the son of a streetcar conductor. He exhibited extreme despotism. Everything that he wanted had to be done precisely. For example, when he walked along the street with his mother, he wanted her to pick up a paper that was lying on the ground, although he did not need the paper at all. The child was brought to us with a complaint about his fits. When his wishes are denied, he throws himself on the floor, begins to scream wildly and pound with his hands and feet. But these are not pathological convulsions, but a form of behavior that some authors evaluate as a regression to the reaction of infancy when the child cries, arms and legs flailing. In the child we were observing, these were incidents of helpless anger when he was not in a state to protest otherwise and made a scene. I am giving this as an example of complications of the crisis at age three that make up the second layer of symptoms: they do not belong to the basic traits of the crisis, but are one link—from the difficult rearing within the family to that state which produces neurotic, psychopathic symptoms.

We will make some theoretical conclusions, that is, we will try to determine what kinds of events occur in the development of the child and what the significance is of the symptoms described. This attempt to present the crisis at age three theoretically is an initial and rough attempt based on certain factual material and on some personal observations (because the crisis is connected with a difficult childhood which I had the opportunity to study) and on certain attempts at critically processing a little of what has been proposed in the theory on these age levels. Our attempt is very preliminary and to a certain degree subjective, and has no pretensions to becoming the theory of critical age levels.

In reviewing the symptoms of the age-three crisis, we have already noted that an internal reconstruction occurs along the axis of social relations. We indicated that the negative reaction that the child of three exhibits must be distinguished from simple disobedience; stubbornness that appears here as a trait of the crisis must also be clearly distinguished from the child's persistence.

1. The negative reaction appears at the moment when the child is neutral with respect to your request, or even when he wants to do what he is asked, but nev-

ertheless refuses. The motive for refusal, the motive for his action, lies not in the content of the activity itself which he is asked to do, but in relations to you.

2. The negative reaction is apparent not in the child's refusal to do something he is asked to do, but in the fact that *you ask him*. For this reason the true essence of the child's negative attitude consists in doing the opposite, that is, in a display of an act of independence of behavior with respect to what he is *asked* to do.

The same thing is true for stubbornness. Mothers complain of difficult children, frequently saying that they are stubborn and persistent. But stubbornness and persistence are different things. If the child wants something very much and persistently tries to get it, this has nothing to do with stubbornness. In stubbornness, the child insists on something that he does not want very much or does not want at all, or has long since stopped wanting in order that the force of his demand be met. The child insists not according to the content of what he wants, but because *he said so*, that is, a social motivation is operating here.

The so-called seven experiences of symptoms of the crisis show that new traits are always connected with the fact that the child's acts begin to be motivated not by the content of the situation itself, but by relations with other people.

If we generalize the actual picture of the crisis at age three, then we cannot but agree with investigators who maintain that the crisis, essentially speaking, occurs mostly as a crisis of the child's social relations.

What is essentially restructured during the crisis? The social position of the child with respect to the people around him and to the authority of the mother and father. There is also a crisis of the personality—of the "I," that is, a series of acts takes place, the motive for which is connected with the development of the child's personality and not with a given, instantaneous desire; motive is differentiated from the situation. To put it more simply, the crisis occurs along the axis of a reconstruction of social interrelations of the child's personality and the people around him.

Chapter 11
THE CRISIS AT AGE SEVEN[1]

School age, like all other age levels, opens with a critical or turning-point period; this was described in the literature as the crisis at age seven before the other age levels were described. It was noted for a long time that in making the transition from preschool to school age, the child changes abruptly and becomes more difficult with respect to rearing than he was previously. This is a kind of transitional stage—he is no longer a preschooler and not yet a school child.

Recently a number of studies on this age have appeared. The results of the studies can be expressed graphically: more than anything, the loss of childlike directness distinguishes the child at seven years of age. The proximate cause of childlike directness is an inadequate differentiation of internal and external life. The experiences of the child, his desires and expressed desires, that is, behavior and activity, usually are an inadequately differentiated whole in the preschooler. In us, this is all very definitely differentiated, and for this reason, the behavior of the adult does not make as direct and naive an impression as the behavior of the child.

When the preschooler enters the crisis, even the most experienced observer is struck by the fact that the child suddenly loses naiveté and directness; in his behavior and in relations with those around him, he becomes less understandable in all aspects than he was formerly.

Everyone knows that the seven-year-old child grows taller rapidly, which indicates a number of changes in the organism. This age is the age during which teeth are replaced and the age of stretching up. Actually the child changes abruptly, and the changes are more profound and more complex than the changes that were observed during the crisis at age three. It would take a long time to enumerate all the symptoms of the crisis under consideration since it is multifaceted. It is sufficient to indicate the general impression that investigators and observers usually convey. I shall elaborate on two traits that are observed in almost all seven-year-olds, especially those who have a difficult childhood and experience the crisis in a concentrated form. The child begins to behave affectedly and capriciously and to behave not as he had previously. Something deliberate, ridiculous, and artificial, some kind of frivolousness, clownishness, and playing the fool appears in his behavior; the child makes himself a jester. Even before the age of seven, the child may play the fool, but at that time, people would not say the same things about him that they would say at this point. Why is this unmotivated clowning so striking? When the child looks at the samovar, on the surface of which he sees a distorted image, or makes faces before a mirror, he is simply playing. But when the child walks into a room with a funny gait, and talks in a squeaky voice, this is not motivated and it is striking. No one is surprised when a preschool child talks nonsense, jokes, plays, but if the child makes a fool of himself and elicits censure and not laughter, this leaves the impression of unmotivated behavior.

The traits indicated point to a loss of the directness and naiveté which were traits of the preschooler. I think that the impression is correct that the external, distinguishing trait of the seven-year-old is the loss of childlike directness and the appearance of oddities that are hard to understand. He exhibits behavior that is somewhat fanciful, artificial, mannered, and forced.

The most essential trait of the crisis at age seven might be called the beginning of the differentiation of the internal and external aspects of the child's personality.

What is concealed behind the impression of naiveté and directness in the child's behavior prior to this crisis? Naiveté and directness indicate that the child is the same inwardly as he is outwardly. The inward quietly makes a transition to the outward, and we regard the one as a disclosure of the other. What kinds of acts do we regard as direct? There is very little childlike naiveté and directness in adults, and if adults exhibit them, they leave a comical impression. For example, the comic actor, Charlie Chaplin, reflects this when, in playing serious people, he begins to behave with unusual childlike naiveté and directness. This is the main point of his comedy.

The loss of directness signifies the introduction of the intellectual factor into our acts, and this wedges itself between experience and the direct act, which is the direct opposite of the naive and direct action proper to the child. This does not mean that the crisis at age seven leads from direct, naive, nondifferentiated experience to the opposite pole, but only that a certain intellectual factor appears in each experience, in each of its manifestations.

One of the most complex problems of contemporary psychology and psychopathology of the personality, which I will try to elucidate with an example, is the problem that might be called experience of meaning.

I will try to approach this problem using the analogy to the problem of external perception. Then it will be clearer. The essential distinction of human perception is its intelligence and its objectivity. We realize the perceived complex of impressions simultaneously and together with external impressions. For example, I see immediately that this is a clock. In order to comprehend the characteristic of human perception, we must compare it with the perception of a patient who has lost this characteristic as a result of a nervous brain disease. If such a patient is shown a clock, he will not recognize it. He sees the clock, but does not know what it is. When you begin to wind the clock, or place it to your ear to see whether it is running, or look at it to see what time it is, the patient will say what it is, that it is a clock. He guesses that what he sees is a clock. For you and for me, what we see and the fact that it is a clock is a single act of realization.

Thus, perception does not occur separately from visual thinking. The process of visual thinking is done in unity with intellectual designation of the thing. When I say: this thing is a clock and then see some other kind of clock on a tower that does not resemble the first clock at all, but is also called a clock, this means that I perceive this thing as a representative of a certain class of things, that is, I generalize them. In short, a generalization is made in each perception. To say that our perception is intellectual perception is to say that all of our perception is generalized perception. This may be elucidated as follows: if I should look at a room without generalizing, that is, look the way an agnostic or an animal might, then the impressions of the things would appear in relation to each other as they appear in the visual field. But since I generalize them, I perceive the clock not only within the structure of the things that are together with it, but also within the structure of what a clock is, within the structure of the generalization in which I see it.

The development of intellectual perception in man may be compared to how a child sees a chessboard or plays on it while just learning, but not knowing how to play. The child, not knowing how to play, may amuse himself with the chess pieces, sort them according to color, etc., but the movement of the pieces will not be structurally determined. The child who learned to play chess will proceed differently. For the first child, the black knight and the white pawn have no connection with each other, but the second child, knowing the moves of the knight, understands that an attacking move by the knight threatens his pawn. For him, the knight and the pawn are a unit. In precisely this way, a good player can be distinguished from a poor player by the fact that he sees the chess field differently.

An essential trait of perception is structural quality, that is, perception is not made up of separate atoms, but represents an image within which there are various parts. Depending on what the position of the pieces on the chessboard is, I see it differently.

We perceive surrounding reality the way a chess player perceives a chessboard: we perceive not only the neighborhood of the objects or their contiguity, but also the whole reality with its intellectual connections and relations. In speech, there are not only names, but also meanings of objects. Quite early, the child develops the ability to express in speech not only the meanings of objects, but also his own actions and the actions of others and his own internal states ("I'm sleepy," "I'm hungry," "I'm cold"). Speech as a means of communication leads to naming and connecting our internal states to words. However, the connection to words never signifies the formation of a simple associative connection, but always signifies a generalization. Every word signifies more than one thing. If we say that it is cold now, and can say the same thing a day later, this means that every single feeling of cold has also been generalized. Thus, a generalization of an internal process is developed.

In an infant, there is no intellectual perception: he perceives a room but does not separately perceive chairs, a table, etc.; he will perceive everything as an undivided whole in contrast to the adult, who sees figures against a background. How does a child perceive his own movements in early childhood? He is happy, unhappy, but does not know that he is happy, just as an infant when he is hungry does not know that he is hungry. There is a great difference between feeling hunger and knowing that I am hungry. In early childhood, the child does not know his own experiences.

At the age level of seven years, we are dealing with the onset of the appearance of a structure of experience in which the child begins to understand what it means when he says: "I'm happy," "I'm unhappy," "I'm angry," "I'm good," "I'm bad," that is, he is developing an intellectual orientation in his own experiences. Precisely as a three-year-old child discovers his relation to other people, a seven-year-old discovers the fact of his own experiences. Because of this, certain features characterizing the crisis at age seven appear.

1. Experiences acquire meaning (an angry child understands that he is angry), and because of this, the child develops new relations to himself that were impossible before the generalization of experiences. As on a chessboard, where completely new connections between the pieces develop with each move, so here also completely new connections appear between experiences when they acquire a certain sense. Consequently, the whole character of experiences of the child is reconstructed at the seventh year the way the chessboard was when the child learned to play chess.

2. Generalizations of experiences or affective generalization, logic of feelings, appears at the beginning of the crisis at age seven. There are deeply retarded children who experience failure at every step: normal children play, the abnormal child tries to join them, but they reject him and he goes along the street and is laughed

at. In a word, he loses at every step. In each separate case, he has a reaction to his own inadequacy, but after a minute, you will see—he is completely satisfied with himself. A thousand separate failures, and there is no general sense of his worthlessness, he does not generalize what happened many times. In a school-age child, there is generalization of feelings, that is, if this kind of situation had happened to him many times, an affective formation would have developed, the character of which would relate to a single experience or affect the way understanding relates to a single perception or recollection. For example, a preschool child has no real self-evaluation, self-love. The level of our demands of ourselves, of our success, of our position, arises specifically in connection with the crisis at age seven.

A child of preschool age likes himself, but self-love as a generalized relation to himself which remains constant in various situations, self-evaluation as such, generalized relations to those around him and understanding his own value, is something a child of this age does not have. Consequently, toward the seventh year, a number of complex formations develop that lead to an abrupt and radical change in the difficulties of behavior that are fundamentally different from the difficulties of the preschool age.

Neoformations such as self-love and self-evaluation remain, but the symptoms of the crisis (affectation, posing) are transitional. In the crisis at age seven, because of the fact that a differentiation of the internal and external develops and intellectual experience first appears, a sharp conflict of experiences also develops. The child who does not know which candy to choose—the bigger or the sweeter—finds himself in a state of internal conflict even as he vacillates. The internal conflict (contradiction of experiences and selection of his own experiences) becomes possible only at this time.

There are typical forms of difficulties in rearing that are never encountered during the preschool age. These include conflicts and contradictory experiences, unresolved contradictions. As a matter of fact, where this internal division of experiences is possible, where first the child understands his experiences, where internal relations arise, there also occurs a change in experiences indispensable for the school-age level. To say that in the crisis at age seven, preschool experiences change to school experiences, is to say that a new unity of environmental and personal factors has appeared that makes the new stage of development possible—school age. For the child, his relation to the environment has changed, and this means that the environment itself has changed, it means that the course of the child's development has changed and that a new period in development has started.

It is necessary to introduce into science a concept, little used in the study of the social development of the child: we have studied inadequately the internal relation of the child to those around him, and we have not considered him as an active participant in the social situation. We admit in words that it is necessary to study the personality and the environment of the child as a unit. But we must not think that the influence of the personality is on one side and the influence of the environment, on the other, that the one and the other act the way external forces do. However, exactly this is actually done frequently: wishing to study the unity, preliminarily investigators break it down, then try to unite one thing with another.

Even in the study of difficult childhood, we cannot go beyond the limits of this formulation of the question: what played the main role, constitution or environmental conditions, psychopathic conditions of a genetic character or conditions of external circumstances of development? This brings us to two basic problems that must be elucidated on the plane of the internal relation of the child to the environment during the periods of crises.

The first principal inadequacy in practical and theoretical study of the environment is that we study the environment in its absolute characteristics. Whoever is involved in practical study of difficult cases knows this very well. You are given a social, life-style investigation report on the child's environment in which the cubic capacity of the living area is explained, whether the child has his own bed, how many times he goes to the bath house, when he changes his underwear, whether the family reads papers, and what the mother's and father's education was. The investigation is always the same, regardless of the child and his age. We study some absolute indicators of the environment as circumstances, trusting that knowing these indicators, we will know their role in the development of the child. Some Soviet scientists have made a principle of this absolute study of the environment. In a textbook edited by A. B. Zalkind, you will find a statement that the social environment of the child remains basically unchanged over the whole course of his development. Keeping in mind the absolute indicators of the environment, we can agree with this to a certain degree. In actual fact, this is completely false from both the practical and theoretical points of view. Of course, the essential difference between the child's environment and that of an animal is that the human environment is a social environment, that the child is a part of a living environment and that the environment never is external to the child. If the child is a social being and his environment is a social environment, then it follows from this that the child himself is a part of this social environment.

Consequently, the most essential turn-around that must be made in the study of the environment is the transition from absolute to relative indicators; the environment of the child must be studied: most of all, we must study what it means for the child, what the child's relation to the separate aspects of this environment is. Let us say that the child does not talk before he is a year old. When he starts to talk, the speech environment of those around him remains unchanged. And for the year before and the year after, in absolute indicators, the speech culture of those around him did not change at all. But I think that everyone will agree that from the minute the child began to understand the first words, when he began to pronounce the first deliberate words, his relation to speech factors in the environment, the role of speech in relation to the child changed a great deal.

Every step in his movement changes the influence of the environment on the child. From the point of view of development, the environment becomes entirely different from the minute the child moves from one age level to another. Consequently, we may say that perception of the environment must change in the most substantial way in comparison with the way we have usually treated it in practice thus far. The environment must be studied not as such, not in its absolute indicators, but in relation to the child. An environment that is the very same in absolute indicators is completely different for a child at age one, three, seven, or twelve. Dynamic change in the environment, its relation, is brought to the forefront. But, naturally, where we speak of relation, another factor develops: the relation is never purely external relation between the child and the environment taken separately. One of the important methodological problems is the problem of how the study of unity is really approached in theory and in research. Unity of personality and environment, unity of mental and physical development, and unity of speech and thinking are spoken of frequently. What does it really mean in theory and in research to approach the study of some unity and all properties that are pertinent to this unity as such? It means finding the principal unity every time, that is, finding the proportions in which the properties of the unity as such are combined. For example, when the relation of speech and thinking is studied, speech is artificially separated from thinking and thinking from speech, and then the question is raised as to what speech does for thinking and thinking for speech. The matter is presented in this way, as if these were two different liquids that could be mixed. If you want to know how a unity developed, how it changes, how it affects the course of the child's development, it is important not to break down the unity into its component parts because when this is done, the essential properties of specifically this unity are lost; the unity, for example, in the relation of speech and thinking, must be taken as a unity. Recently, an attempt has been made to isolate such a unity; take meaning, for example. Meaning of a word is a part of the word, a speech formation, because a word without meaning is not a word. Since all meaning of a word is a generalization, it is a product of the intellectual activity of the child. Thus, the meaning of a word is a unity of speech and thinking that cannot be broken down further.

A unity can be noted in the study of personality and environment. This unity in psychopathology and psychology has been called experience. The child's experience is also this kind of very simple unity about which we must not say that in itself it represents the influence of the environment on the child or the individuality of the child himself; experience is the unity of the personality and the environment as it is represented in development. Thus, in development, the unity of environmental and personality factors is achieved in a series of experiences of the child. Experience must be understood as the external relation of the child as a person to one factor or another of reality. All experience is always experience of something. There is no experience that would not be experience of something just as there is no act of consciousness that would not be an act of being conscious of something. But every experience is my experience. In modern theory, experience is introduced as a unity of consciousness, that is, a unity in which the basic properties of consciousness are given as such, while in attention and in thinking, the connection of consciousness is not given. Attention is not a unity of consciousness, but is an element of consciousness in which there is no series of other elements, while the unity of consciousness as such disappears, and experience is the actual dynamics of the unity of consciousness, that is, the whole which comprises consciousness.

Experience has a biosocial orientation; it is what lies between the personality and the environment that defines the relation of the personality to the environment, that shows what a given factor of the environment is for the personality. Experience is determining from the point of view of how one environmental factor or another affects the child's development. This, in any case, is confirmed at every step in the teaching on difficult childhood. Any analysis of a difficult child shows that what is essential is not the situation in itself taken in its absolute indicators, but how the child experiences the situation. In one and the same family, in one family situation, we find different changes in development in different children because different children experience one and the same situation differently.

Consequently, on the one hand, in experience, environment is given in its relation to me, how I experience this environment; on the other hand, features of the development of my personality have an effect. My experience is affected by the extent to which all my properties and how they came about in the course of development participate here at a given moment.

To state a certain, general, formal position, it would be correct to say that the environment determines the development of the child through experience of the environment. Most essential, therefore, is rejection of absolute indicators of the environment; the child is a part of the social situation, and the relation of the child to the environment and the environment to the child occurs through experience and activity of the child himself; the forces of the environment acquire a controlling significance because the child experiences them. This mandates a penetrating internal analysis of the experiences of the child, that is, a study of the environment which is transferred to a significant degree to within the child himself and is not reduced to a study of the external circumstances of his life.

Analysis becomes very complex, and we are confronted here with tremendous theoretical difficulties. Nevertheless, with respect to separate problems of development of character, critical age levels, and difficult childhood, separate factors connected with the analysis of experiences become somewhat more clear and visible.

Careful study of the critical age levels shows that changes in the child's basic experiences occur in them. The crisis is most of all a turning point that is expressed in the fact that the child passes from one method of experiencing the environment to another. The environment as such does not change for the child at the age of three. The parents continue to earn as much as they did before, and for every mouth there is the same budgeted minimum and maximum as before, there are subscriptions to the same number of papers as before, underwear is changed as frequently as before, the living area is the same, and the parents have not changed their relations to the child. Observers who study the crisis say that without any reason, the child who behaved so well, was obedient and affectionate, is suddenly capricious, bad and stubborn.

All bourgeois investigators emphasize the internal character of the crisis. Most of them explain the internal character of the crisis with biological causes. One of the most widespread theories for explaining the crisis at age thirteen is that there is a parallel between sexual maturation and the crisis, and internally established biological maturation of the child is seen as the basis of the crisis.

Other authors, like A. Busemann, who want to emphasize the significance of the social environment, correctly point to the fact that the crisis may have a completely different course depending on the environment in which it occurs. But Busemann's point of view does not differ essentially from the point of view that considers the crisis as a phenomenon due to purely exogenous causes. Busemann considers the crisis, like all features in the child not established as biological features, as a manifestation of changes in a changed environment. The idea arises that bourgeois research is wholly incorrect, or incorrect to some extent at least. Let us start with the factual aspect. It seems to me that the bourgeois investigators have a very limited range of observations, that is, they always observe the child in conditions of the bourgeois family with a certain type of rearing. Facts show that in other conditions of rearing, the crisis occurs differently. In children who go from nursery school to kindergarten, the crisis occurs differently than it does in children who go into kindergarten from the family. However, the crisis occurs in all normally proceeding child development; the age of three and the age of seven will always be turning points in development: there will always be a state of things where the internal course of the child's development will conclude a cycle, and the transition to the next cycle will necessarily be a turning point. One age level is reconstructed in some way in order to allow a new stage of development to begin.

The observers' most general, naive impression that the child has somewhat suddenly, unrecognizably changed is correct: over the course of three to six months, the child has become different from what he was before; the crisis passes as a process that is little understood by those around the child since it is not connected with changes that occur around the child. To put it more simply, the crisis is a chain of internal changes of the child with relatively insignificant external changes. For example, when the child enters school, he changes over the course of school age from year to year, and this does not surprise us since the whole situation in which the child grows, all the circumstances of his development, change. When the child moves from nursery school to kindergarten, it does not surprise us that the preschooler changes, and here the changes of the child are connected with the changes that occur in the conditions of his development. But essential to every crisis is the fact that the internal changes occur in a much greater dimension than the changes in the external circumstances, and for this reason they always cause impressions of an internal crisis.

It is my impression that the crises actually have an internal source and consist in changes of an internal nature. There is no precise correspondence here between external and internal changes. The child enters the crisis. What has changed so abruptly outwardly? Nothing. Why has the child changed so abruptly in such a short time?

Our idea is that we must object not to the bourgeois theories of the critical age levels, or the idea that the crisis is a very profound process interwoven into the course of the child's development, but we must object to the understanding of the internal nature itself of the process of development. If, in general, everything that is internal in development is understood as biological, then of necessity, it will be the change in glands of internal secretion. In this sense, I would not call the critical ages the ages of internal development. But I think that internal development always occurs in such a way that there is a unity of personality and environmental factors, that is, every new step in development is directly determined by the preceding step, by all that has already happened and appeared in development at the preceding stage. True, this means that development must be understood as a process where all subsequent change is connected with what went before and with the present in which the features of personality that have developed previously are now manifested and now act. If we understand the nature of the internal process of development correctly, then there will be no theoretical objections to understanding the crisis as an internal crisis.

It seems to me that behind every experience, there is a real, dynamic action of the environment with respect to the child. From this point of view, the essence of every crisis is a reconstruction of the internal experience, a reconstruction that is rooted in the change of the basic factor that determines the relation of the child to the environment, specifically, in the change in needs and motives that control the behavior of the child. Growth and change in needs and motives are the least conscious and least voluntary part of the personality, and in the transition from age level to age level, new incentives and new motives develop in the child; in other words, the motive forces of his activity undergo a reevaluation. That which was essentially important, controlling, for the child becomes relative and unimportant at the subsequent stage.

The restructuring of needs and motives and the reevaluation of values are basic factors in the transition from age level to age level. Here, the environment also changes, that is, the relation of the child to the environment. Other things begin to interest the child, he develops other activity, and his consciousness is restructured, if we understand consciousness as the relation of the child to the environment.

EPILOGUE

1

Lev Semenovich Vygotsky was first of all a specialist in the area of general psychology and a methodologist in psychology. He saw as his scientific vocation the construction of a scientific system of psychology, the basis of which would be dialectical and historical materialism. The historical method and systemics are the main principles of his approach to studying psychological reality and especially consciousness and its specifically human forms. He mastered Marxism and its method in the course of his own theoretical and experimental research, constantly turning to the works of Marxist-Leninist classics. Specifically because of this, Marxism, historical materialism, and dialectics are so organic in the works of Vygotsky.

L. S. Vygotsky took only the first, most difficult steps in the new direction, leaving a number of interesting hypotheses for future investigators and, what is the main thing, the historical method and systemics in the study of problems of psychology, which is the principle according to which almost all of his theoretical and experimental studies are constructed.

Sometimes we come upon the opinion that Vygotsky was the main exponent of child psychology. This opinion is based on the fact that he and his colleagues did most of the major experimental studies working with children. True, almost all the studies are connected with the construction of a theory of development of higher mental functions, experimentally carried out with children, including one of the basic books published immediately after Vygotsky's death, *Thinking and Speech* (1934). But it does not follow from this that in the studies mentioned, Vygotsky acted as a child psychologist. The basic subject of his research was the history of the origin, development, and disintegration of specific human higher forms of activity of consciousness (its functions). He was the creator of a method, which he himself called an experimental-genetic method; by this method, neoformations are brought to life or experimentally created—psychological processes that did not exist—and in this way, an experimental model of their origin and development is created and patterns of this process are revealed. In this case, children are the most suitable material for creating an experimental model of development of neoformations, but not the subject of research. To study the disintegration of these processes, Vygotsky used special studies and observations in neurological and psychiatric clinics. His work on the development of higher mental functions does not pertain to the area of child (developmental) psychology proper in the same way that a study of disintegration pertains to the area of psychopathology.

We must emphasize very firmly that specifically Vygotsky's general theoretical studies served as the basis on which he developed his special studies in the area of child (developmental) psychology proper.

297

Vygotsky's path in child psychology was not simple. He approached the problems of child (developmental) psychology mainly from demands of practice (before undertaking psychology, he was a teacher, and problems of pedagogical psychology interested him even before he devoted himself to the solving of general questions in psychology).

L. S. Vygotsky not only carefully followed the changes that occurred in the course of the construction of the Soviet system of education and rearing, but, as a future member of the GUSa,[1] he also took an active part in its construction. There is no doubt that the resolution of problems of teaching and development played an important role in the formation of the author's general psychological views and was the most direct form connected with the radical reconstruction of the system of education that followed the decree of the TsK VKP(b) [Central Committee of the All-Union Communist Party of the Bolsheviks] "On the Primary and Middle School," 1931, and determined the transition from a complex to a subject system of teaching in school.

One cannot understand Vygotsky's deep interest in problems of child (developmental) psychology if one does not also take into account the fact that he was a theoretician and, what is especially important, a practitioner in the area of anomalous mental development. For many years, he was the scientific director of a number of studies done at the Experimental-Defectology Institute (EDI) and systematically took a leading role in consultations with children. Hundreds of children with various deviations in psychological development were the subjects of the consultations. Vygotsky considered the analysis of every case of one anomaly or another as a concrete expression of some general problem. As early as 1928, he published a paper, "Defect and Overcompensation," in which he presented a systemic analysis of the anomaly of mental development; in 1931, he wrote a major work, "Diagnostics of Development and the Pedological Clinic for Difficult Childhood" (published in 1936, Vol. 5, pp. 257-321), in which he analyzed critically and in detail the state of diagnostics of that time and noted paths for its development.

The strategy of his studies was constructed in such a way that purely methodological problems of psychology and problems of the historical origin of human consciousness—its structure, ontogenetic development, and anomalies in the process of development—were combined into one whole. Vygotsky himself frequently called this combination the unity of genetic, structural, and functional analysis of consciousness.

2

The works of L. S. Vygotsky on child (developmental) psychology included the term "pedology" in the titles. In his understanding, this was a special science of the child, part of which was child psychology. Vygotsky himself began his scientific life and continued it to the very end as a psychologist. Specifically methodological problems of psychology as sciences were at the center of both his theoretical and experimental studies. His studies pertaining to the child also had an essentially psychological character, but during the period of his scientific work, problems of the psychological development of the child pertained to pedology. He wrote: "Pedology is the science of the child. The subject of its study is the child, the natural whole that, despite what is an exceptionally important object of theoretical knowledge,

[1]State Scientific Council—Methodological Center of the People's Commissariat of Education (1919-1932).

like the world of stars and our planet, is, nevertheless, an object of the influence of teaching and rearing which pertain specifically to the child as a whole. This is why pedology is a science of the child as a single whole" (*Pedology of the Adolescent*, 1931, p. 17).

Here Vygotsky, like many pedologists, makes a methodological mistake. Sciences cannot be divided into separate objects. But this is a problem of the study of science, and we will not deal with it.

At the center of Vygotsky's attention was explaining the basic patterns of the mental development of the child. In this respect, he did tremendous critical work on a review of the views of the process of mental development that dominated foreign child psychology and influenced the views of Soviet pedologists. In its scope and significance, this work is similar to that which Vygotsky carried out and organized on methodological problems in psychology, published for the first time in the present Collection of Works in the treatise, "The Historical Meaning of the Crisis in Psychology" (Vol. 1, pp. 291-436). Unfortunately, Vygotsky himself did not succeed in collecting his theoretical studies on the problem of mental development in a special work, but left only its fragments contained in critical introductions to books by K. Bühler, J. Piaget, K. Koffka, and A. Gesell, and in his previously unpublished manuscripts and lectures. (Shorthand transcriptions of some lectures are published in this volume; introductions to books by Bühler and Koffka were published in Vol. 1; a critical analysis of the concepts of Piaget was a substantial part of the book *Thinking and Speech*, published in Vol. 2).

Resolving the central problem of child psychology—the problem of driving forces and conditions of mental development during childhood, the development of consciousness and personality of the child—was merged for Vygotsky into a single whole with his general methodological research. Even in his early works on the development of higher mental functions, he formulated the hypothesis of their origin and, consequently, of their nature. There are many such formulations. We will present only one of them: "Every mental function was external because it was social before it became one's own internal mental function; it was first a social relation of two people."

Even in this hypothesis, dating back to 1930-1931, there is a completely different representation of the role of the social environment in development: interaction of the child with reality, mainly social, with an adult, is not a factor of development, not what acts from outside on what is already there, but is a source of development. This, of course, was not in any way connected with the theory of the two factors (which are the basis of the pedology contemporaneous with Vygotsky) according to which the development of the organism and the mind of the child are determined by two factors, heredity and environment.

The problem of the driving causes of development could not but be at the center of Vygotsky's scientific interests. Having considered the different points of view that existed in psychology in other countries, he evaluated them critically. Vygotsky espoused the position of Blonsky when Blonsky indicated that heredity is not a simple biological phenomenon: we must distinguish the social heredity of the conditions of life and social position from the chromatin of heredity. On the basis of social, class heredity, dynasties are also formed. Vygotsky continues the idea: "Possible only on the soil of the deepest mixing of biological and social heredity are such scientific misunderstandings as the positions of K. Bühler on the inheritance of 'criminal inclinations,' Peters' heredity of good marks in school, and Galton's heredity of ministry and judicial posts and the learned professions. For example, a hereditary biological trait passed on from forebears to progeny with the same regularity as a certain eye color could be used instead of analysis of socioeconomic factors that promote criminality, a purely social phenomenon—the product of social inequality and exploitation.

"Under the aegis of merging social and biological heredity, there is also bourgeois eugenics, a new science related to improving and revitalizing the human race by attempting to control the laws of heredity and subjecting them to its power" (*Pedology of the Adolescent*, p. 11).

In the introduction to A. Gesell's book, *Pedology of Early Childhood* (1932), Vygotsky presents a more solidly based criticism of the theories of development that were widely represented in bourgeois child psychology of that time.

Vygotsky has a high regard for Gesell's studies because they "contain, in a consistent and undeviating pursuit, the idea of development as the only key to all the problems of child psychology. . . . But as to the very basic problem, the key problem—the problem of development—Gesell solves things halfway . . . The stamp of duality on these studies is the stamp of methodological crisis being experienced by science, which in its factual studies outgrew its methodological bases" (see A. Gesell, 1932, p. 5). (We note that Gesell's book, entitled *Pedology of Early Childhood*, is considered by Vygotsky to be a book on child psychology, that is, pertaining to the solution of questions of the mental development of the child.)

Emphasizing what was said with an example, Vygotsky continues: "With the higher genetic law, Gesell formulates the basic idea of his book, and this is evidently the following: *all growth in the present is based on growth in the past. Development is not a simple function determined by X units of heredity plus Y units of environment; it is a historical complex that reflects at each given stage the past that is included in it.* In other words, the artificial dualism of environment and heredity leads us to a false path; it hides from us the fact that development is a continuous self-promoted process and not a marionette controlled by pulling two strings" (ibid.).

Vygotsky continues: "We must look attentively at how Gesell represents the comparative sections of development in order to be convinced that this is a kind of series of still photographs from which the main thing is absent—there is no *movement*, to say nothing of self-movement, there is no process of transition from stage to stage and *no development itself* even in the sense that the author himself theoretically deduced as being obligatory. How the transition is made from one level to another, what the internal connection is between one stage and another, how growth in the present is based on preceding growth—specifically, none of this is demonstrated" (ibid., p. 6).

We believe that all of this is the result of the purely quantitative understanding of the processes themselves of development and the method used by Gesell to study them, the method which entered the history of child psychology as the method of sections, which is, unfortunately, dominant thus far. Gesell considers the process of child development approximately as he considers the movement of a body, for example, the movement of a train along a certain segment of track. The measure of such movement is velocity. For Gesell, the basic index for development is always the rate of development over a certain interval of time, and the law based on this consists of a gradual deceleration. It is greatest at the initial stages and least at the final stages. Gesell seems to eliminate the problem of environment and heredity in general and replaces it with the problem of rate or tempo of growth or development. (Gesell uses the latter two concepts as synonymous.)

However, as Vygotsky shows, behind this replacement is hidden a certain solution to the problem nevertheless. It is uncovered when Gesell considers the specifics of the human in child development. As Vygotsky notes, Gesell categorically rejects the line of theoretical studies generated by Bühler, permeated with tendencies of zoomorphism, that consider the whole period of child development from the point of view of an analogy to the behavior of the chimpanzee.

In a critical note, analyzing the child's primary sociability proclaimed by Gesell, Vygotsky shows that Gesell, however, understands this same sociability as a special biology. Vygotsky writes: "More than that: the very process of personality formation that Gesell considers as the result of social development, he reduced, in essence, to purely biological and purely organic, consequently, to zoological processes of connection between the organism of the child and the organisms of the people around him. Here the biologism of American psychology reaches its apogee, here it celebrates its greatest triumph, gains its latest victory: *discovering the social as simply a variety of the biological.* A paradoxical situation develops in which the highest evaluation of the social in the process of child development is admitting the initially social character of the process and disclosing the social as the habitat of the secret of human personality—all of this is a somewhat pompous hymn in honor of the sociability required only for the greater celebration of the biological principle that, due to this, acquires a universal, absolute, almost metaphysical significance designated as the 'life cycle.'

"And, guided by this principle, Gesell begins, step by step, to take back for the biological what he himself had just given to the social. This understandable theoretical movement is accomplished along a very simple scheme: *the personality of the child from the very beginning is social, but sociability itself consists in nothing other than the biological interaction of organisms.* Sociability does not lead us beyond the limits of biology; it leads even deeper into the core of the 'life cycle'" (ibid., p. 9).

L. S. Vygotsky indicates that in the works of Gesell, removing the dualism of heredity and environment "*is attained by biologizing the social, by reducing to a common denominator both the hereditary and social factors in the development of the child.* Unity this time is frankly purchased for the price of a complete dissolving of the social in the biological" (ibid., p. 11).

Summarizing the critical analysis of Gesell's theory, Vygotsky describes it as empirical evolutionism: "It cannot be called anything else except the *theory of empirical evolutionism.* From the theory of evolution, from a somewhat changed teaching of Darwin, are deduced both the philosophy of nature and the philosophy of history. The principle of evolution appears to be universal. This is obvious in two factors: first, in the extension of natural limits of application of this principle, indicated above, and extending its meaning to the whole area of formation of the child's personality; second, in the very understanding and disclosure of the nature of development. Typically, the evolutionistic understanding of this process is the nucleus of the antidialectics of all the constructs of Gesell. He seems to repeat the known antidialectical law of Bühler, which he recently advanced in application to child psychology: 'Nature is not spasmodic. Development always occurs gradually.' From this comes the lack of understanding of what is basic in the process of development: *the appearance of neoformations.* Development is considered as the realization and modification of hereditary properties" (ibid., p. 12).

Vygotsky continues: "After all that has been said, is it necessary to speak of the fact that Gesell's theoretical system is inseparably connected with the whole methodology of the critical period that bourgeois psychology is now experiencing and in this way is opposed, as has already been said, to dialectical-materialistic understanding of the nature of the child's development? Is it necessary to speak further of the fact that this ultrabiologism, this empirical evolutionism in the teaching on the development of the child that subjects the whole course of the child's development to the eternal laws of nature and does not leave room for understanding the class nature of child development in a class society, itself has a completely determined class sense, closely tied to the teaching on class neutrality of childhood, with essentially reactionary tendencies toward discovery of the 'always of the child' (in the expression of another psychologist), with the tendencies of bourgeois pedagogy to mask the class nature of rearing? 'Children—always children'—as Gesell himself expresses this idea of his on the child in general, of the 'always of the child' in the introduction to the Russian translation of another of his books. In this universality of the traits of childhood, he says, we see the reflection of so much promise for the future of the beneficial solidarity of the whole human race" (ibid., p.13).

We have considered in such detail Vygotsky's critical appraisal of Gesell's theory for two reasons: first, the critique of Gesell's theory is an excellent example of how Vygotsky analyzed theoretical concepts of development, how he was able to disclose the real methodological sources of theoretical errors behind the outward appearance and phraseology which at first glance seemed to be true; second, the critique of Gesell's theoretical views even today sounds very contemporary in comparison with the theories of American child psychology, in which much is said about the social and its role in the development of the child.

3

We stress: Vygotsky did not leave a definitive theory of mental development. He simply did not have time, although in the last months of his life, he tried to do so.

In the fifty years since Vygotsky's death, much has changed in both world and Soviet child psychology. Many facts to which Vygotsky refers have become obsolete and new facts have appeared. Theories existing in his time have been replaced by new concepts that require critical consideration. Nevertheless, thorough knowledge of the enormous work that Vygotsky did is of more than historical interest. His work contains a method of approach to the study of mental development and to the theoretical concepts of development, and, if we may say so, "prolegomena" for future scientific theory of mental development.

When he lived and even after death, Vygotsky was sometimes reproached with the fact that foreign psychologists influenced him greatly. Vygotsky would probably respond to these reproaches thus: "We do not need to be Ivans who do not remember our ancestry; we are not suffering from megalomania, thinking that history begins with us; we do not want history to give us a pure and dull name; we want a name on which the dust of the ages has settled. This is what we see as our historical right, the indication of our historical role, the claim to establishing psychology as a science. We must consider ourselves in connection with and relation to the past; even rejecting it, we depend on it." (Vol. 1, p. 428).

We can divide Vygotsky's interest in problems of child (developmental) psychology proper into two periods: the first (1926-1931), in which there was intense work on the problem of mediation of mental processes that represented for Vygotsky, as is very well known, the central link in the development of higher mental processes; and the second (1931-1934), when experimental study of the problem of the development of higher mental processes was finished and Vygotsky was working on the problem of semantic structure of consciousness and a general theory of child development. During this period, as authors of the epilogue to Volume 1 note, "without exaggerating, it can be said that the problem of development and primarily, *'the drama of the mental development of the child'* (my italics—D. E.) occupies the center of Vygotsky's thinking (ibid., p. 447). Both periods are presented in the present volume of *Collected Works*.

In 1928, Vygotsky published a course of study entitled, "School-Age Pedology." Experimental studies of higher mental functions were just beginning; therefore studies of mediated mental processes, mainly of memory, were presented in the course in the form of a general outline. There are notes on natural and learned arithmetic and a description of the first experiments with counting with the help of signs. All of these data are presented only as first attempts.

Moreover, in "School-Age Pedology," there are already some notes on the historical origin of periods of childhood. This is of undoubted interest. Considering the process of transition to development in adolescence, Vygotsky wrote: "It may be assumed that the period of sexual maturation at one time concluded the process of child development and coincided with the end of childhood in general and with the onset of general organic maturity. The connection between general organic and sexual maturity is biologically completely understandable. A function such as increase and continuation of the genus, bearing an infant and nourishing it, can be based only on an already mature and formed organism that completed its own development. At that time, the period of sexual maturation had a completely different significance than it does now.

"Now the period of sexual maturation is characterized by the fact that the definitive factors of sexual maturation, general maturation, and formation of the human personality do not coincide. Humanity has won for itself a long childhood; it stretched the line of development far beyond the period of sexual maturation; it postponed the mature state with a period of youth or a period of definitive formation of the personality.

"Depending on this, three factors of maturation of the human personality— sexual maturation, general organic maturation, and sociocultural maturation—do not coincide. This lack of coincidence is the root cause of all the difficulties and contradictions of the transitional period. Sexual maturation occurs in man before general organic maturation, the growth of the organism, is concluded. Sexual instinct matures earlier than the organism is definitively ready for the function of multiplying and continuing the genus. Sexual maturation also precedes sociocultural maturation and definitive formation of the human personality" (1928, pp. 6-7).

The development of these positions, especially the position on the lack of coincidence of the three factors of maturation during adolescence, was continued in Vygotsky's book *Pedology of the Adolescent*. We will speak of this later. Now we would like to note that although certain positions expressed by Vygotsky and Blonsky are at present debatable, and perhaps even simply untrue, of essence is the fact that already at the end of the 1920s, in Soviet psychology, the question was posed on the historical origin of periods of childhood, on the history of childhood as a whole, on the connection of the history of childhood with the history of society. The history of childhood has not been studied sufficiently and has not been written, but the formulation of the question itself is important. It is important because certain key problems of the theory of the mental development of the child, while still not resolved definitively, may at least be elucidated, specifically in the light of the history of childhood. These include one of the most important problems—the problem of the factors of mental development, and together with it, the question of the role of maturation of the organism in mental development.

The question of specific features of mental development of the child and its difference from the development of the offspring of even a species of humanlike apes closest to man is one of these problems. Finally, it is essentially important that this historical approach put an end to the search for the "always of the child," typical for various biologizing conceptions of mental development and replace it with a study of the *"historically of the child."* (We will not make it part of our task to explain who had the priority in formulating the question on the historicity of childhood. On the whole, the first thoughts on this were expressed by Blonsky. For us, it is important that Vygotsky did not bypass this, but in studies on child psychology and on adolescence, he extended this concept.)

We have already said that not everything was decided correctly in formulating the question in this way. It is doubtful, for example, that historically, the separate periods of childhood were simply constructed one above another. There is a basis for assuming a significantly more complex process of development of the separate periods. Doubtful also is the comparison of level of development of children in remote periods of life in society and of contemporary children. To say that a three-year-old child in the remote past was younger than a contemporary three-year-old would scarcely be correct. These were simply completely different children; for example, in the level of independence, our children who are three years old are much less independent than their Polynesian peers described by N. N. Miklukho-Maclay.

Enormous ethnographic material accumulated from the time of the publication of Vygotsky makes us think that the very lack of coincidence between sexual maturation, general maturation, and the formation of personality about which Vygotsky speaks must be considered from a more general point of view, from the point of view of the historical change of the place of the child in society, as a part of this society, and a change, in connection with this, of the whole system of interrelations of children and adults. Without going into detail on this question, we shall only stress that the historical point of view of processes of mental development of the child was accepted as equipment in Soviet child psychology although it is obviously still not sufficiently developed.

4

In 1929-1931, different editions of Vygotsky's textbook, *Pedology of the Adolescent*, were published. The present volume includes that part of it that pertains to mental development proper at this age level. Vygotsky himself singled out this part of the book, calling it, "Psychology of the Adolescent." Parts of the textbook on general questions of the transitional period and problems of sexual maturation were not part of the present *Collected Works*, although some sections, for example, the review of the main theories of the transitional age, are of interest to specialists. The factual material contained in those parts of the book is definitely obsolete, and the theories of the late 1920s have been replaced by new theoretical concepts.

Vygotsky's book was designed as a textbook for correspondence courses. Naturally, the question arises as to whether the book is simply a textbook or whether it was a monograph in which the theoretical conceptions of the author are reflected that developed in the course of theoretical and experimental work. Vygotsky himself considered the book as a study. He begins the final chapter with the words: *"We are coming to the end of our research"* (my italics—D.E.) (1931, p. 481). Why the author selected this form of presentation for his studies, we do not know precisely. Probably there were reasons of a purely external character and a profound internal basis as well for writing this kind of book, and for the book to be specifically on adolescence.

Before writing this textbook, Vygotsky concluded basic experimental studies on the development of higher mental processes. The studies were formulated into a long paper, *Tool and Sign in the Development of the Child* (Vol. 6) and the monograph, *The History of the Development of Higher Mental Functions* (Vol. 3). Neither work was published in the lifetime of the author. Most likely, this was because specifically at that time, the theory promulgated by Vygotsky was being subjected to serious criticism.

It seems to us that there was still another serious circumstance. In the experimental-genetic studies communicated in these manuscripts, functions of perception, attention, memory, and practical intellect were analyzed. The mediated character of all these processes was demonstrated. It was not just a study of one of the most important processes, the process of formation of concepts and transition to thinking in concepts. In this connection, the whole theory of higher mental processes as mediated and one of the most important positions of the theory on systemic relations between mental processes and changes of these relations in the course of development remained as if unfinished. For a relative completeness of the theory, there was insufficient research, first, on the appearance and development of the process of formation of concepts and, second, of the ontogenetic (age-related) study of the process of appearance and change in systemic relations of mental processes.

The study of the formation of concepts was undertaken under the direction of Vygotsky by his closest student, L. S. Sakharov, and after his untimely death, was concluded by Yu. V. Kotelova and E. I. Pashkovskaya. This study showed, first, that the formation of concepts is a process mediated by the word, and, second (and no less important), that the meanings of words (generalizations) develop. The results of the study were first published in the book, *Pedology of the Adolescent*, and were later part of Vygotsky's monograph, *Thinking and Speech* (Vol. 2, Chap. 5). This work provided the lacking link in the study of higher mental functions. At the same time, the possibility opened for considering the problem of what kind of changes in relations between separate processes are introduced by the formation of concepts during adolescence.

L. S. Vygotsky posed the question even more broadly, including it in the more general problem of development and disintegration of the *system* of mental functions. This is covered in Chapter 11 [Chapter 3 in this translation], "Development of Higher Mental Functions during the Transitional Age" (*Pedology of the Adolescent*). In it, citing his own experimental material as well as the materials of other investigators, he systematically considers the development of all the basic mental functions—perception, attention, memory, and practical intellect—over the course of ontogenesis, paying particular attention to changes of systemic relations between mental functions during periods preceding adolescence and especially at that age. Thus, in the first section of *Pedology of the Adolescent*, one of the central problems that interested Vygotsky is considered in a brief and concentrated form.

Even in early experimental studies on the problem of mediation, he proposed as a hypothetical conception that, taken in isolation, mental function has no history and that the development of each separate function is determined by the development of the whole system and the place that the separate function occupies in this system. Experimental-genetic studies could not give an unequivocal answer to the question that interested Vygotsky. The answer to it was obtained in a consideration of development in ontogenesis. However, the evidence obtained in an ontogenetic consideration of development of the systemic organization of mental processes seemed to Vygotsky to be insufficient, and he brought in material from various areas of neurology and psychiatry to consider the processes of disintegration of systemic relations between mental functions.

For a comparative study, Vygotsky selected three diseases: hysteria, aphasia, and schizophrenia, made a detailed analysis of the process of disintegration in these diseases, and found the required evidence.

In analyzing these two chapters of the monograph on the adolescent, which we believe are central, we wanted to show Vygotsky's methodology in studying the processes of mental development. It can be described very briefly as *the historical method and systemics as a unity of the functional-genetic, ontogenetic, and structural approach* to the processes of mental development. In this regard, the analyzed studies remain an unsurpassed example. There is no doubt that empirical data on the features of the thinking of the adolescent and their relatedness to chronological boundaries must be reconsidered. We must remember that the studies were done when a complex system of teaching prevailed in the primary classes, and due to this, a complex system of meanings of words was also typical for the younger school age. It is entirely natural that the formation of concepts was moved downward at present as is apparent, for example, from the research of V. V. Davydov and his colleagues. We must remember that Vygotsky himself considered the mental features not "always of the child" but "historically of the child."

Chapter 16 [Chapter 5 in this book], "Dynamics and Structure of the Adolescent's Personality," is very interesting and has not lost its significance even now. It opens with a summary of studies of the development of higher mental functions. Vygotsky attempts to established the basic laws of their development and considers adolescence as a period in which the process of development of higher mental functions is completed. He gives much attention to the development of self-consciousness in the adolescent and concludes the consideration of the development of higher mental functions with two important ideas: (1) during this period, "a new acting persona enters the drama of development, a new, qualitatively unique factor—the personality of the adolescent himself. We have before us the very complex structure of this personality" (Vol. 4, p. 238) [Chapter 5, p. 180]; and (2) "Self-consciousness is social consciousness transferred within" (ibid., p. 239) [Chapter 5, p. 182]. With these ideas, Vygotsky as if summarizes the studies of higher mental processes for the development of which there is a single pattern: "what were at one time relations between people became mental relations transferred to the personality" (ibid.) [Chapter 5, p. 182].

Our task does not include presenting Vygotsky's views of the adolescent period of development. The reader can become familiar with them directly in the psychological section of the book, *Pedology of the Adolescent.*

It is important to determine the place that this research occupied in the whole creative path of the author. It seems to us that this book is a unique transitional stage in Vygotsky's work. On the one hand, Vygotsky summarized his studies and the studies of his colleagues on the problem of development of higher mental functions and the systemic structure of consciousness, and verified the generalizations and hypotheses with much material of other scientists, showing how factual data accumulated in child psychology may be elucidated from a new point of view. This book closes an important period in Vygotsky's work, a period in which he appears primarily as a general, genetic psychologist using ontogenetic studies and simultaneously realizing in them his theory of general psychology. On the other hand, *Pedology of the Adolescent* is a transition to a new stage in the work, a new cycle of studies, related to the data of experimental study on the formation of concepts first published in this book specifically. This work laid a foundation for the study of the semantic structure of consciousness. In the agenda, the question arose of the interrelation of the systemic and semantic structure of consciousness. Thus, the further development of Vygotsky's views was directed, first, toward extending the study of the semantic structure of consciousness, which found its expression in the monograph, *Thinking and Speech,* and, second, toward elucidating the connections of the systemic and semantic structure of consciousness during individual development.

It must be noted that studies on the formation of concepts had two aspects. On the one hand, they confirmed that the formation of concepts arises on the basis of the word—the basic means for their formation—and on the other hand, they disclosed the ontogenetic path of development of concepts. Another aspect—establishing the stage of development of generalizations—had the character of factual description, not going beyond the limits of a statement. Attempts to elucidate the transitions from one stage of development of word meanings to another evidently did not satisfy the author himself. The elucidation settled on the presence of a contradiction between the object reference of words on the basis of which understanding between adults and children was possible and their meaning, different for the adult and the child. The idea that meanings of words develop on the basis of speech contact of the child with adults can scarcely be considered as sufficient. In it, the main thing is absent—the real, practical connection of the child with reality, with the world of human objects. Absence of any acceptable explanations of the transitions of the semantic and systemic structure of consciousness from one stage to another made it necessary for Vygotsky to resolve this very important problem. Its solution also constituted the content of studies of the next stage in his work.

5

The last period of Vygotsky's work includes the years 1931-1934. During this time, just as always, he worked extremely hard and productively.

At the center of his interests were problems of mental development in childhood. Specifically during this time, he wrote critical introductions to translations of books of foreign psychologists, representatives of basic directions in child psychology. The papers served as a basis for developing the general theory of mental development in childhood, and were a unique preparatory work for "the significance of crisis" in child psychology. Similar work was done in connection with the problem of crisis in general psychology. Through all the papers passes the red thread of the struggle between Vygotsky and biologizing tendencies that dominated child psychology abroad and an elaboration of the bases of the historical approach to problems of development of the mind in childhood. Unfortunately, Vygotsky himself did not have time to correlate this work and did not leave any finished theory of mental development in the course of ontogenesis. In one of the lectures, Vygotsky considered the specific features of mental development and, comparing it with other types of development (embryonal, geological, historical, etc.), said: "Can one imagine . . . that when the most primitive man just arrived on Earth, simultaneously with this initial form there existed a higher, final form—"man of the future" and that this ideal form somehow directly affected the first steps that primitive man took? This is impossible to imagine. . . . Not in any type of development that we know did it happen that at the moment when the initial form appears . . . a higher, ideal form is present that appears at the end of development, and that it would directly interact with the first steps that a child takes along the path of development of this initial, or primitive, form. In this lies the greatest uniqueness of child development in contrast to other types of development among which we never find and cannot find such an arrangement of things . . ." Vygotsky continues: "Consequently, this means that the environment acts in the development of the child, in the sense of development of the personality and its specific, human properties, in the role of a source of development, that is, in this case, the environment plays the role not of circumstance, but of source of development" (Fundamentals of Pedology. Stenographic transcript of a lecture, 1934, pp. 112-113).

These considerations have a central significance for the conception of mental development worked out by Vygotsky. Implicitly they were already contained in the studies of the development of higher mental functions, but acquired a completely different resonance and proof after Vygotsky studied teaching and development directly related to the problem. To formulate and resolve this problem, central to understanding the processes of mental development, Vygotsky was influenced on the one hand by the logic of his own studies and on the other, by the need to solve certain major, although purely practical problems that confronted the school at just this period.

Specifically in these years after the 1931 resolution "On the Primary and Middle School" of the TsK VKP(b), an important reconstruction of the whole system of national education took place—a transition from the complex system of teaching in the primary classes to an objective system of teaching in which the assimilation of a system of scientific information and scientific concepts was central as early as in the primary school. The reconstruction of education was in clear contradiction to the features established by Vygotsky as well as other investigators for children's thinking during early school age, thinking based on a complex system of generalization and complex meaning of words. The problem stood thus: if thinking based on complex generalizations is actually proper to children of primary school age, then a complex system of teaching is specifically most appropriate to these features of the children. But this conception contradicted Vygotsky's hypothesis on the environment, and, consequently, on teaching as a source of development. The need arose for overcoming the dominating points of view on the relation between teaching and mental development in general and intellectual development in particular.

As always, Vygotsky combined experimental work with a criticism of the views of this problem of leading foreign psychologists. The views of E. Thorndike, J. Piaget, and K. Koffka were subjected to critical analysis. Here, Vygotsky shows the connection between the general psychological theory of development developed by these authors and their views on the connection between teaching and development.

L. S. Vygotsky contrasts his own point of view with all of these theories and shows the dependence of the process of development on the character and content of the teaching process itself, and, theoretically, also experimentally confirms the thesis on the leading role of teaching in the intellectual development of children. In this case, also completely possible is teaching that has no influence on the processes of development or even has an inhibiting effect. On the basis of theoretical and experimental studies, Vygotsky shows that that teaching is good which anticipates development and is oriented not toward already completed cycles of development, but toward those that are developing. Teaching, according to Vygotsky's thinking, has a progenerative significance for the process of development.

During 1931-1934, Vygotsky undertook a cycle of experimental studies for the purpose of disclosing the complex interrelations between teaching and development when children are taught concrete segments of school work. These studies are presented in the book *Thinking and Speech* (Vol. 2, Chap. 6).

At the very beginning of the 1930s, there was no other possibility for confirming the hypothesis proposed by Vygotsky on the leading role of teaching in mental development except for the method he selected. This position was fully confirmed only in connection with the experimental studies started at the end of the 1950s and continuing to this day when special experimental schools were established in which the content of teaching could be constructed along new principles and the development of the children studying according to experimental programs could be compared with that of children of the same age studying according to the usual programs used in school.[2]

The studies Vygotsky conducted at the very beginning of the 1930s were important not only as concrete results, but in the general methodological approach to the problem. In his studies, as well as in those being carried out at present, the question of the psychological mechanisms of assimilation that lead to the appearance of completely new mental processes or to a substantial change in processes that developed earlier is inadequately explained. This is one of the more difficult problems. It seems to us that the approach to its solution is more boldly expressed by Vygotsky in studies on the child's mastery of the written language and grammar. Although Vygotsky himself did not formulate the principles of his approach anywhere, they seem to us to be pellucidly clear. According to Vygotsky's idea, in every historically developed human acquisition of culture, human capabilities (mental processes of a certain level of organization) were formed and materialized that were historically accumulated in the course of the process. Without historical and logical-psychological analysis of the structure of human capabilities that were formed in one acquisition or another of human culture and the methods of their exploitation by contemporary man, we cannot imagine the process of mastery by an individual man or child of those achievements of culture as a process of his developing those same capabilities. Thus, teaching may be evolving only if the logic of historical development of one system of capabilities or another finds its realization in it. It must be stressed that we are speaking of internal psychological logic of this history. Thus, in the course of a complex process, contemporary sound-letter writing developed from pictographic writing in which the written word reflected the object signified directly in a graphic form. The external sound form of the word was perceived in this case as a single indivisible sound complex, the internal structure of which the speaker and the writer could not detect. Subsequently, through a series of stages, writing began to represent the sound form itself of the word—at first its articulation-pronunciation syllable composition, then the purely sound (phonemic) composition. Phonemic writing developed in which every separate phoneme was signified by a special sign—a letter or combination of letters. The basis for contemporary writing of most languages of the world is a completely new, historically developed mental function—phonematic distinction and generalization. The developing role of the very beginning of teaching literacy (reading and writing) may be carried out only under the condition that the teaching is oriented toward the formation of the historically developed function. Special experimental studies showed that with this kind of orientation the indicated mental processes develop optimally and, together with this, practical efficiency of teaching language increases significantly.

During the same period, Vygotsky also provided an analysis of children's play from the point of view of the influence that it has on the processes of mental development during the preschool period. He compares the role of play in mental development during the preschool age with the role of teaching in mental development during primary school age. In a stenographic transcript of the lecture, "The Role of Play in Mental Development of the Child" (1933), Vygotsky first speaks of play specifically as the leading type of activity during the preschool age and

[2]At the beginning of the study, quite a few papers were already published on this problem. The studies were connected mainly with the names of P. Ya. Galperin, V. V. Davydov, and their colleagues.

discloses its significance for the development of basic neoformations of this period. In a paper at the All-Russia Conference on Preschool Rearing, "The Problem of Teaching and Intellectual Development during School Age" (1934), he deals in detail with the questions of the relation of teaching and development during the preschool years and shows how during this period prerequisites appear for the transition to school teaching constructed according to the logic of the sciences that start to be presented in school.

The works of Vygotsky pertaining to teaching and development during the preschool and school years have not lost their significance even now. A series of problems is formulated in them that only recently have started to be developed in Soviet child psychology. All of these works were published, some even several times, and for this reason are not contained in the present *Collected Works*. For a full picture of Vygotsky's views, it would be useful to the reader of this volume to recall from memory or read again his works on the problem of teaching and development during the preschool and school years. Without this, some questions may remain not entirely clear.[3]

6

We have already indicated that the study of mental development during adolescence has a special significance for Vygotsky. Thus, in the study, the semantic structure of consciousness and the character and content of the generalizations which serve as a base of the adolescent's construction of a world view was described for the first time. Because of this work, the possibility arose for considering the development of a systemic and semantic structure of consciousness as a unity. At the same time, the study contained a description of the point of development of consciousness that is attained toward the end of adolescence—the establishment of a developed semantic and systemic structure of consciousness and the appearance of self-consciousness of personality. From the result of the studies of the adolescent, for Vygotsky, the problem arose completely naturally of tracing the whole course of individual mental development of the child and explaining the basic patterns of the transition from one stage of development to another, which is the main thing. This was one of the main problems that Vygotsky was resolving in the last years of his life.

Judging by the material that he left, he was preparing to write a book on child (developmental) psychology. Everything would be contained in it that he had done in developing a new theory of mental development based on critically overcoming the various theories that existed at that time. Fragments of this theory are written in his critical notes. There is a basis for assuming that the book would include some of his lectures on the fundamentals of pedology which he gave at the Second Moscow Medical Institute and which were published after his death. These materials would comprise an introduction to a consideration of problems of mental development during different periods of childhood. The second part of the prospective

---

[3]"The Prehistory of Written Speech" (1929), in: L. S. Vygotsky, *Intellectual Development of Children in the Process of Teaching,* Moscow–Leningrad, 1935; "Dynamics of Intellectual Development of the Schoolchild in Connection with Teaching" (1933), ibid.; "Play and Its Role in the Mental Development of the Child" (1933), Vopr. Psikhologii [Problems in Psychology], 1966, No. 6; "A Study of the Development of Scientific Concepts during Childhood" (1933), *Collected Works,* Vol. 3, Moscow, 1983; "Teaching and Development during the Preschool Years" (1934), in: L. S. Vygotsky, *Intellectual Development of Children. . .* ; "The Problem of Teaching and Intellectual Development during the School Years" (1934), ibid.

book would open with a chapter on general problems of dividing childhood into periods and elucidating the principles of analyzing the processes of mental development in different periods and the transitions from one period of development to the next. Then there would be chapters on description and analysis of processes of development in different periods of childhood. Probably in considering the mental development during the preschool years, material would be used on play and the problem of teaching and development during this period, and in a consideration of mental development during school age, materials on the development of scientific concepts and on teaching and development at this age. On the basis of extant materials, such would be the proposed construction of the book Vygotsky did not have time to write.

Fragments for this [prospective] book make up the second part of the present volume. It contains chapters written by Vygotsky for the prospective book, "The Problem of Age," and "Infancy" and stenographic transcripts of lectures he gave on child psychology. Several facts should be kept in mind in becoming familiar with these materials.

First, at that time, in the system of Soviet psychology, child psychology was not yet identified as an independent area of psychological science and did not have civic rights. Its fundamentals were only being established. There were still very few concrete psychological studies, and these were carried out from the most various positions. Problems of child psychology were developed intensively by the remarkable and thoroughgoing psychologist, M. Ya. Basov, and his colleagues, mainly on a plan of organization of separate mental processes (M. Ya. Basov, 1932). Basov did not touch on problems of age levels proper in child psychology. Significantly more attention was given to problems of age levels of development and their features by the well-known pedagogue, P. P. Blonsky, who constructed his books on the age principle. Thus, he wrote: "The aggregate of age-level changes, that is, changes connected with time of life, we will agree to call the age-level symptom-complex. These changes may occur abruptly, critically, or may occur gradually, lytically" (1930, p. 7). Thus, among Soviet child psychologists, Blonsky was the first to call attention to the need to identify periods of child development separated by critical periods. From reflexological positions, important facts pertaining to the development of children during the first year of life were obtained by N. M. Shchelovanov and his colleagues, M. P. Denisova and N. L. Figurin (1929).

Second, fifty years have passed since that time. It is natural that the positions put forward by Vygotsky, very frequently being in the nature of hypotheses, must be compared with new facts—made more precise and augmented, and perhaps, refuted if there is sufficient basis for this.

Finally, third, the preserved fragments and hypotheses, although connected by one idea, sometimes are insufficiently detailed. These should be taken for what they are, the property of history or what is timely for contemporary development of science.

The chapter, "The Problem of Age," was written by Vygotsky as a preliminary consideration of the dynamics of development during separate age levels. In the first paragraph, he subjects to criticism the attempts at periodization that existed in his time as well as the theories of development that were its basis. The criticism proceeded in two directions. On the one hand, it proceeded in the direction of analyzing the criteria that served as the basis for periodization. Speaking against monosymptomatic criteria and the attempts of Blonsky to characterize the period according to a symptom-complex, Vygotsky develops neoformations that appear at one period of development or another as a criterion, that is, that which is new that appears in the structure of consciousness at a certain period. This point of view logically continues Vygotsky's ideas on the change in the course of development of the content and character of generalizations (the semantic aspect of consciousness) and, connected with this, the changes in functional relations (systemic structure of consciousness).

On the other hand, Vygotsky considers especially the problem of continuity and discontinuity of the processes of development. Subjecting to criticism the theory of continuity as proceeding from purely quantitative conceptions of mental development and from conceptions of "empirical evolutionism," he considers the process of mental development as a discontinuous process, fraught with crises and transitional periods. Specifically for this reason, he gave special attention to transitional or critical periods. For Vygotsky, they were indicators of *discontinuity* of the process of mental development. He wrote, "If the critical ages had not been discovered through purely empirical means, the conception of them would have to be introduced into the pattern of development on the basis of theoretical analysis. Now it remains for theory only to become cognizant of and comprehend what has already been established by empirical studies (Vol. 4, p. 252) [Chapter 6, p. 193].

In recent years, a number of attempts have been made at periodization of mental development. We note the periodization of H. Wallon and J. Piaget, Freudians, and others. All of them attempted a critical analysis, and the criteria that Vygotsky used in evaluating them may be very useful. In Soviet child psychology, attempts have also been made to expand and develop the conception of periodization proposed by Vygotsky (L. I. Bozhovich, 1968; D. B. Elkonin, 1971). The problem of periodization, posed in its main points by Vygotsky, is still timely.

As we have already indicated, Vygotsky was interested in the transitions from one period of development to another. He believed that studying the transitions would make it possible to disclose the internal contradictions of development. He presents his general views on this problem and the plan for considering the internal structure of processes of mental development at specific age levels from this angle in the second paragraph of the chapter, "Structure and Dynamics of Age Level." For Vygotsky, the central point in considering the dynamics of mental development at this or any period in the life of the child was the analysis of the *social* situation of development (Vol. 4, p. 258) [Chapter 6, p. 198].

According to Vygotsky's thinking, the disintegration of the old and appearance of bases of the new social situation of development is the main content of the critical age levels.

The last and third paragraph of the chapter, "The Problem of Age Level and Dynamics of Development," deals with the problems of practice. Vygotsky believed the problem of age level to be not only the central problem of child psychology, but also the key to all the problems of practice. This problem is in direct and close connection with diagnostics of age-level development of the child. Vygotsky undertakes criticism of the traditional approaches to diagnostics and advances the problem of diagnostics of the "zone of proximal development," which makes possible prognosis and scientific basing of practical prescriptions. These ideas sound completely contemporary and must be taken into account in the development of a system and methods of diagnostics. (For more detailed consideration of problems of diagnostics, see Vol. 5, p. 257.)

Central in this chapter is the plan of analysis of mental development at different age periods proposed by Vygotsky. According to this plan, the analysis must (a) elucidate the critical period that opens an age level and its basic neoformation; (b) this must be followed by an analysis of the appearance and establishment of the new social situation and its internal contradictions; (c) after that, the genesis of the basic neoformation must be considered; (d) finally, the neoformation itself must be considered as well as the prerequisites it contains for the disintegration of the social situation of the age level.

In itself, the development of this kind of plan was a significant step forward. Even now a description of development at one stage or another frequently is a simple enumeration of features of separate mental processes (perception, memory, etc.) that are not connected with each other in any way. Vygotsky was not able to carry out an analysis of all the age levels of development according to the plan he proposed.

The chapter, "Infancy," is an attempt to realize the plan he outlined for separate age periods. The chapter opens with a paragraph on the newborn period,[4] which was considered by the author as critical—transitional from intrauterine to exouterine, to individual existence, to individual life. Much attention is given to evidence of the transitional character of the period. Analyzing the social situation during this period of development and the external forms of the manifestation of the life of the newborn, Vygotsky expresses the hypothesis that the basic neoformation of the period is the appearance of individual mental life that consists in isolating from a general amorphous background of the whole situation a more or less defined phenomenon that appears as a figure against this background.

L. S. Vygotsky indicates that such an isolated figure against a general undifferentiated background is the adult. In a regular pattern, the hypothesis is developed that supplements Vygotsky's basic idea that the very first, still completely undifferentiated forms of the child's mental life are social in origin. Many studies of child development during the first two months of life, especially those done by M. I. Lisina and her colleagues (M. I. Lisina, 1974), although they were not directly aimed at elucidating the problem posed by Vygotsky, contain material that confirms his hypothesis.

We will turn our attention to certain points of the methodology of analysis. First, in the analysis of the social situation, Vygotsky identifies the main internal contradiction, the development of which determines the genesis of the basic neoformation. Vygotsky writes: "By the whole organization of life, he (the infant—D. E.) is forced into maximum interaction with adults. But this interaction is nonverbal interaction, frequently silent interaction of a completely unique type. The basis for all the child's development during infancy is laid down in the contradiction between maximum sociability of the infant (the situation in which the infant finds himself) and minimum capability for interaction" (Vol. 4, p. 282) [Chapter 7, p. 216].

Most likely from inaccessibility of appropriate factual material at that time, L. S. Vygotsky did not pay sufficient attention to the development of pre-speech forms of sociability of the infant with adults. In other works (see Vol. 3), he indicated, for example, the fact that the pointing gesture develops from grasping and becomes a means of pre-speech sociability. The original contradiction, according to Vygotsky's thinking, develops due to the enriched sphere of the child's socializing with the adult and the ever greater inadequacy of his pre-speech means of socializing.

Further, on the basis of materials at his disposal, Vygotsky established that "first, for the infant, the center of every object situation is another person who changes its significance and sense, second, that the relation to the object and the relation to the person have not yet been separated in the infant" (Vol. 4, p. 308) [Chapter 7, p. 235]. For the investigator, these ideas were central to isolating and describing the basic neoformation of the period—the consciousness of the infant. "In the mind of the infant, from the first moment of his conscious life, appears the fact that his life is included in common life with other people . . . . The child

[4]This paragraph is designated as paragraph two; the content of paragraph one has not been established.

is not so much in contact with a world of lifeless, external stimuli as across and through it to a much more internal, although primitive, communication with the personalities that surround him" (ibid., p. 309) [Chapter 7, p. 236]. Borrowing a term from the German literature, Vygotsky designates this consciousness of the infant as the "great-we." Thus, in the chapter analyzed, despite the various biologizing conceptions in the atmosphere of which Vygotsky lived, he convincingly shows how the inception of individual mental life at the end of the newborn period, as well as the form of consciousness that arises toward the end of infancy, are social in origin; they arise from the child's socializing with adults around him and this socializing is their source, although Vygotsky's hypothesis itself on the nature of the construction of consciousness that appears at the end of infancy is at present disputed. In studies done in the last twenty years, the whole system of relations of the child and the adult has been subjected to careful study in the works of M. I. Lisina and her colleagues (M. I. Lisina, 1974). Vygotsky's methodology is clearly presented in the material in the chapters written. In them, the method of analysis of age-level (ontogenetic) development of consciousness and the child's personality is demonstrated. We may assume that the remaining chapters of the book would be constructed according to the same method of analysis.

7

Immediately following these chapters, the present volume contains stenographic transcripts of lectures given by Vygotsky in 1933-1934. The lectures were not subjected to the author's editing and proofing. In preparing them for print, we retained the style of oral speech and eliminated only definite repetitions. In reading them, one must keep in mind that these are fragments of future chapters—individual paragraphs for them or parts of paragraphs. For their correct understanding, one must imagine to which paragraph of which chapter these fragments may pertain according to Vygotsky's plan of analysis of one age level or another.

The basic problem discussed in the lecture on the crisis of the first year of life is the problem of the development of speech and its features that clearly appear during the period of transition from infancy to early childhood. This resulted from the internal contradiction contained in the social situation of the infant's development. According to Vygotsky's thinking, the contradiction consists in a maximum dependence of the child on the adult with a simultaneous absence of adequate means of socializing and is resolved with the appearance of speech that, during this period, has the character of so-called autonomous speech. Vygotsky believed that the mutual lack of understanding between the adult and the child that arises on the basis of the features of this speech leads to hypobulic reactions that also are one of the important symptoms of the crisis of the first year of life. Unfortunately, Vygotsky pays very little attention to hypobulic reactions. They are inadequately studied even at the present time. Meanwhile, their study might cast light on the appearance of the first, still little differentiated form of consciousness (manifested in the disintegration of the social situation of development), and the system of new relations of the child and the adults that develops over the course of infancy.

Vygotsky's special attention to autonomous speech is connected with the fact that it can be used very easily to demonstrate the transitional character of development in critical periods. Also, Vygotsky pays much attention to the development of meanings of words, and he found it very important to elucidate how these meanings appear at the initial stage of speech development. Unfortunately, it still remains to be established that, regardless of the appearance in Soviet psychology of a large number of studies on the socializing of the infant with adults, the problem of the uniqueness of the means of socializing, and specifically oral socializing, has been inadequately treated.

In the lecture on early childhood, Vygotsky attempts to analyze the processes of development at this stage, to elucidate the genesis of the basic neoformation of the period and, in this way, to confirm once more the plan that he developed for studying the processes of development. Although the analysis Vygotsky made cannot be considered conclusive (many questions remained beyond the limits of the investigation), in the stenographic transcript, the course of the author's thinking and the difficulties which he encountered in the first attempt at describing scientifically and analyzing the process of development in one of the most important periods of childhood are very clear. For the author, early childhood is important primarily because, according to his thinking, specifically at this age level, there is the first differentiation of mental functions, the special function of perception appears and on its basis, the systemic and semantic structure of consciousness.

Thinking aloud (and Vygotsky's lectures always had the character of such thinking), he first presents an external picture of the child's behavior at this period, then he explains the features of the behavior with a sensory-motor unity or a unity of affective perception and action; later he proposes a hypothesis on the appearance of the first differentiation by the child of his own "I." Only after this, Vygotsky says: "Now we shall consider the basic types of activity of the child at the stage of early childhood. This is one of the most difficult problems and, it seems to me, the least developed theoretically" (Vol. 4, p. 347) [Chapter 9, p. 266].

Regardless of how Vygotsky solved this problem, its very formulation is of great interest. There is every basis to assume that he felt the absence of some link that would lead from the contradictions in the social situation to the appearance of basic neoformations. Vygotsky took only the first step to isolating this activity. He gave it a negative value, comparing it to the extended form of play of a child during the following period and establishing that this *was not play*. To designate this kind of activity, he used the term, "serious play," borrowed from German authors. Vygotsky did not give a positive description to this type of activity. Neither did he attempt to connect the development of this activity with the basic neoformations of the period. To explain mental development, Vygotsky brings in the development of speech. Analyzing the development of speech during this period, he develops two theses that to this day have not lost their significance. First, the thesis that development of speech, especially at this period, must not be considered out of context, outside the child's socializing with adults and interacting with "ideal" forms of oral socializing, that is, outside the language of adults in which the speech of the child himself mingles; second, the thesis that "the sound aspect of children's speech develops in direct functional dependence on the semantic aspect of children's speech, that is, it is subordinate to it" (ibid., p. 356) [Chapter 9, p. 272]. Of course, we must not consider the development of mental processes outside the development of speech, and at the same time explain the development of perception only by the child's achievement in the sphere of language; leaving aside the child's real practical mastery of human subjects is hardly right. And Vygotsky did undoubtedly make an attempt at such explanation. Probably at that time there could be no other attempts.

Several decades have passed since the lectures were given. Much new material on the development of speech, object actions, and forms of socializing with adults and with other children has been accumulated in child psychology, but all of these materials lie as if in a row. The stenographic transcript included in this book shows an example of how separate information on development of various aspects of the child's mind can be connected into one picture at a certain age level of development. Soviet psychologists face solving the problem on the basis of new materials and showing the dynamics of development in early childhood. And here such stenographic transcripts which express a special approach to mental development may be useful.

In correlating all the material accumulated after Vygotsky's death, as far as possible, we must verify and retain the basic hypotheses that Vygotsky formulated: first, the idea that in early childhood, the function of perception is differentiated first and systemic and semantic consciousness develops, and, second, the idea of the development of a special form of personal consciousness, an external "I myself" toward the end of this period, that is, of a primary separation of the child from the adult, which leads to the disintegration of the formerly constituted social situation of development.

The stenographic transcript of lectures on the crisis at age three is a review of studies, mainly foreign, and the author's own observations in the clinic operated under his direction at the Experimental-Defectology Institute. In the stenographic transcript there is reference to observations of the critical period by C. Bühler, and a mention of the first "age of obstinacy" by O. Kroh (1926). It is not so important as to who first isolated this period as special; what is important is that Vygotsky called attention to this period and analyzed its nature thoroughly. He subjected the symptoms of this period to careful analysis. It is particularly necessary to stress how behind one and the same symptom of disobedience or insubordination to adults, Vygotsky saw completely different bases according to their mental nature. A specifically detailed analysis of the mental nature of various manifestations that characterize the behavior of the child during this period formed the basis for Vygotsky's important hypothesis that the crisis occurs along an axis of reconstruction of social relations of the child and the people around him. It seems to us essentially important that Vygotsky's analysis is a basis for the idea that in this crisis two interrelated tendencies are intertwined—the tendency toward emancipation, toward separation from the adult and a tendency not toward an affective, but toward a volitional form of behavior.

Many authors considered the critical periods as periods connected with authoritarian rearing and its rigidity. This is true, but only partially. Evidently, only obstinacy is such a general reaction to the system of rearing. It is also true that with a rigid system of rearing, the symptoms of the crisis are manifested more sharply, but this does not at all mean that with the most gentle system of rearing, there will not be a critical period with its difficulties. Certain facts show that in a relatively gentle system of relations, the critical period passes more gently. But in these cases, the children themselves sometimes actively look for the possibility to oppose an adult, and such opposition is internally necessary for them.

Meanwhile, materials proposed by Vygotsky for the analysis of the nature of the crisis at age three also present a number of important problems. We will indicate only one of these. Is not the tendency toward independence, toward emancipation from the adult a necessary prerequisite and the other side of the construction of a new system of relations between the child and adults; is not all emancipation of the child from adults, moreover, a form of a deeper connection of the child with society, with adults?

If we follow the logic of mental development, then after the indicated stenographic transcript, we should place Vygotsky's works on development during preschool age. These were published earlier and were not a part of the *Collected Works*.[5]

[5]L. S. Vygotsky, "Teaching and Development during School Age," in: *Intellectual Development of Children in the Process of Teaching*, Moscow–Leningrad, 1935; "Play and Its Role in Mental Development of the Child," Vopr. Psikhologii [Problems of Psychology], No. 6 (1966).

The next stenographic transcript covers the crisis at age seven. Like the preceding one, it is Vygotsky's correlation of material he knew from the literature and from clinical practice on the prerequisites for the transition from preschool age to primary school age. Vygotsky's ideas are of much interest even today in connection with the discussion of the problem of when teaching in school should start. In the stenographic transcript, there are no indications of the sources that the author used. The central idea of the lecture is that the child's loss of directness lies behind the external manifestations, the affectations, mannerisms, and capriciousness which is observed at this age.

L. S. Vygotsky develops the hypothesis that this loss of directness is the result of the initial differentiation of external and internal life. Differentiation becomes possible only when generalization of one's experiences appears. The preschooler also has experiences, and he experiences each reaction of an adult as either a good or bad evaluation, as a good or bad relation to him on the part of the adults or peers. However, these experiences are of that moment, exist as separate moments of life and pass relatively quickly. At age seven, generalization of an isolated experience of socializing appears that is connected mainly with relations with adults. On the basis of this generalization, the child first develops a self-evaluation, and the child enters a new period of life in which the first instants of self-consciousness begin to be formed.

The whole second part of the stenographic transcript has a more general sense and pertains to the problem of how a psychologist should study the child. It is directed against the study of the environment as unchanging or the circumstances of development and the living environment as changing very slowly. Here Vygotsky poses the question of a unit that would contain a unity of environment and the child's personality. The author proposes adopting experience as such a unity. Among contemporary psychologists, this problem is being developed by one of Vygotsky's students, L. I. Bozhovich (1968).

It should be noted that the problem of transitional or critical periods still requires study, which, unfortunately, clearly lags behind the study of other periods of childhood. We would propose that the study of critical periods requires a radical change in strategy and methods of study. Needed here, obviously, are long-term individual studies of individual children, studies which alone can serve to disclose both the detailed symptoms of development in critical periods and the mental reconstruction through which the child passes during these periods. The strategy of sections that is applied in ordinary studies with a subsequent mathematical processing in which features of the transition from one period to another are lost can scarcely be suitable for a study of this problem.

Do we proceed correctly in publishing these lectures? Perhaps it would have been well to leave them to the "gnawing criticism of the mice?" We think that not one psychologist working in the area of child (developmental) psychology will disregard these materials, but will, perhaps, follow the hypotheses of Vygotsky and even follow the methodological principles of analysis of age-level development advanced by him, or turn his attention to the critical periods. The latter is especially important since in the study of development in these periods, at the center of attention, of necessity, is the individual child and not an abstract statistical average value.

—D. B. Elkonin

NOTES TO THE RUSSIAN EDITION

Pedology of the Adolescent
Selected Chapters

1. In the period from 1928 to 1931, L. S. Vygotsky published a number of hand-books for correspondence courses. From this came *School-Age Pedology* (1928), *Pedology of Youth* (1929), and *Pedology of the Adolescent* (1930-1931). The present *Collected Works* contains chapters from the latter book. The handbook was published in separate sections, each of which included several chapters. The first part contained four chapters: "The Concept of Pedology," "Methods in Pedology," "A Brief Review of the Principal Periods of Child Development," and "A Review of the Principal Theories of the Transitional Age." The second part consisted of five chapters: "A General Description of the Transitional Age," "Anatomical-Physiological Features of the Adolescent," "Sexual Maturation," "The Psychology of Sexual Maturation," and "Conflicts and Complications of the Transitional Age." Both these parts were published in 1930 under the imprint, "Office for Correspondence Courses at the Pedagogical Faculty of the Second Moscow State University." Parts three and four were published in 1931 in one book under the imprint, "Central Institute for Higher Qualification of Personnel of National Education. Correspondence Courses." The handbook was published according to the laws covering manuscripts. Each chapter was supplied with a plan for studying the assignment and a list of recommended literature. Naturally, in the new edition, we thought it desirable to omit the plans for studying the assignments and to include the recommended literature in a general list of literature, marking it with an asterisk (*).

    Chapters are included in the *Collected Works* that pertain to psychological development proper during adolescence.

    L. S. Vygotsky literally picks up crumbs in the studies of foreign authors, monographs and separate journal articles, materials that confirm his point of view of the mental development of adolescents. For this reason, there are many references in the book to foreign authors, but since this was a textbook, the sources are not indicated. More than fifty years have passed since the writing of the book, and it was impossible to establish all the sources Vygotsky used, especially the separate papers. Vygotsky frequently cited foreign authors and did his own translations. Such citations in the present volume are given in the form of indirect speech.

    In the second half of the 1920s in our country, an increased interest developed in the problems of the adolescent period closely connected with the problems confronting society. All studies were being extended from the pedological approach and, in connection with this, strictly psychological features of that age received very little attention. There were mainly physiological-hygienic or social-pedagogical studies. At just this time, a series of works appeared that referred to foreign studies and theories. Such works included the books of V. E. Smirnov (1929), M. M. Rubinstein (1926), and P. L. Zagorovsky (1928) as well as Vygotsky's *Pedology of the Adolescent*, which P. P. Blonsky evaluated as the most acceptable.

    Remarkable primarily is the fact that Vygotsky begins the consideration of mental development during adolescence with a consideration of interests. In understanding the nature of interests, he goes beyond the limits of the conceptions that prevailed at that time, and even here makes an attempt to distinguish two lines in the process of the child's development.

2. *Antigenetic*—here in the meaning, "contradicting the principle of development."
3. At the time this book was written, many authors called all of adolescence transitional, using these terms as equivalent and having in mind the transition from childhood to adulthood. Vygotsky too followed this tradition. Later, he introduced a distinction (see Vol. 4, p. 256). Moreover, during that time, the ages of adolescence and of the older child were considered together, which Vygotsky believed to be wrong.
4. Here we have in mind the younger school age, a pupil of the primary school.
5. *Bühler, Charlotte* (1893-?), Austrian psychologist, wife and associate of K. Bühler. Mainly, she developed problems of child psychology (problems of periodization and child development at different periods, and development of social behavior) and the ideas of K. Bühler. She directed many studies on early childhood, play, and adolescence; she gathered around her a group of investigators (H. Hetzer, K. Reininger, B. Tudor-Hart, E. Köhler, and others). C. Bühler made the first attempt to construct a theory of the transitional age, and the author proceeds from maturation of sexual function as the basic process; other aspects of development are considered in this light. According to the ideas of C. Bühler, sexual function is represented in consciousness as a "need to be met." The period of puberty is a period in which this need awakens.
6. *Herbart, Johann* (1776-1841), see Vol. 1, p. 466.
7. *Lipps, Theodor* (1851-1914), see Vol. 1, p. 465.
8. *Thorndike, Edward* (1874-1949), eminent American psychologist. Founder of objective psychology as a behavioral science. For the attitude of Vygotsky to Thorndike during the period of enthusiasm for reactology, see Vol. 1, pp. 176-196. He gave much attention to the development of the problem of learning, considering learning to be an acquisition of habits constructed over innate forms of behavior on the basis of trial and error, positively and negatively reinforced. He considered the development of the child to be a process of purely quantitative accumulation of habits and equated development with teaching. Vygotsky considered the problem of teaching and development and criticized theory that equated them (Vol. 2, pp. 231-234).
9. *Lewin, Kurt* (1890-1947), German psychologist, representative of Gestalt psychology. He extended the principles of Gestalt psychology to experimental study of personality: its needs, affects, will. He worked on problems of child psychology in close connection with the solving of problems in general psychology that interested him. In 1931-1932, he gave a course in child psychology at the Psychological Institute of the University of Berlin. Lewin's general methodological aims were not suitable for Soviet psychology, and his theory of structure of the field as determining behavior is an extension of the principle of structural quality to analysis of the determination of all of behavior and the

dynamics of needs and motives. All of the criticism to which Vygotsky subjected Gestalt psychology wholly applies to Lewin (Vol. 1, pp. 210-238). Vygotsky highly prized Lewin's experimental studies and used some of his methodological devices and facts, being critical of the absence of the genetic approach and the break between development of affect and intellect (Vol. 5, pp. 231-256). Lewin came to the USSR and was familiar with L. S. Vygotsky and A. R. Luria. After the establishment of fascism in Germany, he emigrated to the U.S.

10. Here we are speaking of the theory of K. Lewin.

11. *Hegel, Georg Wilhelm Friedrich* (1770-1831), see Vol. 1, p. 464.

12. The structure of the field in Lewin's theory includes not simply the things that surround us as physical bodies, but also the stimulating forces that arise when we are confronted by needs. His development of the problem of stimulating forces arising in things was inadequate. It may be assumed that the tendency toward certain actions with things arises in the course of mastering socially developed methods of dealing with them.

13. " . . . in one of the preceding chapters": we are speaking of a chapter not in the *Collected Works* in which the author developed the historical point of view of the processes of mental development during childhood and specifically during adolescence.

14. Evidence of the fact that in the book Vygotsky considered the whole adolescent period as transitional and used the terms "adolescent" and "transitional" as equivalents.

15. " . . . in one of the first chapters of our course"—the subject here is Chapter I, which is not included in the *Collected Works*.

16. *Baldwin, James Mark* (1861-1934), see Vol. 2, p. 483.

17. *Kroh, Oswald* (1887-?), German psychologist working in child psychology, mainly in the psychology of the juvenile and the adolescent. In the next chapter, Vygotsky frequently refers to his work in connection with the transition from visual thinking to thinking in concepts (O. Kroh, 1922, 1926, 1928).

18. The term "alienation" is used incorrectly here. Kroh, like certain other investigators, did not see that behind the so-called alienation, that is, exit from the environment, lies a reconstruction of social relations of the adolescent, the appearance of a new and perhaps closer connection with social reality. An analogy between the transition from early childhood to preschool age (approximately at the age of three) and the transition from primary school age to adolescence (approximately at thirteen years of age) is purely external, connected with certain phenomena (negativism, stubbornness, etc.). Vygotsky proposed the hypothesis that every transitional or critical period, and not just the two indicated, turns on an axis of social relations (see Vol. 4, p. 260).

19. *Zagorovsky, Pavel Leonidovich* (?), Soviet psychologist and pedagogue. He worked mainly in the area of adolescent (youth) psychology. In this case, we have in mind his paper, "On the So-Called Negative Phase in Adolescence" (1928).

20. *Hall, Stanley* (1844-1924), American psychologist. One of the founders of the study of youth, the author of a two-volume monograph on youth (S. Hall, 1904), a partisan of the biogenetic law, considered child development, specifically in adolescence, as a maturation of instincts.

21. We are speaking of the German school and adolescents of that time, that is, the mid-1920s.

22. *Tolstoy, Lev Nikolaevich* (1828-1910), classical writer of Russian literature. He is the author of the autobiographical trilogy: *Childhood, Boyhood,* and *Youth.*

He writes about the desert of adolescence in Chapter 20 of *Boyhood:* "I involuntarily want to get through the desert of boyhood and reach that happy time when again a truly tender, noble feeling of friendship will illuminate the end of this age with a bright light and begin a new time of youth full of wonder and poetry."

23. *Tumlirz, Otto* (?), Austrian psychologist who tried to unite various points of view of adolescence.

24. The authors to whom Vygotsky refers: K. Reininger, L. Večerka, and H. Hetzer were of the Vienna group working under the direction of C. Bühler (see References).

25. *Zalkind, Aron Borisovich* (1888-1936), Soviet psychologist, pedologist, and pedagogue. He was an active participant in the struggle for a reconstruction of the whole range of psychoneurological sciences on the basis of Marxism. He was an ideologue with a sociogenetic inclination in pedology with respect to the processes of development in childhood in which adaptation and equilibrium of the organism with the environment is a determining factor. The environment was a mechanically acting, unchanging, and fatefully determining factor in development. He wrote much on the development of adolescents and sex education. Zalkind's views are marked by an eclectic combination of behaviorism, reflexology, and Freudianism and were criticized in discussions over the last part of the 1920s and beginning of the 1930s. Criticism of the theory of fatalistic dependence of children's fate on heredity and unchangeable environment, and at the same time criticism also of sociogenetic control was concluded by a resolution of the Central Committee of the All-Union Communist Party (of Bolsheviks), "Pedological Perversions in the System of the People's Commissariat of Education" (1936). Vygotsky uses Zalkind's paper, "Basic Features of the Transitional Age" (1930) insufficiently critically, following this author in equating the psychological concept of interest with the physiological mechanism of a dominant.

26. The opinion of A. Biedl is mentioned in Chapter 7 of *Pedology of the Adolescent* (1930, pp. 116-117). Biedl distinguishes the stages depending on which glands of internal secretion occupy the major position at each period.

27. *Stern, William* (1871-1938), German philosopher and psychologist, a representative of the conception of personalism in psychology. Vygotsky frequently criticized his philosophical-psychological views (Vol. 1, pp. 291-436). He did much work in the area of child psychology. In his approach to mental development of the child, he enlarged on a variation of two factors—the theory of convergence, ascribing a determining significance to the internal factor (innate forms of behavior—instincts and drives). His work on the development of speech is especially well known. Vygotsky critically analyzed Stern's views on development of speech (Vol. 2, pp. 80-89). Stern worked on problems of development of perception. On the basis of children's descriptions of pictures, he established stages of development of perception (subject, action, traits, relations). Vygotsky did a critical experimental study on this problem (Vol. 4, p. 116). According to recollections of A. V. Zaporozhets, the experiments were shown to Stern when he came to Moscow, and he agreed with Vygotsky's criticism. In connection with the conception of personalism, Stern turns to the psychology of the transitional age, a period that has special significance in the development of personality. For understanding the changes that occur at that time, Stern develops the theory of "serious play." At present, this theory is being criticized more fundamentally, particularly in connection with the deep understanding of play itself. He was also known as a psychologist interested in the problems of giftedness.

28. *Groos, Karl* (1861-1946), German philosopher and psychologist. He was known mainly for work on the theory of play (1899), which is obsolete at present, although the idea of the developmental meaning of play retains its significance. Groos also did the studies on the thinking of the adolescent used by Vygotsky in this volume (p. 64).

29. This is one of the central chapters of the book. The results of an experimental study of the formation of concepts are published here for the first time; a part of this book was later included in Vygotsky's *Thinking and Speech* (1934). The chapter was written before 1931, that is, before the transition from a complex to a subject system of teaching in the primary classes and before Vygotsky did research on the problem of teaching and development. To a significant degree these studies resulted from the radical changes in the system of education. We must regard critically the characteristics of thinking provided by Vygotsky for the different age periods and keep in mind that in connection with existing changes in the content of teaching, changes also occurred in concrete characteristics of thinking in both the primary school period and in the adolescent period. Absolute characteristics are not as important here as the approach to considering the processes of development in adolescence.

30. Vygotsky uses *maturation* not in the sense of biological maturing of hereditarily fixed properties but in the general meaning of development and the appearance of new qualitative features.

31. *Bühler, Karl* (1879-1963), eminent Austrian psychologist. He worked on problems of mental (psychical) development in childhood. He was a partisan of biological dependence of development in childhood, particularly the hereditary nature of abilities. He is the author of the theory of three stages in the development of the child (instinct, habit, intellect) in which he attempted to synthesize conceptions of the behaviorists who were his contemporaries on the formation of habits and W. Köhler's data on the study of intellect of humanlike apes. According to Bühler's theory, over the course of the first years of life, the child passes through the same stages that sequentially occurred in the evolution of forms of animal behavior. Equating the object-tool actions of young children with the intellectual operations of the chimpanzee, Bühler called this period of childhood the chimpanzee-like age. He considered children's play as activity accompanied by functional satisfaction, that is, satisfaction in the process itself. Vygotsky frequently considered critically Bühler's views on various questions (Vol. 1, pp. 196-209).

32. In this context, the *pupil* is a child in the primary classes. In the period when the book was written, an adolescent was not necessarily a student in a general education school. He could participate directly in productive work and could study in professional educational institutions of the ShKM [Kolkhoz Youth School] or the FZU [Factory Training School], which he entered after finishing the first stages of school (primary school).

33. *Rubinstein, Moisei Matveevich* (1878-1953), Soviet pedagogue and psychologist. His basic circle of interests was age-related and pedagogical psychology. He did much work on problems of psychology and pedagogy of adolescents. P. P. Blonsky believed that his views were greatly influenced by bourgeois trends. Vygotsky criticizes Rubinstein's views on development of thinking in adolescence, having in mind his joint work with V. E. Ignatev (1926).

34. *Meumann, Ernst* (1862-1915), German psychologist and pedagogue, founder of experimental pedagogy. He made an attempt to use the results of psychological studies as a basis for the theory and practice of teaching (1914-1917).

35. *Spranger, Edward* (1882-1939), German philosopher and psychologist, one of the principal representatives of idealistic trends in descriptive or conceptual psychology of the mind, a follower of W. Dilthey (Vol. 1, p. 465). Vygotsky criticized his theory on adolescence in Chapter 4 of *Pedology of the Adolescent* (pp. 65-67).

36. We are speaking here of the systems of tests for measuring mental development that were widely used at that time. The first such system was created in France and was named after its authors, A. Binet and T. Simon. It was subsequently subjected to various modifications. C. Burt, an English psychologist, brought out a new edition of this system and P. P. Blonsky, an edition adapted for Russian children. The measurement of mental development using a system of tests of the Binet type was criticized in Soviet psychology by both progressive psychologists and pedagogues in capitalist countries. Vygotsky severely criticized this system.

37. *Blonsky, Pavel Petrovich* (1884-1941), eminent Soviet pedagogue and psychologist. One of the founders of constructing psychology on the basis of Marxist philosophy. He developed the theory of the trade school and took an active part in its construction. His interests centered around the study of childhood. At initial stages, he overestimated the significance of maturing of the organism and its energy resources for the development of the child. The views of Vygotsky on some questions (on the historical approach to the study of behavior and origin of periods of childhood; on the presence of critical ages; on interfunctional connections and their significance for understanding mental development, and others) were close to those of Blonsky.

38. Evidently Vygotsky has in mind the monograph, *The History of the Development of Higher Mental Functions,* which he wrote at that time (1930-1931), but which was not published while he lived. It was published in full in *Collected Works,* Vol. 3.

39. *Ach, Narciss* (1871-1946), see Vol. 2, p. 483.

40. *Jaensch, Erich* (1883-1940), see Vol. 1, p. 464.

41. *Gesell, Arnold* (1880-1961), American doctor, one of the founders of child psychology in the United States. He was the first to use the strategy of transverse sections for comparative-genetic studies. In the 1930s, only his studies of the early period of development were known. Vygotsky prized highly the research strategy proposed by Gesell. This evaluation, however, contradicts the strategy and method of study of higher mental functions developed by Vygotsky himself, which he called the experimental-genetic method. The strategy of sections, although it provides a conception of quantitative changes that occur in the course of development, does not allow penetration into the internal mechanism of the transition itself from one level of development to another. The essence of the experimental-genetic method is disclosed by Vygotsky in *The History of the Development of Higher Mental Functions* (Vol. 4). The general theoretical views of Gesell on the processes of development and the method of sections were criticized by Vygotsky in the foreword to Gesell's book (1934).

42. . . . *genetic explanation*—in this case, the explanation of the whole preceding history of the adolescent, especially the history of the instruction he received.

43. Materials of these studies and a short description of methods and results are included in the table taken from the book of K. Groos (1916, pp. 224 and 240-241).

44. Humboldt, Wilhelm (1767-1835), see Vol. 2, p. 488.

45. Here Vygotsky once again contrasts his thinking with the views of authors (C. Bühler and others) who took idealistic positions and believed that the infant

possesses the highest forms of consciousness (self-consciousness) from the beginning. Here Vygotsky uses the word "consciousness" in the sense of an undifferentiated mass of sensory impressions.

46. *Potebnya, Aleksandr Afanasevich* (1835-1891), see Vol. 2, p. 486; Vol. 3, p. 349.
47. See Vol. 2, p. 180.
48. See Vol. 2, p. 183.
49. This idea was formulated by K. Marx thus: "For this, neither a microscope nor chemical reagents should be used in analyzing economic forms. The one and the other should be replaced by the power of abstraction." K. Marx and F. Engels, *Works*, Vol. 23, p. 6.
50. *Galton, Francis* (1822-1911), see Vol. 1, p. 464.
51. *Stumpf, Karl* (1848-1936), see Vol. 1, p. 461.
52. These problems are presented in detail in J. Piaget's book, *Speech and Thought*. For Vygotsky's analysis of them, see Vol. 2, pp. 147-175.
53. *Uznadze, Dmitrii Nikolaevich* (1886-1950), founder of the Georgian school of psychologists and author of the theory of attitude. He gave much attention to problems of child psychology and made the first attempt to describe the basic types of children's activity, the theory of children's play, and the development of the problem of readiness for school. Vygotsky uses the data obtained by Uznadze in his early experimental studies on the development of concepts during the preschool age published in German journals (see also Vol. 2, p. 486).
54. *Piaget, Jean* (1896-1980), see Vol. 1, p. 464; Vol. 2, p. 482. In this work, Vygotsky uses materials obtained by Piaget in earlier studies of the development of thinking. In these facts, Vygotsky finds confirmation of his hypothesis on the development of logical thinking with the transition from primary school age to adolescence. Here, the material of the two volumes used is combined in the Russian edition into one book: *Speech and Thinking of the Child*. Vygotsky wrote the introduction to this book, "The Problem of Speech and Thinking of the Child in the Teaching of J. Piaget," (Vol. 2, pp. 23-79); here he provided a critical analysis of Piaget's whole conception of child development. Vygotsky wrote *Pedology of the Adolescent* before he wrote the critical paper. Vygotsky did not agree with Piaget's views on a number of problems, although he valued his studies greatly and spoke highly of them. Vygotsky knew the work Piaget did before 1934 very well. Piaget first became familiar with the views of Vygotsky and his criticism only in 1962 after *Thinking and Speech* was translated into English and felt it necessary to respond to Vygotsky's critical observations. The response was published in a separate brochure, "Comments on Vygotsky's Critical . . . ," and, evidently this brochure was inserted into an edition of Vygotsky's book in English. Piaget agreed with certain of Vygotsky's observations.
55. The Binet–Simon test on three brothers consists in the child's solving a contradiction between the existence of three brothers in a family and the proposition: "I have three brothers: Paul, Ernst, and me" (see J. Piaget, 1932, p. 280).
56. *Leontev, Aleksei Nikolaevich* (1903-1979), Vygotsky's closest comrade-in-arms in developing the theory of the historical origin and the mediating nature of man's higher mental functions. His study, *Development of Memory* (1931), was done specifically during the period of work on this theory. Leontev's study with unfinished sentences (§34) and proverbs (§35), from which Vygotsky used data, was not published. In developing methods, a form proposed by Piaget was used that contained sentences and proverbs modified and adapted to the experience of Russian children (Vol. 2, p. 483).

57. The term *mass child* was introduced by P. P. Blonsky: ". . . pedology prefers to be based on a study not of the individual random child, but on the mass of children. Pedology wants to think not in units, but in masses. Its point of departure is the mass child, the mass of children" (1930, p. 9).

58. Piaget said: "Thus, things do not lead the intellect to the need for verification: things in themselves are, of course, processed by the intellect. Moreover, the child never actually enters into real contact with things because he does not work. He plays with things, he relies on them without analyzing them" (1932, p. 373). Piaget's idea that the child never enters into real contact with things is at least debatable. Of course the child does not work, but he masters the world of common objects, assimilates commonly developed methods of their use, and has some understanding of their properties. This is a form of his social practice.

59. *Wertheimer, Max* (1880-1943), see Vol. 1, p. 460.

60. L. S. Vygotsky looks for factual evidence for his hypothesis that, in the transition from primary school age to adolescence, substantial qualitative shifts occur in the development of thinking. In Soviet psychology, there were very few such studies at that time. He specially organized the efforts of colleagues (A. N. Leontev) for such comparative-genetic studies and undertook a careful analysis of the data obtained in Piaget's studies. Vygotsky carefully collected and systematized foreign material that contained facts relative to the problem on which he was working. V. E. Smirnov and P. L. Zagorovsky refer to some of these materials in their books. However, in the studies of foreign authors, these materials appear as a simple description of features of thinking at very early age levels with no connection to the appearance at adolescence of the formation of concepts, with no conception of the development in this important period. Factual materials to which Vygotsky refers were taken from publications of J. Piaget, R. Rossello, H. Roloff, M. Vogel, H. Schüssler, H. Eng, H. Ormian, G. Müller, E. Monchamps, and E. Moritz (see References).

61. One of the central chapters of the monograph in which Vygotsky generalized the material on the study of higher mental functions, presenting them as the development of interfunctional connections. Of special interest is Vygotsky's general methodological principle in which morphological, genetic, and functional approaches were united into a single whole representing the systemic study of processes of mental development during adolescence, which was characteristic of Vygotsky.

62. *Kretschmer, Ernst* (1888-1924), known mainly for his work on the connection between body build (constitution) and character traits (1924). In this chapter, Vygotsky uses his general neurological views and studies of hysteria (1927, 1928). See also Vol. 1, p. 464; Vol. 2, p. 486.

63. *Hering, Ewald* (1834-1918), see Vol. 2, p. 490.

64. *Helmholtz, Herman* (1821-1894), see Vol. 2, p. 490.

65. *Volkelt, Hans* (?), German child psychologist, outstanding representative of the so-called Leipzig school; the basic concept of this school for explaining mental life and its point of origin was whole life experience (*Ganzheiterlebnis*), a diffuse whole in which perception and its sensual coloring were merged into one with a certain meaning of the sensory-emotional experience. These are the idealistic points of the conception. Volkelt is known as a subtle experimenter working in the area of child perception (1930).

66. *Claparède, Edward* (1873-1940), see Vol. 1, p. 463; Vol. 2, p. 482.

67. *Koffka, Kurt* (1873-1941), see Vol. 1, p. 460.

68. *Eidetic tendency* is the tendency toward preserving an image of an object or situation for a certain time in a visual, concrete form. Vygotsky had a negative attitude toward eidetic psychology as to a special trend, believing it to be idealistic; nevertheless he was interested in eidetic phenomena and confirmed their presence; one of his colleagues, K. I. Veresotskaya, even conducted a special study in this area.

69. *Binet-Bobertag*, a variant of Binet's test systems.

70. The experiments refer to a period of conflict of the Würzburg school with associationism, in which K. Bühler participated.

71. Vygotsky describes the methodology with insufficient clarity. The second series, presented after a recess, consisted of sentences connected in sense with those presented in the first series or of parts of sentences connected with fragments of ideas contained in the first series.

72. *Ribot, Theophil* (1839-1916), one of the founders of scientific psychology in France. He applied himself to the study of higher mental processes and personality. Working in a clinic with pathological material, he believed that psychopathology supplies the psychologist with experimental facts provided by nature itself. He established the tradition of studying pathological material, which many French psychologists continued. See also Vol. 2, p. 491.

73. Before this book appeared (A. N. Leontev, *Development of Memory*), research materials were published in: L. S. Vygotsky, *Development of Active Attention during Childhood* (1929, pp. 112-142). This same paper, entitled, "Development of Higher Forms of Attention," was published in 1956 in the book: L. S. Vygotsky, *Collected Psychological Studies.* Vygotsky's paper and the chapter in Leontev's book are far from identical. In Vygotsky's paper, data obtained by Leontev occupy a limited place; most of it pertains to experiments with complex selection. The publication of Leontev's book was delayed, and it was published simultaneously with Vygotsky's book, *Pedology of the Adolescent* (1931). There is every basis for assuming that the factual data, tables, and graphs presented in this section were taken from Leontev's manuscript.

74. The graph for this volume is taken from A. N. Leontev's book, *Development of Memory* (p. 175). It presents data from two series of experiments. In each series, the child answered 18 questions; among these, seven critical questions required an answer on the color of an object (for example: "What color is the doctor's smock?" or "What color are tomatoes?)" In both series, it was forbidden to, first, name a certain color, and, second, repeat already named colors in answers to subsequent questions. The second series was conducted in the form of a simple conversation, a game with rules; in the third series, the child was given nine colored cards which he could use as a means to help him carry out the instruction. The number of correct answers to the seven control questions is given along the ordinate in the table. Figure 3 presents the efficiency of remembering a series of fifteen words by subjects of different ages without the use of auxiliary means (the second series is direct remembering) and with the use of means—cards (the third series is mediated remembering). The number of correctly reproduced words is presented along the ordinate. This was printed in A. N. Leontev's book, *Development of Memory* (p. 89). This same table is presented in A. N. Leontev's book, *Problems of Mental Development* (Moscow, 1981, p. 468).

75. The term was introduced by Leontev: " . . . in their main expression, the curves of the two lines of development may be represented specifically in the form of a complete parallelogram inclined with one of its angles toward the abscissa" (1931, p. 91).

76. *Titchener, Edward* (1867-1927), see Vol. 1, p. 471.
77. *. . . during the period of first childhood* has in mind primary school age.
78. P. L. Zagorovsky refers to the paper of H. Meyer and G. Pfahler, 1926.
79. Experiments were conducted in a wooden construction, "Matador," very popular at that time in Vienna.
80. There is reason to believe that the table in the form as given by Vygotsky is taken from the book of P. L. Zagorovsky (1929, p. 143). Vygotsky regarded critically the direct connection between the third stage of technical images and experiences evoked by sexual maturation of adolescents established by Smirnov.
81. The tasks set out by these studies basically reproduced Köhler's experiments with minor changes and were reduced to the children's getting attractive objects with the help of a tool.
82. *S. A. Shapiro* and *E. D. Gerke* were colleagues of M. Ya. Basov and worked under his direction in the Leningrad Institute of Scientific Pedagogy. The results of their studies were published in the paper, "The Process of Adaptation to Conditions of the Environment in the Behavior of the Child" (1930).
83. The results of the studies were not published. They were described in relatively good detail in Vygotsky's manuscript, "Tools and the Sign in the Development of the Child" (1930), first published in Vol. 6. In his experiments, Vygotsky paid most attention to the connection between speech and tool activity. Certain considerations of this can be found in the book, *Thinking and Speech* (Vol. 2, pp. 89-118).
84. K. Marx says: ". . . he also accomplishes his conscious purpose which, like a law, determines the method and character of his activity and to which he must subordinate his will" (K. Marx and F. Engels, *Works*, Vol. 23, p. 189).
85. *Sepp, Evgenii Konstantinovich* (1878-1957), Soviet neuropathologist.
86. Coincidence refers to animals. On this, Vygotsky wrote: "We are inclined for this reason to assume that in animals, as a rule, both these points—completion of general organic development and sexual maturation—coincide" (*Pedology of the Adolescent*, 1930, p. 71). Vygotsky was developing the hypothesis that the basis of all features of the transitional period is the lack of coincidence in the course of historical development, or a divergence of three points of development—the general organic, sexual, and cultural. "We might say . . . that cultural growth not only reinforces the critical nature of the transitional age, but that culture in general first creates this crisis. Outside cultural development, we cannot speak at all about the crisis of the transitional age. This culture, this historical development of humanity, breaks down the biological harmony of maturation, separating it into three separate peaks and forming the basic contradiction of the whole age" (ibid., p. 75).
87. In Chapter 4, Vygotsky wrote on Spranger's theory as follows: "Thus, for Spranger, a mental change occurs simply approximately simultaneously with the bodily, but he does not know how to connect the one with the other. Spranger's teaching is an extreme expression of the idealistic and dualistic psychology which developed in the last decades" (*Pedology of the Adolescent*, p. 66).
88. *Wernicke, Carl* (1848-1905), German psychiatrist. In 1874, he published a description of cases of loss of the ability to understand the spoken word connected with injury to a part of the temporal gyrus of the left hemisphere. Several years before this, in 1861, the French anatomist, Paul Broca (1824-1880), described a patient who understood speech, but could not speak, and Broca established the connection of this disruption with damage to a part of the lower frontal gyrus of the hemisphere. Broca and Wernicke were founders of a fine localization movement in understanding the connection between mental functions and certain segments of the brain.

89. *Monakow, Constantin* (1853-1930), Swiss neurologist, anatomist, and physiologist.
90. Vygotsky objected decisively to the analogies made by authors (Kretschmer, Blonsky) between symptoms of schizophrenia and certain features of adolescent behavior.
91. *Bleuler, Eigen* (1857-1939), see Vol. 2, p. 482.
92. The chapter closes with a consideration of the development of separate mental processes and interfunctional connections as bases of their development. It is the final chapter in the part of the book that Vygotsky called *"Psychology of the Adolescent."* At the same time, this chapter seems to continue the small book of Vygotsky, *Imagination and Creativity during Childhood* (1930).
93. The conception of the children's collective by authors to which Vygotsky refers is the conception of a group of children cooperating with each other and entering into various interrelations. At that time no study was yet done that showed that such cooperation can be found at various levels of development and that groups of children acting together may not be a collective in the strict meaning of that term. The idea that children's logical thinking develops parallel to the development of the children's social life was connected by Piaget with the view that "we have no other criterion for truth except the agreement of minds with each other" (1932, p. 401). Vygotsky frequently criticized this, one of the original positions of Piaget (Vol. 2, pp. 70-74).
94. *Janet, Pierre* (1859-1947), see Vol. 2, pp. 482-483; Vol. 3, p. 348.
95. *Busemann, A.*, German psychologist. He worked in the area of adolescent psychology.
96. *"Vertebrata"* (Vertebrates—D.E.). "Their essential trait: assembly of the whole body around a nervous system. This makes possible development to self-consciousness, etc." (K. Marx and F. Engels, *Works*, Vol. 20, p. 623).
97. The description of the personality of the adolescent in most German studies of that time, especially those of Spranger, refers to adolescents and youth from educated classes, that is, bourgeois (upper and middle) and bourgeois intelligentsia. There were still very few studies of personality of adolescents of other classes. Busemann's work is interesting because it contains comparative studies of adolescents of different social strata and of urban and village inhabitants. As Vygotsky shows in his careful analysis of Busemann's facts, the investigator himself did not succeed in doing this completely.
98. *Deborin* (Ioffe) *Abram Moiseevich* (1881-1963), Soviet philosopher.
99. *Politzer, Jean* (1903-1942), French philosopher-Marxist and psychologist. His work was based on the materialistic position of society and its history. He was killed by the Fascist invaders.
100. *Lévy-Bruhl, Lucien* (1857-1939), see Vol. 1, p. 464; Vol. 2, p. 482.

The Problem of Age

1. A chapter in the book on child (developmental) psychology that L. S. Vygotsky was preparing during the last years of his life (1932-1934). From the archives of the family of the author. The first section of the chapter was published in a somewhat abbreviated form in the journal *Voprosy Psikhologii* [Problems in Psychology], No. 2, 1972. The chapter as a whole is published here for the first time.

2. Vygotsky has in mind the transition from primary school age to adolescence.
3. "All life is at the same time also a dying (F. Engels)" has in mind the idea of Engels: "To live means to die" (K. Marx and F. Engels, *Works*, Vol. 20, p. 611).
4. It is interesting to note that in the chapters of the book, *Pedology of the Adolescent,* published in this volume, Vygotsky has still not determined the age of adolescence as being stable, frequently using the concepts of "transitional age" and "adolescent age" as synonyms.
5. In the manuscript, Vygotsky's critical periods are presented as consisting of three phases: precritical, critical, and postcritical, and the stable phases as consisting of two stages: the first stage and the second stage.
6. "My relation to my environment is my consciousness." (K. Marx and F. Engels, *Works*, Vol. 3, p. 29).
7. The concept of zones of proximal development introduced by Vygotsky is of extreme importance. It is closely connected with his understanding of the relation between learning and development.

    The methodology of the diagnostics of the zones of proximal development is beginning to be developed in just the last decades, but thus far, it has been developed inadequately.
8. Evidently, Vygotsky planned to treat this problem in a special chapter, but did not have time to do so.
9. Vygotsky presents the problems of diagnostics of development in greater detail in "Diagnostics of Development and the Pedological Clinic for Difficult Childhood" (Vol. 5, pp. 257-321).

Infancy

1. This chapter was written by L. S. Vygotsky in preparation for a book on child (developmental) psychology. From the archives of the author's family. Published here for the first time. The first section of the manuscript is missing. A description of two periods is given in this chapter: the newborn, which Vygotsky considered transitional or critical, and infancy, which the author considered stable. It presents Vygotsky's attempt to realize the principles of considering the dynamics of development that he formulated in the chapter, "The Problem of Age," as applied to a concrete age period.

    It must be kept in mind that during the years when this paper was written, in Soviet science, there were very few studies of the newborn period and infancy and these were mainly the work of N. M. Shchelovanov and his colleagues, representatives of reflexology. Studies of the earliest times of appearance of conditioned reflexes were just beginning; data on the development of the brain during the first year of life at the cellular level were scant. Regardless of this, Vygotsky succeeded in developing a number of productive hypotheses that were partially confirmed, for example, the hypothesis that the upper limit of the newborn period is connected with the appearance of the basic neoformation—the appearance of individual mental life connected with isolating a person as a basic figure in a social situation; this created the possibility for characterizing the social situation of development in infancy and its basic contradictions.

    Studies of premature and postmature newborns conducted after 1932 wholly confirmed Vygotsky's conclusions. However, as studies of the earliest formation of conditioned reflexes have shown, the formation of these reflexes is possible in newborn children as early as during the period between the moment of actual birth and the end of the normal period of pregnancy.

These facts are evidence of the enormous influence of the environment on the maturation of the physiological mechanisms of higher sections of the nervous system (N. I. Kasatkin, 1951).

2. Studies have shown that the earliest conditioned reflexes can be formed by the second to third week of life (N. I. Kasatkin, 1951).

3. *Wallon, Henri* (1879-1962), French psychologist, specialist on child, patho-, and pedagogical psychology. He developed dialectical-materialistic views of mental development during childhood. After the Second World War, he participated in the reform of education in France. In our country, two of his books were translated: *From Action to Thought*, Moscow, 1956, and *Mental Development of the Child*, Moscow, 1967.

4. Vygotsky describes experiments conducted by F. Lebenstein under the direction of H. Volkelt in which the latter frequently participated.

5. See the last section of this chapter: "Basic Theories on Infancy."

6. N. M. Shchelovanov was a primary representative of this theory; he was one of the closest students of the founder of reflexology, V. M. Bekhterev. The founders of infant reflexology were colleagues of Shchelovanov—N. L. Figurin, M. P. Denisova, and N. I. Kasatkin. According to the initiative of V. M. Bekhterev, at the beginning of the 1920s, Shchelovanov organized a special institute in which the development of children from birth to age three was studied. Here, on the basis of daily, systematic observations of children's development and special experiments, important materials were developed on the course of development of children of this age. Even now, the materials have not lost their significance. Subsequently, the institute branched into two: one worked in Leningrad under the direction of Figurin within the Leningrad Medical Pediatric Institute; the other, directed by Shchelovanov in Moscow, became part of the Moscow Pediatric Institute. On the basis of the work of these institutes, a system of rearing young children was developed together with corresponding handbooks for the care givers (*Rearing Young Children in Children's Institutes*, edited by N. M. Shchelovanov and N. M. Aksarina, 3rd ed., Moscow, 1955).

7. This theoretical conception was developed by K. Bühler (1932). Vygotsky frequently considered the theoretical views of Bühler critically on this and on other problems (Vol. 2).

8. K. Koffka was a representative of this theory. For a more detailed criticism of Koffka's views, see Vol. 1, pp. 238-290.

9. This conception was represented, first, by the Freudians, in the person of S. Freud himself, and S. Bernfeld; second, by J. Piaget. For Vygotsky's criticism of the theory of autism and egocentrism, see also Vol. 2, pp. 20-23.

The Crisis of the First Year

1. This is a stenographic transcript of a lecture delivered by L. S. Vygotsky at the A. I. Herzen Leningrad Pedagogical Institute in 1933/34. From the archives of the author's family. Published here for the first time. The transcript reflects the oral speech of the author. Vygotsky's lectures were distinguished by the special expressiveness of sense. They were devoid of any external impact, but were rich in intonation. At the same time, they had the character of thinking

aloud and contained various hypotheses. In his lectures, Vygotsky frequently presented what he was thinking at the time. This course was a course on problems and was not a systematic presentation of all the questions of child psychology. In the lectures, problems were elucidated which the author considered to be central. When the lectures were being given, under Vygotsky's direction, T. E. Konnikova conducted a study on the initial stage of speech development. The study was concluded after Vygotsky died (see T. E. Konnikova, 1947). Some examples given in the lecture were taken from Konnikova's research. Interesting material on the appearance of the child's first words are contained in the paper of Vygotsky's student, F. I. Fradkina, "The Appearance of Speech in the Child" (1955). Important materials on the characteristics of autonomous speech in twins, conditions of retardation of speech at this stage of development, and preventing such retardation are given in the book: A. R. Luria and F. Ya. Yudovich, *Speech and Development of Mental Processes in the Child*, Moscow, 1956.

2. We are speaking here of the personalistic theory developed by Stern (Vol. 2, pp. 80-89, 484).

3. This seems to be a contradiction. Vygotsky calls this stage of speech development autonomous speech, and in the lecture, he says that this language cannot be considered as autonomous. In this case, Vygotsky wants to emphasize that the indicated form of language nevertheless develops on a base of the developed language of adults and in interaction with them.

4. The Experimental-Defectological Institute (EDI) is at present the Scientific Research Institute of Defectology of the Academy of Pedological Sciences of the USSR.

5. *Rau, Fedor Andreevich* (1868-1957), eminent Soviet teacher of the deaf and speech therapist. For many years, he worked in the Scientific Research Institute of Defectology.

6. See: K. Marx and F. Engels, *Works*, Vol. 3, p. 29: "Where there is any relation, it exists for me; an animal does not '*relate*' to anything and does not, in general, '*relate*'; for an animal, its relation to others does not exist as relation. Consciousness, therefore, is from the very beginning a social product and remains as such as long as there are any people. Consciousness is, of course, in the beginning, consciousness of the *closest*, sensorily perceived environment and consciousness of a limited connection with other people and things that are outside the individual who is beginning to be conscious of himself . . ."

Early Childhood

1. Stenographic transcript of a lecture delivered by L. S. Vygotsky at the A. I. Herzen Leningrad Pedagogical Institute during the 1933/34 academic year. From the archives of the A. I. Herzen Leningrad Pedagogical Institute. Published here for the first time.

2. Under Vygotsky's direction at the Psychology Laboratory of the Academy of Communist Education, there was, at the end of the 1920s, a group of young psychologists, including L. I. Bozhovich, A. N. Leontev (1903-1979), A. V. Zaporozhets (1905-1981), R. E. Levina (b. 1908), N. G. Morozova (b. 1906), and L. S. Slavina (b. 1906); in 1931, in connection with the liquidation of the laboratory and moving of some of the colleagues (A. N. Leontev, A. R. Luria,

L. I. Bozhovich, and A. V. Zaporozhets) to Kharkov, the group disintegrated. Studies by L. S. Slavina were not published.

3. *The Leipzig school,* a trend in German psychology promulgated by F. Krueger, the director of the Leipzig Psychology Institute. For this trend, the principal concept in explaining mental life was the concept of initial whole mental experience. The views of the school have an idealistic character—the mind is reduced to a sensory-like experience and points of reflection of objective reality are excluded from it.

4. *Sechenov, Ivan Mikhailovich* (1829-1905), see Vol. 2, 488.

5. Vygotsky uses the word "activity" quite frequently, but in a very general sense. Here he resorts to a concrete description and analysis of a child's activity at an early age.

6. For more detailed information on Vygotsky's views of play, see "Play and Its Role in the Mental Development of the Child," *Vopr. Psikhologii* [Problems in Psychology], No. 6, 1966.

7. *Phonology,* see Vol. 2, p. 482.

8. On Vygotsky's distinguishing two types of analyses, see Vol. 2, pp. 13-15.

9. Vygotsky has in mind the idea: ". . . he (L. Feuerbach—D.E.) does not notice that the sensory world around him is not at all a certain given, directly given by the age, always the same kind of thing, but that he is the product of industry and the social state, and in the sense that this is a historical product, the result of activity of a whole series of generations, each of which stood on the shoulders of the preceding . . . " (K. Marx and F. Engels, *Works,* Vol. 3, p. 42).

10. Morozova's studies were not published.

11. Here Vygotsky states the position: "Language is as old as consciousness; language *is* practical, existing also for other people and only in this way existing also for me alone, real consciousness; like consciousness, language develops only from need, from a persistent need to communicate with other people" (K. Marx and F. Engels, *Works,* Vol. 3, p. 29).

The Crisis at Age Three

1. The stenographic transcript of a lecture delivered by L. S. Vygotsky during the 1933/34 academic year at the A. I. Herzen Leningrad Pedagogical Institute. From the archives of the author's family. Published here for the first time. No sources are indicated in the lecture for the factual material Vygotsky used for his generalizations. We shall indicate only certain possible sources: E. Köhler, *Die Personlichkeit des dreiyärigen Kindes,* Vienna, 1926.

The Crisis at Age Seven

1. The stenographic transcript of a lecture delivered by L. S. Vygotsky during the 1933/34 academic year at the A. I. Herzen Leningrad Pedagogical Institute. From the archives of the author's family. Published here for the first time.

REFERENCES[1]

Marx, K., and Engels, F., Works, Vols. 3, 20, 21, 23, 25, Part II.
Lenin, V. I., Complete Works, Vols. 18, 29.

* * *

Ament, W. (1908). *Dusha Rebenka* [The Mind of the Child]. St. Petersburg.
*Ananin, S. A. (1915). *Interes po Ucheniju Sovremennoj Psikhologii i Pedagogiki* [Interest in the Teaching of Contemporary Psychology and Pedagogy]. Kiev.
*Arjamov, I. A. (1928). *Rabochij Podrostok* [The Working Adolescent]. Moscow.
*Arjamov, I. A. (1928). Osobennosti povedenija sovremennogo podrostka [Behavioral features of the contemporary adolescent]. *Pedologija, 1.*
*Arjamov, I. A. (1929). Osnovnye Voprosy Pedologii Podrostka [Basic Problems in Adolescent Pedology]. *Trudy 2-go Mosk. Gos. Universiteta* [Proceedings of the Second Moscow State University], Vol. 1.
*Arjamov, I. A. (1930). *Osnovy Pedologii* [Fundamentals of Pedology]. Moscow. (4th edition).
*Arkin, E. A. (1924). *Doshkol'nyj Vozrast* [The Preschool Age]. Moscow. (2nd edition).
Baldwin, J. (1904). *Psikhologija v ee Primenenii k Vospitaniju* [Psychology and Its Application to Education]. Moscow.
Baldwin, J. *Dukhovnoe Razvitie Detskogo Individuuma i Chelovecheskogo Roda* [Mental Development of the Child as an Individual and of the Human Race]. Moscow. (Vol. I, 1911; Vol. II, 1912).
*Basov, M. Ja. (1926). *Metodika Psikhologicheskikh Nabljudenij nad Det'mi* [Methods of Psychological Observation of Children]. Moscow–Leningrad.
*Basov, M. Ja. (1928). *Obshchie Osnovy Pedologii* [General Fundamentals of Pedology]. Moscow.
Bekhterev, V. M. (1926). *Obshchie Osnovy Refleksologii Cheloveka* [General Fundamentals of Human Reflexology]. Leningrad.
Bernfeld, S. (1931). Psikhologija Junosti E. Shprangera [The Psychology of Youth of E. Spranger]. In I. A. Arjamov (Ed.), *Pedologija Junosti* [Pedology of Youth]. Moscow–Leningrad.
Biedl, A. K. (1931). K kharakteristike perioda polovogo sozrevanija [Toward a description of the period of sexual maturation]. In I. A. Arjamov (Ed.), *Pedologija Junosti* [Pedology of Youth]. Moscow–Leningrad.
Binet, A. (1889). *Psikhologija Umozakljuchenija na Osnovanii Eksperimental'nykh Issledovanij Posledstvom Gipnoza* [The Psychology of Deduction Based on Experimental Studies of Hypnosis]. Moscow.
Binet, A. (1894). *Mekhanizm Myshlenija* [Mechanism of Thinking]. Odessa.
Binet, A. (1910). *Sovremennye Idei o Detjakh* [Contemporary Ideas about Children]. Moscow.
Bleuler, E. (1927). *Autisticheskoe Myshlenie* [Autistic Thinking]. Odessa.
*Blonsky, P. P. (1925). *Osnovy Pedagogiki* [Fundamentals of Pedagogy]. Moscow.
*Blonsky, P. P. (1925). *Pedologija* [Pedology]. Moscow.
*Blonsky, P. P. (1927). *Pedologija v Massovoj Shkole I Stupeni* [Pedology in a Mass School in Grade I]. Moscow.
Blonsky, P. P. (1927). *Psikhologicheskie Ocherki* [Essays in Psychology]. Moscow.
Blonsky, P. P. (1930). *Vozvratnaja Pedologija* [Reflexive Pedology]. Moscow–Leningrad.

[1]An asterisk (*) before a reference denotes works recommended by L. S. Vygotsky as supplementary literature to the course he gave.
Publisher's note: The references consist of two parts in the Russian edition. The first part is given in the Cyrillic alphabet, and the second part, which begins on page 339, is given in the Roman alphabet. Cyrillic titles in the first part are transliterated, followed by their translation.

335

Blonsky, P. P. (1930). *Osnovy Pedologii* [Fundamentals of Pedology]. Moscow.
*Blonsky, P. P., Ionova, M., Levinskij, V., and Shejman, M. (1927). *Metodika Pedologicheskogo Obsledovanija Detej Shkol'nogo Vozrasta* [Methodology of Pedological Examination of School-age Children]. Moscow–Leningrad.
Bühler, C., Tudor-Hart, B., and Hetzer, H. (1931). *Sotsial'no-psikhologicheskoe Izuchenie Rebenka Pervogo Goda Zhizni* [Sociopsychological Study of the Child during the First Year of Life]. Moscow.
Bühler, K. (1924). *Dukhovnoe Razvitie Rebenka* [Mental Development of the Child]. Moscow.
Bühler, K. (1930). *Ocherk Dukhovnogo Razvitija Rebenka* [Outline of the Mental Development of the Child]. Moscow.
Claparède, E. (1911). *Psikhologija Rebenka i Eksperimental'naja Pedgogika* [Child Psychology and Experimental Pedagogy]. St. Petersburg.
Claparède, E. (1932). Predislovie k knige Zh. Piaget *Rech' i Myshlenie Rebenka* [Introduction to J. Piaget's book, *Speech and Thinking of the Child*]. Moscow–Leningrad.
Compayré, G. (1910). *Otrochestvo, Ego Psikholkogija i Pedagogija* [Adolescence, Its Psychology and Pedagogy]. St. Petersburg.
Compayré, G. (1912). *Umstvennoe i Nravstvennoe Razvitie Rebenka* [Intellectual and Moral Development of the Child]. Moscow.
Darwin, C. (1881). *Nabljudenija nad Zhizn'ju Rebenka* [Observations of the Life of a Child]. St. Petersburg.
Deborin, A. M. (1923). *Vvedenie v Filosofiju Dialekticheskogo Materializma* [Introduction to the Philosophy of Dialectical Materialism]. Moscow.
Deborin, A. M. (1929). *Dialektika i Estestvoznanie* [Dialectics and Natural Science]. Moscow–Leningrad.
Denisova, M. P., and Figurin, N. L. (1925). Opyt refleksologicheskogo izuchenija novorozhdennogo [Research on reflexological study of the newborn]. In *Novoe v Refleksologii i Fiziologii Nervnoj Sistemy* [What's New in Reflexology and the Physiology of the Nervous System]. (1st edition). Leningrad.
Denisova, M. P., and Figurin, N. L. (1929). Eksperimental'noe izuchenie reaktsii na novoe u rebenka do odnogo goda [Experimental study of reaction to the new in a child younger than one year]. In *Voprosy geneticheskoj refleksologii i Pedologii Mladenchestva* [Problems of Genetic Reflexology and Pedology in Infancy]. Moscow–Leningrad.
*Dewey, J. (1915). *Psikhologija i Pedagogika Myshlenija* [The Psychology and Pedagogy of Thinking]. Moscow.
Figurin, N. L., and Denisova, M. P. (1926). Kratkaya diagnosticheskaya skhema razvitiya rebenka do 1 goda [A brief diagnostic plan of the child's development up to age one]. In *Novoe v Refleksologii i Fiziologii Nervnoi Sistemy: Sb. Vtoroi* [What's New in Reflexology and the Physiology of the Nervous System]. (2nd collection). Leningrad.
Figurin, N. L., and Denisova, M. P. (1929). *Etapy razvitija povedenija rebenka ot rozhdenija do odnogo goda* [Stages of development of child behavior from birth to age one]. In *Voprosy Geneticheskoj Refleksologii i Pedologii Mladenchestva. Sb. Pervij* [Problems of Genetic Reflexology and Pedology, First Collection]. Moscow–Leningrad.
Freud, S. (1923). *Vlechenija i Ikh Sud'ba* [Drives and Their Fate]. Berlin; Moscow.
Freud, S. (1923). *Psikhoanaliz Detskikh Nevrozov* [Analysis of Childhood Neuroses]. Moscow.
Freud, S. (1924). *Ja i Ono* [I and It]. Leningrad.
Freud, S. (1925). *Po Tu Storonu Printsipa Udovol'stvija* [This Side of the Pleasure Principle]. Moscow.
Galton, F. (1875). *Nasledstvennost' Talanta* [Inheritance of Talent]. St. Petersburg.
*Gellerstein, S. G. (1926). Psikhotekhnika [Psychotechnique]. Moscow.
*Gel'man, I. G. (1923). *Polovoja Zhizn' Sovremennoj Molodezhi: Opyt Social'no-biologicheskogo Obsledovanija* [Sex Life of Contemporary Youth: Results of Social-Biological Study] Moscow–Petrograd.
Gesell, A. (1930). *Umstvennoe Razvitie Rebenka* [Intellectual Development of the Child]. Moscow–Leningrad.
Gesell, A. (1932). *Pedologija Rannego Vozrasta* [Pedology of Early Childhood]. Moscow; Leningrad.
Groos, K. (1916). *Dushevnaja Zhizn' Rebenka* [Mental Life of the Child]. Kiev.
Hall, S. (1912). *Sobranie Statej po Pedologii i Pedagogike* [Collected Papers on Pedology and Pedagogy]. Moscow.
*Hall, S. (1920). *Instinkty i Chuvstva v Junosheskom Vózraste* [Instincts and Feelings in Adolescence]. Petrograd.
Herbart, J. F. (1906). *Izbrannye Pedagogicheskie Sochinenija* [Collected Pedagogical Works]. Moscow.
Jerusalem, W. (1911). *Uchebnik Psikhologii* [Psychology Text]. (translation of the 4th German edition). Moscow.
Jung, K. (1909). *Psikhoz i Ego Soderzhanie* [Psychosis and Its Content]. St. Petersburg.
Jung, K. (1924). *Psikhologicheskie Tipy* [Psychological Types]. Moscow.
Koffka, K. (1934). *Osnovy Psikhicheskogo Razvitija* [Fundamentals of Mental Development]. Moscow–Leningrad.

Köhler, W. (1930). *Issledovanie Intellekta Chelovekopodobnykh Obez'jan* [Study of the Intellect of Human-like Apes]. Moscow.

*Kolodnaja, A. I. (1929). *Interesy Rabochego Podrostka* [Interests of the Working Adolescent]. Moscow.

*Kornilov, K. N. (1928). Biogeneticheskij princip [The Biogenetic Principle]. In S. M. Vasilejsky (Ed.), *Osnovnye Voprosy Pedologii v Izbrannykh Stat'jakh* [Basic Problems of Pedology in Selected Papers]. Moscow–Leningrad.

Kretschmer, E. (1924). *Stroenie Tela i Kharakter* [Body Structure and Character]. Kiev.

Kretschmer, E. (1927). *Meditsinskaja Psikhologija* [Medical Psychology]. Moscow.

*Kretschmer, E. (1928). *Histerija* [Hysteria]. Moscow.

Kroh, O. (1931). Intellectual'noe razvitie v period sozrevanija [Intellectual development during maturation]. In I. Arjamov (Ed.), *Pedologija Junosti* [Pedology of Youth]. Moscow–Leningrad.

Külpe, O. (1914). Sovremennaja psikhologija myshlenija [Modern psychology of thinking]. *Novye Idei v Filosofii, 16* [New Ideas in Philosophy, 16].

Lashley, K. (1930). Osnovnye nervnye mekhanizmy povedenija [Basic nerve mechanisms of behavior]. *Psikhologija, 3*, 3 [Psychology, 3, No. 3].

Lay, W. A. (1909). *Eksperimenmtal'naja Pedagogika* [Experimental Pedagogy]. Moscow.

Lay, W. A. (1910). *Eksperimental'naja Didaktika* [Experimental Didactics]. St. Petersburg.

*Leontev, A. N. (1931). *Razvitie Pamjati* [Development of Memory]. Moscow.

Lévy-Bruhl, L. (1930). *Pervobytnoe Myshlenie* [Primitive Thinking]. Moscow.

Lipps, Th. (1907). *Rukovodstvo k Psikhologii* [Psychology Handbook]. St. Petersburg.

*Luria, A. R. (1929). Puti razvitija detskogo myshlenija [Ways of developing children's thinking]. *Estestvoznanie i Marksizm, 2* [Natural Science and Marxism, 2].

Maslov, M. S. (1926-27). *Osnovy Uchenija o Rebenke i ob Osobennostjakh Ego Zabolevanij* [Fundamentals of Teaching on the Child and the Features of His Illnesses]. Leningrad.

Meumann, E. (1914-17). *Lektsii po Ekspermental'noj Pedagogike, ch. 1-3* [Lectures on Experimental Pedagogy, Parts 1-3]. Moscow.

*Nikolaev, L. P. (1925). *Vlijanie Sotsial'nykh Faktorov na Fizicheskoe Razvitie Detej* [Influence of Social Factors on Physical Development of Children]. Kharkov.

O'Shea, M. (1910). *Rol' Aktivnosti v Zhizni Rebenka* [The Role of Activity in the Life of the Child]. Moscow.

Pavlov, I. P. (1932). Probnaja ekskursija fiziologa v oblast' psikhiatrii [A trial excursion of a physiologist into the area of psychiatry]. In *Dvadtsatiletnij Opyt Ob'ektivnogo Izuchenija Vysshej Nervnoj Dejatel'nosti (Povedenija) Zhivotnykh* [Twenty-Year Experiment in Objective Study of Higher Nervous Activity (Behavior) of Animals]. Leningrad.

*Pedologija, 1(7). (1930).

Peiper, A. (1929). *Funktsija Mozga Grudnogo Rebenka* [Brain Function in the Nursing Child]. Moscow.

*Piaget, J. (1932). *Rech' i Myshlenie Rebenka* [Speech and Thinking of the Child]. Moscow–Leningrad.

Potebnya, A. A. (1922). *Mysl' i Jazyk (Vol. 1)* [Thinking and Language (Vol. 1)]. Odessa.

Preyer, W. (1894). *Dukhovnoe Razvitie v Pervom Detstve* [Mental Development in Earliest Childhood]. St. Petersburg.

Preyer, W. (1912). *Dusha Rebenka* [The Mind of the Child]. St. Petersburg.

Ribot, Th. (1892). *Psikhologija Vnimanija* [The Psychology of Attention]. St. Petersburg.

*Ribot, Th. (1901). *Opyt Issledovanija Tvorcheskogo Voobrazhenija* [A Study of Creative Imagination]. St. Petersburg.

*Rubinstein, M. M. and Ignatev, V. E. (1926). *Psikhologija, Pedagogika i Gigiena Junosti* [Psychology, Pedagogy and Hygiene of Youth]. Moscow.

*Ruele, O. (1923). *Proletarskoe Ditja* [Proletarian Children]. Moscow.

*Sakharov, L. S. (1930). O metodakh issledovanija ponjatij [Methods for studying concepts]. *Psikhologija, 3*, 1 [Psychology, 3:1].

Shapiro, S. A., and Gerke, E. D. (1930). *Protsess prisposoblenija k uslovijam sredy v povedenii rebenka* [The process of adaptation to conditions of the environment in the behavior of the child]. In *Ocherednye Voprosy Pedologii* [Immediate Problems of Pedology]. Moscow–Leningrad.

Shchelovanov, N. M. (1926). *Nekotorye otlichitel'nye osobennosti v razvitii nervnoj dejatel'nosti cheloveka po dannym sravnitel'nogo izuchenija rannikh stadij ontogeneza povedenija cheloveka i zhivotnykh* [Certain distinguishing features in the development of nervous activity in man according to data from comparative study of early stages of the ontogenesis of behavior of man and animals]. *Trudy Vtorogo Vsesojuznogo S'ezda Fiziologov* [Proceedings of the Second All-Union Congress of Physiologists]. Moscow–Leningrad.

Shchelovanov, N. M., Figurin, N. L., and Denisova, M. N. (1928). *Osobennosti rebenka rannego vozrasta po dannym geneticheskoj refleksologii* [Characteristics of the child at an early age according to data of genetic reflexology]. In *Pedologija i Vospitanie* [Pedology and Education]. Moscow.

*Smirnov, V. E. (1929). *Psikhologiya Junosheskogo Vozrasta* [Psychology of Youth]. Moscow–Leningrad.

Stern, W. (1922). *Psikhologija Rannego Detstva do Shestiletnego Vozrasta: S Ispol'zovaniem v Kachestve Materiala Nenapechatannykh Dnevnikov Klary Stern* [Psychology of Early Childhood up to Age Sixteen Using Unpublished Diaries of Clara Stern as Material]. Petrograd.

Stern, W. (1926). *Odarennost' Detej i Podrostkov i Metody Ee Issledovanija* [Giftedness of Children and Adolescents and Methods for Studying It]. Kharkov.

*Storch, A. (1930). *Arkhaicheski-Primitivnoe Perezhivanie i Myshlenie Shizofrenikov* [Archaic-Primitive Experience and Thinking of Schizophrenics]. Moscow.

Sully, J. (1901). *Ocherki po Psikhologii Detstva* [Essays on the Psychology of Childhood]. Moscow.

Taine, H. (1872). *Ob Ume i Poznanii* [The Mind and Perception] St. Petersburg.

Thorndike, E. (1926). *Printsipy Obuchenija, Osnovannye na Psikhologii* [Principles of Teaching Based on Psychology]. Moscow.

Titchener, E. (1898). *Ocherki Psikhologii* [Essays in Psychology]. St. Petersburg.

Titchener, E. (1914). *Uchebnik Psikhologii, ch. 1, 2* [Psychology Textbook, Parts 1, 2]. St. Petersburg.

Tolstoy, L. N. (1958). *Detstvo. Otrochestvo. Junost'. Sobr. Soch., Vol. 1* [Childhood. Boyhood. Youth. Collected Works, Vol. 1]. Moscow.

Tumlirz, O. (1931). *Edinstvo psikhologii i ego znachenie dlja teorii perekhodnogo vozrasta* [Unity of psychology and its significance for the theory of the transitional age. In I. Arjamov, *Pedologija Junosti* [Pedology of Youth]. Moscow–Leningrad.

*Veselovskaja, K. P. (1924). *Pedologicheskij Praktikum: Posobie dlja Prakticheskikh Zanjatij po Pedologii* [Pedological Laboratory Manual: Handbook for Practical Exercises in Pedology]. Moscow.

*Veselovskaja, K. P. (1926). *Pedologicheskie Osnovy Polovogo Vospitanija* [Pedological Bases for Sex Education]. Moscow.

Volkelt, H. (1930). *Eksperimental'naja Psikhologija Doshkol'nika* [Experimental Psychology with the Preschool Child]. Moscow.

Volpin, L. L. (1902). *Vesovye Dannye o Roste Golovnogo Mozga u Detej* [Weight Data on Growth of the Brain in Children].

Vyazemsky, N. V. (1901). *Izmenenie Organizma v Period Sformirovanija* [Change in the Organism during the Period of Formation]. St. Petersburg.

Vygotsky, L. S. (1926). *Pedagogicheskaja Psikhologija* [Pedagogical Psychology]. Moscow.

*Vygotsky, L. S. (1928). *Pedologija Shkol'nogo Vozrasta* [School-Age Pedology]. Moscow.

*Vygotsky, L. S. (1929). Struktura interesov v perekhodnom vozraste i interesy rabochego podrostka [The structure of interests during the transitional age and interests of the working adolescent]. In *Voprosy Pedologii Rabochego Podrostka* [Problems in the Pedology of the Working Adolescent]. Moscow.

*Vygotsky, L. S. (1929). Geneticheskie korni myshlenija i rechi [Genetic roots of thinking and speech]. *Estestvoznanie i Marksizm, 1* [Natural Science and Marxism, 1].

Vygotsky, L. S. (1929). Razvite activnogo vnimanija v detskom vozraste [Development of active attention during childhood]. In *Voprosy Marksistskoj Pedagogiki, vyp. 1* [Problems of Marxist Pedagogy] (1st edition). Moscow.

Vygotsky, L. S. (1930). *Voobrazhenie i Tvorchestvo v Detskom Vozraste* [Imagination and Creativity during Childhood]. Moscow–Leningrad.

Vygotsky, L. S. (1929-1931). *Pedologija Podrostka* [Pedology of the Adolescent]. (1929). *Zadanija 1-4* [Assignments 1-4]. Moscow; (1930). *Zadanija 5-8* [Assignments 5-8]. Moscow. (1931). *Zadanija 9-16* [Assignments 9-16]. Moscow–Leningrad.

Vygotsky, L. S. (1932). *K Probleme Psikhologii Shizofrenii. Sovetskaja Nevropatologija, Psikhiatrija, Psikhogigiena* [On the Problem of the Psychology of Schizophrenia. Soviet Neuropathology, Psychiatry, Psychohygiene], Vol. 1. (8th edition). St. Petersburg.

Watson, J. (1926). *Psikhologija kak Nauka o Povedenii* [Psychology as a Behavioral Science]. Moscow–Leningrad.

Watson, J. (1929). *Psikhologicheskij Ukhod za Rebenkom* [The Psychological Care of Children]. Moscow.

Wundt, W. (1897). *Ocherk Psikhologii* [Outline of Psychology]. St. Petersburg.

Wundt, W. (1914). *Fantazija kak Osnova Iskusstv* [Fantasy as a Basis for the Arts]. St. Petersburg.

*Zagorovsky, P. L. (1928). O tak nazyvaemoj negativnoj faze v podrostnichestve [On the so-called negative phase in adolescence]. *Pedologija, I, 1.*

Zagorovsky, P. L. (1929). *Vtoroe Shkol'noe Detstvo i Osobennosti Ego Sotsial'nogo Povedenija* [The Second School Childhood and Features of Its Social Behavior]. Voronezh.

*Zalkind, A. B. (1925). *Revoljutsija i Molodezh'* [Revolution and Youth]. Sverdlovsk.

*Zalkind, A. B. (1926). *Voprosy Sovetskoj Pedagogiki* [Problems of Soviet Pedagogy]. Leningrad.

*Zalkind, A. B. (1927). *Osnovnye Voprosy Pedologii* [Basic Problems of Pedology]. Moscow.

*Zalkind, A. B. (1928). *Polovoe Vospitanie* [Sex Education]. Moscow.

*Zalkind, A. B. (1929). Pedologicheskie osnovy vospitatel'noj raboty s podrostkovym vozrastom [Pedological Bases for Educational Work with Adolescents]. In *Voprosy Pedologii Rabochego Podrostka* [Problems in Pedology of the Working Adolescent]. Moscow.

*Zalkind, A. B. (1929). *Pedologija v SSSR* [Pedology in the USSR]. Moscow.

Zalkind, A. B. (1930). Osnovnye osobennosti perekhodnogo vozrasta [Basic features of the transitional age]. *Pedologija, 1* [Pedology, 1].

*Zavadovsky, B. I. (1923). *Problemy Starosti i Omolozhenija* [Problems of Age and Rejuvenation]. Moscow.

Ziehen, T. (1909). *Fiziologicheskaja Psikhologija v 15 Lektsijakh* [Physiological Psychology in 15 Lectures]. St. Petersburg.

Ziehen, T. (1924). *Dushevnaja i Polovaja Zhizn' Junoshestva* [Mental and Sexual Life of Youth]. Moscow.

* * *

Ach, N. (1921). *Über die Begriffsbildung.* Bamberg.

Ament, W. (1899). *Die Entwicklung von Sprechen und Denken beim Kinde.* Leipzig.

Berger, F. (1929). Beitrage zum probleme der kategorialen wahrnehmung und ihren pädagogischen bedeutung. *Z. Psychol.,* B. 110, 111.

Bernfeld, S. (1925). *Psychologie der Saüglings.*Wien.

Busemann, A. (1925). Kollektive selbsterziehung in kindheit und jugend. *Z. Pädagogische Psychol.*

Busemann, A. (1926). *Die Jugend im Eigenem Urteil.* Langensalz.

Busemann, A.(1927). Die erregungsphasen. *Z. Kinderforsch.,* No. 2.

Busemann, A. (1927). *Pädagogische Milienkunde.* Halle.

Bühler, Ch. (1923). *Das Seelenleben des Jugendlichen.* Jena.

Bühler, Ch. (1926). Die schwarmerei als phase der reifezeit. *Z. Pädagogische Psychol.,* B.100.

Bühler, Ch. (1928). *Kindheit und Jugend.* Leipzig.

Bühler, Ch. (1929). Das Märchen und die Phantasie des Kindes. *Beiheft 17 zur Z. Angew Psychol.* Leipzig.

Bühler, K. (1907, 1908). Tatsachen und probleme zu einer psychologie der denkvorgänge. *Arch. Gesamte Psychol.,* 9, 12.

Bühler, K. (1908). Uber das Sprachverstandnis vom Standpunkt der Normalpsychologie aus. (Sammelreferat). 3. Monograf. Exp. Psych.

Bühler, K. (1913). *Die Gestaltwahrnemungen. 1 Experimentelle Untersuchungen zur Psychologischen und Ästhetischen Analyse der Raum- und Zeitanschauung.* Stuttgart.

Bühler, K. (1922). *Die Theorie der Perzeption.* Jena.

Canestrini, D. (1913). Über das sinnesleben des neugeborenen. *Monograf. aus dem Gesamtgebiet der Neurol. u. Psychiatrie,* 5, Heft.

Cassirer, E.(1923). La pathologie de conscience symbolique. *J. Psychol.,* Nos. 5-8.

Claparède, E. (1916). *Psychologie de lEnfant.* Geneve.

Claparède, E. (1918). La conscience de la ressemblance et de la difference chez lenfant. *Arch. Psych.,* XVII, S. 1.

Comments in Vygotskys critical remarks concerning "The Language and Thought of the Child, and Judgment and Reasoning in the Child by Jean Piaget." Massachusetts (1962).

Deuchler, G. (1920). Über schlusversuche insbesondere an kindern und jugendlichen. *Z. Pädagogische Psychol.*

Doflein, Fr. (1920). *Die Fortplanzung die Schwangerschaft und das Gebären der Sängetiere.* Jena.

Edinger, L. (1911). *Vorlesungen über den Bau der Nervosen Zentralorgane der Menschen und der Tiere.* Leipzig.

Edinger, L. (1921). *Einführung in die Lehre vom Bau und den Verrichtungen des Nervensystems.* Leipzig.

Eliasberg, W. (1928). *Über die Autonomische Kindersprache.* Berlin–Wien.

Eng. H, (1914). *Abstracte Begriffe im Sprechen und Denken des Kindes.* Leipzig.

Fajans, S. (1933). Erfolg, ausdauer und aktivität beim säugling und kleinkind. *Psychol. Forsch.*

Fajans, S. (1933). Die bedeutung der entfernung für die stärke eines aufforderungscharakters beim säugling. *Psychol. Forsch.,* Bd. 13, H. 3-4.

Gelb, A. Grundfragen der Wahrnehmungspsychologie. Ber ub. d. VII Kongr. f. exp. Psych. Jena. SS.

Gelb, A. (1920). Über den wegfall der wahrnehmung von "oberflächenfarben," *Z. Psychol.,* No. 84.

Gelb, A. and Goldstein, K. (1920). *Psychologische Analysen Hirnpathologischen Fälle.* Berlin.

Giese, F. (1920). Untersuchung der practischen intelligenz. *Z. Gesamte Neurol. Psychol.,* Bd. 59, 64.

Giese, F. (1922). *Kinderpsychologie. B. 1 abt. 3 (Handbuch der vergl. Psychologie).* München.

Goldstein, K. (1924). Das wesen der amnestischen aphasie. *Dtsch. Z. Nervenheilkunde,* 82.

Goldstein, K. (1926). Über aphasie. *Schweiz. Arch. Neurol. Psychiat.,* 19.

Goldstein, K. (1932). Die pathologischen tatsachen in ihrer bedeutung fur das problem der srpache. *Kongr. D. Ges. Psychol.,* 12.

Goldstein, K., and Gelb, A. (1924). Über farbennahmenamnesie. *Psych. Forsch.,* 6, Berlin.

Gregor, A. (1915). Untersuchungen über die entwicklung eingacherlogischer leistungen. *Z. Angew. Psychol.,* 10.

Groos, K. (1899). *Die Spiele der Menschen.* Jena.

Groos, K. (1907). *Die Spiele der Tiere.* Jena.

Groos, K. (1912). *Zur Psychologie der Reifenden Jugend*. S.L.

Hall, St. (1904). *Adolescence: Its Psychology and Its Relations to Physiology, Anthropology, Sociology, Sex, Crime, Religion, and Education*. New York.

Head, H. (1926). *Aphasia and Kindred Disorders of Speech*, Vols. I, II, Cambridge.

Hering, E. (1920). Grundzüge der Lehre vom Lichtsinn. Handbuch. Bd. III. Berlin.

Hetzer, H. (1927). Sistematische danerbeobachtungen am jugendlichen über der verlauf der negativen phase. *Z. Pädagogische Psychol.*, 2.

Hombergur, A. (1926). *Psychopatologie des Kindes und Jugendalter*. Berlin.

Hombergur, A. (1926). *Psychologie des Kindesalters*. Berlin.

Jaensch, E. R. (1920). *Einige Allgemeinere Fragen der Psychologie und Biologie des Denkens*. Leipzig.

Jaensch, E. (1925). *Über den Aufbau der Wahrnehmungswelt und ihre Strucktur im Jugendalter*. Leipzig.

Jaensch, E. R. (1927). Über eidetick und die typologische forschungsmethode. *Z. Psychol.*, 102.

Jaensch, E. R. (1927). *Über den Aufbau der Wahrnehmungswelt und die Grundlagen der menschlichen Erkenntnis*. Leipzig, Vol. 1.

Jaensch, E. R. (1930). *Eidetic Imagery*. New York.

Janet, P. (1930). *LEvolution Psychologique de la Personnalite*. Paris.

Koffka, K. (1915). Zur grundlegung der wahrnehmungs—Psychologie. *Z. Psychol.*, Bd. 73.

Köhler, W. (1920). *Die Physischen Gestalten in Ruhe und in stazionaren Zustand*. Brunswick.

Köhler, W. (1925). Komplextheorie und gestalttheorie. *Psychol.Forsch.*, 6.

Köhler, W. (1929). *Gestalt Psychology: An Introduction to New Concepts in Modern Psychology*. New York–London.

Köhler, W. (1932). *Probleme der Psychologie*. Berlin.

Kroh, O. (1922). *Subjektive Anschauungsbilder bei Jugendlichen*. Göttingen.

Kroh, O. (1924). Die eidetische anlage bei jugendlichen. *Z. Kinderforsch.*, Bd. 29.

Kroh, O. (1926). *Die Phasen der Jugendentwicklung: Entwicklungspsychologie des Grundschulkindes*. Berlin.

Kroh, O. (1928). *Die Psychologie des Grundschulkindes*. Langensalza.

Kroh, O. (1932). *Psychologie des Oberstufe*. Langensalza.

Krüger, F. (1926). Über psychische ganzheit. *Neue Psychol. Stud.*, 1.

Lashley, K. S. (1929). *Brain Mechanisms and Intelligence*. Chicago.

Lau, E. (1923). *Die Berliner Jugend und ihr Beruf*. Berlin.

Lau, E. (1925). *Beitrage zur Psychologie der Jugendlichen. Moral und Sozialpsychologische Untersuchungen auf Experimenteller Grundlage*. 3 Aufl. Langensalza.

Lewin, K. (1926). *Vorsatz, Wille und Bedürfnis*. Berlin.

Lewin, K. (1929). *Die Entwicklung der Experementellen Willenspsychologie und die Psychotherapie*. Leipzig.

Lindworsky, J. (1916). *Das Schlufolgernde Denken*. Freiburg.

Lindworsky, J. (1918).Wahrnehmmung und vorstellung. *Z. Psychol.*, 80.

Lindworsky, J. (1925). Methoden der Phantasieforschung. In E. Abderhalden (Ed.), *Handbuch der Biologischen Arbeitsmethoden*. Vienna.

Lindworsky, J. (1925). Methoden der Denkforschung. In E. Abderhalden (Ed.), *Handbuch der Biologischen Arbeitsmethoden*. Vienna.

Lipmann, O. (1924). Über begriff und formen der intelligenz. *Z. Angew. Psychol.*, 24.

Lipmann, O., and Bogen H. (1923). *Naive Physik*. Jena.

McDougall, W. (1912). *Psychology, the Study of Behavior*. London.

McDougall, W. (1923). *Outline of Psychology*. New York.

McDougall, W. (1924). Fundamentals of psychology. *Psyche*, 5.

McDougall, W. (1929). *Modern Materialism and Emergent Evolution*. New York.

Meumann, E. (1908). *Die Entstehung der Ersten Wortbedeutungen beim Kinde*. Leipzig.

Meumann, E. (1911-1914). *Vorlesungen zur Einführung in die Experimentelle Paedagogik und ihre Psychologischen Grundlagen*. Leipzig.

Meumann, E. (1925). *Intelligenz und Wille*. Leipzig.

Messer, A. (1906). Experementell-psychologische untersuchungen über das denken. *Arch. Gen. Psychol.*, 8.

Messer, A. (1908). *Empfindung und Denken*. Leipzig.

Meyer, H. and Pfahler, G. (1926). Untersuchung des technisch-praktischen und des technisch-theoretischen verhaltens bei schulkindern. *Z. Angew. Psychol.*, Bd. 27.

Monchamps, E., and Moritz, E. (1927). *Les Ètapes Mentales de lObservation des Images*. Bruxelles.

Müller, G. (1924). *Zur Analyse der Gedachtnistatgkeit und des Vorstellungsverlaufes*. Leipzig.

Müller, G. (1925). Ein beitrag zur prufung logische tatigkeiten. *Arch. Gesam. Psychol.*, Bd. 1.

Müller, G. (1931). Untersuchungen über kindliche schlusprozesse. *Arch. Gesam. Psychol.*, Bd. 78, 79.

Neubauer, V. (1927). Uber die entwicklung der technischen begabung bei kindern. *Z. Angew. Psychol.*, Bd. 29.

Ormian, H. (1926). Das schlufolgernde denken des kindes. *Wiener Arbeiten zur Päd.*, Ps. 4, Wien.

Peters, W. (1923). *Struktur in Jugendalter*. Leipzig.

Peters, W. (1925). *Einführung in das Seelenleben des Jugendlichen*. S.1.

Peters, W. (1927). Die entwicklung von wahrnemungsleistungen beim kinde. *Z. Psychol.*, 103.

Pfister, O. (1903). Gewicht des Gehirns beim Saügling. *Neurol. Zentralblatt. Leipzig.*

Piaget, J. (1921). Une forme verbale de la comparaison chez lenfant. *J. Psych.*, XVIII.

Piaget, J. (1926). La première annèe de lenfant. *Br. J. Psychol.*, 18.

Piaget, J. (1926). *La Reprèsentation du Monde chez lEnfant.* Paris.

Piaget, J. (1927). *La Causalité Physique chez lEnfant.* Paris.

Piaget, J., and Rossello, R. (1922). Notes sur les types de description dimages chez lenfant. *Arch. Psych.*, 71.

Reininger, K. (1924). *Über Soziale Verhaltungsweisen in der Vorpubertat.* Wien.

Revault d'Allones, G. (1923). Lattention. *Traite de Psychologie par. G. Dumas.* V. I., Paris.

Roloff, H. P. (1922). *Vergleichend-psychologische Untersuchungen über Kindlichen Definitionsleistungen.* Leipzig.

Schneider, K. (1930). *Die Psychologie der Schizophrenen und ihre Bedeutung fur die Klinik der Schizophrenie.* Leipzig.

Schüssler, H (1924). Die entwicklung des schlussfolgernden denkens bei kindern und jugendlichen. *Z. Psychol.*,Bd. 23.

Schüssler, H. (1924). 1st die behauptung meumanns richtig: kinder können im allgemeinen vor dem 14 lebenjahre nicht logisch schlieen? *Z. Angew. Psychol.*, Bd. 23, 4.

Spranger, E. (1924). *Psychologie des Jugendalters.* Heidelberg.

Spranger, E. (1928). *Kultur und Erziehung. Gesammelte Pädagogische Aufsätze.* 4 aufl., Leipzig.

Stern, Cl. (1927). *Die Kindersprache: Eine psychologische und Sprachteoretische Untersuchung.* Leipzig.

Stern, W. Psychologie der reifenden jugend. *Z. pädagogische* Psychol., 1.

Stern, W. (1922). Vom ichbewusstsien des jugendlichen. *Z. Pädagogische Psychol.*, No. 1.

Stern, W. (1924). Das "Ernstspiel" in Jugendzeit. *Z. Pädagogische Psychol. Jugenkund.*, No. 25

Stern, W. (1925). *Anfänge der Reifezeit. Ein Knabentagebuch in Psychologischer Bearbeitung.* Leipzig.

Stern, W., and Stern, Cl. (1907). *Monographien über die Seelische Entwicklung des Kindes.* Leipzig.

Sterzinger, O. (1924). Über den stand und die entwicklung von begabungen während der gimnasialzeit. *Arch. Ges. Psychol.*, 49.

Stratz, C. H. (1922). *Der Körper des Kindes und Seine Pflege.* Stuttgart.

Stumpf, K. (1901). Eigenartige sprachliche entwicklung eines kindes. *Z. Pädagogische Psyche Phatalogie*, Bd. 3, H. 6.

Thorndike, E. (1913-1914). *Educational Psychology.* New York.

Thorndike, E. (1932). *The Fundamentals of Learning.* New York.

Tumlirz, O. (1924). *Die Reifejahre.* Leipzig.

Tumlirz, O. (1925). *Einführung in die Jugendkunde.* 2 Aufl. Leipzig. Bd. I, II.

Uznadze, D. N. (1929).Die begriffsbildung im vorschulpflichtigen alter. *Z. Angew. Psychol.*, Bd. 34.

Uznadze, D. N. (1929). Die gruppenbildungsversuche bei vorschulpflichtigen kindern. *Arch. Ges. Psychol.*, Bd. 73.

Vecerka, L. (1926). *Die Soziale Verhalten von Mädchen Wärend des Reifezeit.* Wien.

Vierordt, K. (1877). *Physiologie des Kindesalters.* Tubingen.

Vogel, M. (1911). *Untersuchungen über die Denkbeziehungen in Urteilen der Kinder*, S.1.

Wallon, H. (1925). *Stades et Troubles du Development Psychomoteur et Mental chez lEnfant.* Paris.

Wallon, H. (1925). *LEnfant Turbulent. Etude sur les Retards et les Anomalies du Development Moteur et Mental.* Paris.

Werner, H. (1926). *Einführung in die Entwicklungspsychologie.* Leipzig.

Wertheimer, M. (1912). Uber das denken der naturvölker. 1. zahlen und zahlengebilde. *Z. Psychol.*, 60.

Wertheimer, M. (1922). Untersuchungen zur lehre von der gestalt: 1. Prinzipielle bemerkungen. *Psychol. Forsch.*, 1.

Wertheimer, M. (1925). *Drei Abhandlungen zur Gestalttheorie.* Erlangen.

Woodworth, R. (1918). *Dynamic Psychology.* New York.

Yerkes, R. M. (1927).The mind of a gorilla. *Genet. Psychol. Monogr.*, 2.

Yerkes, R. M., and Learned, B. W. (1925). *Chimpanzee Intelligence and Its Vocal Expression.* Baltimore.

Zillig, M. (1917). Über eidetische anlage und intelligenz. *Forsch. Psychol.*, 5.

AUTHOR INDEX

343

SUBJECT INDEX

ERRATA TO VOLUME 4

p. 7, lines 26–27: "they are linked" should read "they are not linked."

p. 16, line 23: "occurs with a change" should read "occurs without a change."

p. 29, line 2: "this not so" should read "this is not so."

p. 29, last line to p. 30 first line: "historically arising before Wundt" should read "historically going back to Wundt."

p. 30, line 2: "values that comprise it, according to the formal type of structure" should read: "values that comprise it than according to the formal type of structure."

p. 32, line 46: "would actually be applied" should read "could be applied."

p. 40: line 7: "any different regard" should read "any special regard."

p. 53, lines 8–9 from bottom: "uncovered form" should read "bare form."

p. 57, line 16: "the very grandiose" should read "a very grandiose."

p. 58, line 10: "domestic and" should read "domestic animal and."

p. 59, lines 8 and 9: The German quotation is incomplete: The words "*es blitzt*" are missing at the end of the quote.

p. 66. line 6 from bottom: "element" should read "elements."

p. 76, line 20: "simpler" should read "simple."

p. 76, line 25: "with" should read "to."

p. 77, line 10: "present" should read "presents."

p. 79, line 16 from bottom: "As a stimulus" should read "As stimuli."

p. 81, line 23: "work" should read "word."

p. 85, line 27: "may" should read "might."

p. 87, line 32: "Just as" should read "Like."

p. 92, line 4: The period after "lower" should be replaced by a comma.

p. 94, line 10: "of patterns or any specific type" should read "or patterns of any specific type."

p. 102, line 13 from bottom: "passed" should read "passes."

p. 105, line 18: "initially made up of an objective situation" should read "initially created by an objective situation."

p. 106, line 4: "a" should read "an."

p. 108, line 11 from bottom: "conclusion, with" should read "conclusion with."

p. 112, line 24: "habits, are" should read "habits are."

p. 128, line 10 from the bottom: "has" should read "have."

p. 138, line 13 from bottom: "belong" should read "belongs."

p. 142, line 31: "course it might" should read "course might."

p. 148, lines 20, 21: "of writing in the blind, we see" should read "of writing, in the blind we see."

p. 150, line 1: "are participants" should read "are four participants."

p. 161, line 11: "devices may be internal" should read "devices may be external" and "consistently internal" should read "consistently external."

p. 161, line 17: "Revo d'Allon" should read "Revault d'Allones."

p. 181, line 18: "(Fig. 2)" should be "(Fig. 2, p. 79)."

p. 197, last line: "cane and a hook" should read "cane with a hook."

p. 201, line 4 from bottom: "simulation" should read "stimulation."

p. 210, line 5 from bottom: "from which Ramon y Cajal diverts" should read "to which Ramon y Cajal ascribes."

p. 234, line 11: "operation" should read "operations."

p. 242, line 21 from bottom: "with a purely" should read "with the purely."

p. 242, line 20 from bottom: "of a method" should read "of the method."

p. 249, line 2: "used" should read "use."

p. 256, line 4: "in different" should read "in the different."